Organ Donation and Transplantation after Cardiac Death in China

Xiaoshun He • Jiefu Huang
Editors

Organ Donation and Transplantation after Cardiac Death in China

Clinical practice

PMPH PEOPLE'S MEDICAL PUBLISHING HOUSE Springer

Editors
Xiaoshun He
The First Affiliated Hospital of Sun Yat-sen University
Guangzhou
China

Jiefu Huang
Peking Union Medical College Hospital
Beijing
China

ISBN 978-981-16-0814-8 ISBN 978-981-16-0815-5 (eBook)
https://doi.org/10.1007/978-981-16-0815-5

This Springer imprint is published by the registered company Springer Nature Singapore Pte Ltd.
The registered company address is: 152 Beach Road, #21-01/04 Gateway East, Singapore 189721, Singapore

Preface

The development of organ transplantation depends on organ donation. Without organ donation, there would be no organ transplantation. China's organ donation and transplantation have experienced a long and bumpy development process. Under the leadership of the National Health and Family Planning Commission of China and the Chinese Red Cross Society, an organ donation and transplantation system that follows the guidelines of the World Health Organization and conforms to China's national conditions has been initially formed after more than ten years of unremitting efforts. A new development stage in which citizens' voluntary donations are the only source of donation has emerged.

Before 2015, due to the constraints of traditional Chinese culture and related laws, the organ donation standards and procedures adopted abroad could not be implemented in China, and a formal channel for citizens to donate organs voluntarily has not been established at the national level. So that most of the transplantation can only rely on organ donations from executed prisoners. On November 8, 2005, at the World Health Organization (WHO) branch meeting in Manila, the capital of the Philippines, the Chinese government publicly stated to the international community for the first time that most of Chinese transplanted organs come from death row prisoners and promised to regulate organ transplantation and donation as soon as possible. It is hailed as major progress in the field of organ transplantation in China by the domestic and foreign media. In 2006, the National Clinical Application Management Summit of Human Organ Transplant Technology was launched in Guangzhou, opening the prelude to the standardized management of organ transplants. In 2007, the State Council promulgated the "Regulations on Human Organ Transplantation," marking that Chinese organ transplantation has embarked on a legal track. In 2010, the National Ministry of Health formulated the "Basic Principles of Distribution and Sharing of Human Organs and the Distribution and Sharing Policy of Liver and Kidney" in accordance with Chinese conditions on the basis of international standards and related policies study. Based on this, the Chinese Human Organ Distribution and Sharing System has been developed, which is responsible for the distribution of donated organs according to the principles of fairness, justice, and openness. The system had a trial run in March 2011. On April 26, 2011, the Ministry of Health launched the pilot work of organ donation and transplantation of donors after cardiac death and encouraged qualified tertiary-A hospitals to carry out the pilot work after approval by the provincial health administrative department. On August 21, 2013, the National Health and Family Planning Commission announced the "Administrative Regulations on the Acquisition and Distribution of Human Donated Organs (Trial)." From September 1, 2013, donated organs must be distributed through the organ distribution system, and technical means are used to eliminate human intervention to the greatest extent to ensure that organ donation and transplantation are transparent, fair, and traceable. The promulgation of the regulations also means that the most critical link in organ transplantation—the acquisition and distribution of organs—will have clear laws and regulations to follow in China. In order to implement the "Regulations on Human Organ Transplantation" and actively promote the construction of Chinese human organ donation and transplantation work system, the National Clinical Application Committee of Human Organ Transplant Technology established the Organ Acquisition Organization Alliance of Chinese Hospital Association on March 20, 2014 (Chinese Hospital Association OPO). On December 3, 2014, the "2014 Chinese OPO Alliance Seminar" was held in Kunming. The meeting decided that from January 1, 2015, China will stop using organs from death prisoners, and voluntary organ donation after the death of citizens will be the only channel of organ transplants. Organ donation in China has been gradually supported and recognized by the international transplant community. At the Global Organ Donation and Transplantation Conference held on October 17, 2015, the Council unanimously approved China to officially join the international organ transplant family, ending the long history of Chinese transplantation being rejected and isolated. After nearly 10 years of development, organ donation after the death of Chinese citizens has made certain achievements, and it has now become the second largest country in the world for organ donation.

With the increasing demand for transplantation in recent years, organ shortage has become a common problem faced by the global transplant community. In order to expand the source of donors and alleviate the problem of organ shortage, finding a multi-channel source of donor organs has become a top priority for the organ transplant community. There are two main international classifications of organ donation after the death of citizens, namely donation after brain death (DBD) and donation after cardiac death (DCD). In global clinical practice, DCD has received extensive attention from the transplant community and has been recognized as a safe and effective way to expand donor sources. Taking 2015 as an example, DCD accounted for approximately 17% of the total number of organ donations after the death of citizens worldwide. In China, due to the absence of brain death legislation, some unique traditional customs, the current medical environment, and other factors, the clinical application of DCD is more common than in other countries in the world. Currently, the number of donated organs in China ranks first in Asia and second in the world. It is the country with the largest number of DCD cases in a single year in the world. In China, DCD belongs to the second category of Chinese Classification of organ donation after death of Chinese citizens. Although Chinese national conditions are special, with the popularization and regulation of DBD, the proportion of donation after brain death followed by cardiac death (DBCD) has declined in recent years; the overall number of DCD is on the rise.

The Organ Transplant Center of the First Affiliated Hospital of Sun Yat-sen University is one of the earliest organ transplantation units in China and one of the designated organ transplant hospitals in the pilot area of the Ministry of Health. The center established an organ donation office in July 2011, which is responsible for organ donation of citizens. From the pilot project in January 2010 to the present, the center has successfully carried out 242 cases of donation after cardiac death, and carried out liver transplantation, kidney transplantation, heart transplantation, lung transplantation, and multiple-organ transplantation. From 2013 to 2016, the Organ Transplant Center of the First Affiliated Hospital of Sun Yat-sen University organized experts to specially compile the first Chinese popular science book on organ donation *500 Questions on Organ Donation of Chinese Citizen* and the first domestic monograph to introduce and summarize the knowledge of organ donation and transplantation *Theory and Practice of Organ Donation Behind Citizens*.

On this basis, in order to clarify the current status and effect of domestic DCD, our center furthermore organized the compilation of this book. This book aims to analyze and prospect the current status of DCD in China and its impact on the application of organ transplantation. The book is divided into 14 chapters. It provides a systematic introduction to the laws, ethics, donor maintenance, organ function assessment, organ acquisition, and transplantation of DCD in China and abroad. It could try to solve the following problems, namely, how to find potential donors, how to maintain the function of the donor's organs and image, pathological evaluation, exploring the high-risk factors that affect the ischemia–reperfusion injury of the donor's organs and the function, and exploring the best criteria for evaluating the quality of the donor organs. Most of the content of this book comes from our clinical experience and research results. Throughout the book, each chapter has prominent themes, novel content, fluent text, and strong readability. It is very useful for understanding and carrying out DCD application. So, it is highly recommended to colleagues engaged in organ donation and transplantation.

Guangzhou, China

Jiefu Huang
Xiaoshun He

Contents

Legal, Moral, and Ethical Issues Related to Cardiac Death Donation

1

Xiaoshun He and Maogen Chen

Abstract

After 20 years development of organ transplantation project in China, it has successfully transformed from relying on judicial channels to the source of voluntary donation by citizens, and gradually moved toward to institutionalization, standardization and legalization channel. The major breakthrough in citizen organ donation has not only brought great well-being to mankind, but also brought serious ethical challenges. However, the human organ properties, such as social, ethical, and legal issues, are special in the process of organ transplantation, which directly affects the application and development of transplantation technology. The reasons lack of donor organ partially due to the unreasonable and traditional morality concept. China is committed to using the model of DCD to carry out organ donation work, hoping to seek and establish a controlled donation model, which is scientific in line with the current situation. Chinese people have been raised by Confucian culture for many years. The application of DCD mode has rekindled the hope of nearly 1.5 million patients who need organ transplantation, but DCD is worth exploring the legal, moral, and ethical problems that may be encountered in the implementation process of donation.

X. He (✉) · M. Chen
The First Affiliated Hospital of Sun Yat-sen University, Guangzhou, China

1.1 Categories and Features of DCD

Organ transplantation is an effective means to treat all kinds of end-stage organ failure, and is known as "the jewel in the crown of medicine" [1]. With the continuous expansion of transplant demand in recent years, organ shortage is a common problem faced by the global transplant community [2]. In order to expand the sources of donor and alleviate the shortage of organs, finding multichannel sources of organ donation have become an urgent task for the organ transplant community [3]. There are two common international classifications of organ donation after the death of citizens, namely, donation after brain death (DBD), and donation after cardiac death (DCD). In global clinical practice, DCD has received wide attention from the transplant community and has been recognized as a safe and effective way to expand the source of organ suppliers. In 2015, for example, DCD accounts for about 17% of the world's total organ donation after the death of a citizen each year [4, 5]. In China, the clinical application of DCD is more common than in other countries in the world due to the absence of brain death legislation, some unique traditional customs and the current medical environment.

DCD refers to organ donation, also known as non-heart-beating donation, from patients convicted of death according to total circulatory

X. He (ed.), *Organ Donation and Transplantation after Cardiac Death in China*,
https://doi.org/10.1007/978-981-16-0815-5_1

arrest standards [6]. Currently, DCD is divided into five categories by the definition of the 1995 Maastricht International Conference in the Netherlands. This standard was revised in 2003 as following: (1) M-I: The patient was pronounced dead upon arrival at the hospital, with a time less than 45 min, and was an unplanned, unpredicted cardiac arrest. (2) M-II: The heart of a patient stopped beating outside the hospital. And the emergency treatment was invalid by CPR for 10 min after the emergency admission to hospital, declared dead. It was an unplanned and unpredicted cardiac arrest. (3) M-III: Patients suffer from severe incurable injury, usually devastating brain trauma, but not fully meet the criteria for brain death. The patient had the will to donate organs and his life support and treatment was removed in plan by the family's initiative or consent to give up rescue, so that the heart stopped beating due to hypoxia and residual brain cells were inactivated. The whole process is a planned, predictable cardiac arrest. (4) M-IV: Unplanned, unpredicted cardiac arrest occurs after the brain death is established and before organ donation. (5) M-V: (New standards in 2003): The inpatients stopped beating their hearts, mainly for the unplanned and unpredicted cardiac arrest that occurred during ICU rescue [7]. Among 5 categories, M-I, M-II, and M-V are called "Non-controlling DCD," which refers to patients with unplanned cardiac arrest in or outside a hospital who cannot be resuscitated, characterized by a long period of warm ischemic, and low organ utilization; M-III is called a "controllable DCD," including patients who are difficult to sustain, even using mechanical assistance, and die quickly after removing mechanical support, characterized by a relatively short time of warm ischemia, and most organs can be used for transplantation; M-IV is a controllable DCD, however, the preparation time is short and the length of warm ischemia time varies. Accordingly, China's classification of human organ donation standards is published by the Chinese Committee for the Clinical Application of Human Organ Transplant Technology [8], including Chinese category I (C-I), the same as DBD; Chinese category II (C-II), that is, DCD, including M-I ~ M-V in Maastricht Category Criteria; Chinese category III (C-III), donation after brain and cardiac death (DBCD).

1.2 The Historical Background and Global Trends of DCD Development

The Netherlands was the first country to expand the pool of donors and forward to explore DCD based on DBD. The Maastricht classification standard was developed at the first international seminar on DCD issues held in Maastricht, the Netherlands, in 1995 and was revised in 2000 [6, 9]. Based on recipients' safety and organ quality concerns, many national strategies for organ donation are increasing the number of DBDs without missing the opportunities to achieve DCD. The implementation of DCD varies from country to country, since differences in clinical practice, public awareness, national legislation, and medical resources all affect the development of DCD. In some countries (e.g., the Netherlands and the United Kingdom), DCD accounts for a large proportion of all organ donors, while in others (e.g., Germany and Portugal), DCD is almost non-existent. In Australia and the United Kingdom, the number of controlled DCD donors has increased significantly over the past 10 years, accounting for more than one-third of all organ donors [9–11]. In addition, most DCDs in Spain are uncontrollable, while controlled DCDs are mainstreamed in the United States [12, 13].

Globally, the proportion of DCD organs is also increasing year by year. However, in the process of actual operation and popularization of DCD, there are many ethical problems. At the 2009–2010 Geneva Conference, a number of international organizations, including WHO, jointly developed a strategic plan for the development of postmortem organ donation, and stated that "the principle of human organ donation is that living organ donation takes precedence over donation after death and DBD has priority over DCD." Brain death is now considered one of the scientific criteria for judging death in more than 90 countries [14].

Brain death is the basic prerequisite of organ donation. In the mid-1980s, Chinese experts drafted the "Brain Death Determination Standard (Draft)." In 2003, the National Health and Family Planning Commission issued the "Brain Death Determination Standards (Adults) (Draft for Comments)"and "Technical Specifications for The Determination of Brain Deaths (Draft for Comments)" [15]. However, since the traditional concept of cardiac arrest death was deeply rooted in our country, and there were differences in diagnosis, treatment, and testing equipment at different medical institutions, DBD could not be widely accepted in our country for a long time. China had to adopt the following death standards: Chinese category II (C-II), also as DCD, which could serve as a breakthrough to unseal organ donation. During the popularization of DCD, the Chinese category III (C-III) has gradually proposed and endowed with more national characteristics. It is important to be clear that, regardless of the criteria used for death determination, organ donation must be strictly followed by the law that donation can only be implemented after death.

On January 1, 2015, China completely bans the sources of organs from prisoners sentenced to death. The domestic organ transplantation industry relies entirely on the channels of organ donation after citizen death, and establishes a system of human organ donation throughout the country, involving the Red Cross organization as a third party to participate in the donation process, insist and advocate the principle of voluntariness and freedom for organ donation, and strive to achieve the fairness and transparency in organ distribution. Organ transplantation with institutionalization, standardization and legalization has been achieved. Up to August 19, 2015, the number of voluntary organ donations in China has reached 4737. At present, China has the highest number of organ donations in Asia, ranked second in the world. China is the world's largest country for the single-year implementation of DCD cases and the annual organ donation rate per million population reached about 2.0 [16]. Despite the specialized national conditions of our country, the proportion of DBCD has decreased in recent years followed by the popularity and regulation of DBD, while the overall number of DCD is on the rise.

1.3 WHO Legal of Organ Donation

The WHO resolution WHA63.22 (2010), a guiding principle on human organ transplantation, has influenced the creation and modification of laws, legislation, and regulations in some 60 countries, and has served as a model for improving or building donation and transplantation programs globally. The guiding principles are helping WHO member states to combat commercial transplantation more effectively and simplify donation after brain- and cardiocirculatory death, as well as increasing protection for living donors. WHO member states and international partners were requested to develop a global consensus on guiding ethical principles for the donation and management of all medical products of human origin including tissue and organ transplantation. The safety issues for donors include the need to ensure organ quality, traceability, vigilance, surveillance, and equitable access. According to the resolution WHA63.22, 10 new guiding principles were proposed at the Seventieth World Health Assembly. WHO assisted member states in developing their donation programs in line with those guiding principles. Data on donation activities and practices are collected by the Global Observatory on Donation and Transplantation (http://www.transplant-observatory.org), a collaborative project between WHO and the Spanish National Transplant Organization. The practice of organ transplantation is increasing worldwide, and is currently carried out in over 110 countries, with a significant increase of around 50% in Latin American countries. Despite this growth, donations still fall far short of meeting actual needs. The Notify Library (http://www.notifylibrary.org), developed jointly by WHO and the Italian National Transplant Centre, has updated the Notify Booklet, which targets clinicians and health authorities, to provide a better didactic overview of vigilance and surveillance related to human organ donation.

1.4 Ethical Supervision in the DCD Donation Process

Ethics supervision is the key step in organ donation workflow. For controllable DCD, a reporting approval department should be designated as generally the organ donation ethics committee or equivalent management department of the institution where the Organ Procurement Organization (OPO) is located. After review and approval, no less than two clinical medical experts in various disciplines (including but not limited to neurology, neurosurgery, anesthesiology, ICU, and emergency department) conduct independent consultations. Evaluation includes etiology, consultation, neurological examination, circulatory maintenance, Glasgow score, and whether or not irreversible injury. The experts record the UW scores and report the results to the Ethics Committee, the OPO. After obtaining unanimous agreement from donor family, they discuss the acquisition time together [17].

In practice, the DCD procedure would be started according to OPO's human resources and the requirements of different transplant centers at the time of warm ischemia. From the perspective of maximizing donation, it is recommended not to miss the opportunity to implement DCD. ICU and OPO should formulate DCD-related clinical procedures, and specify the follow-up measures if the patient does not die within a given time after withdrawal of life support system. When communicating with patients' family members, OPO should explain the various possibilities of failing to achieve DCD and ensure that the family members agree with and sign the letter of consent. The OPO should also reach a consensus with family members on the follow-up measures and nursing expenses when such situations occur. Once such a situation leads to unsuccessful donation, appropriate care should be provided to the family.

1.5 Ethical Considerations on the Development of DCD

In 2010, China adopted the DCD donation model to carry out organ donation work, focusing on the norms and practices of controllable DCD. In May 2010, the Ministry of Health, the Red Cross Society of China, and relevant experts have formed the "Guide to Donation of Cardiac Death" (hereinafter referred to as the "Guide"). In November 2011, the Ministry of Health issued a statement "Donation of organs after Cardiac Death will be fully implemented nationwide starting in January 2012." Regardless of the type of donation, the social individual's value tradeoff is the final judgment that determines whether to donate. The introduction of the advanced Western model must go through the process of localization. At this time, you need to think about DCD behavior with local ethics.

Religious culture and superstitious thinking affect people's attitude toward organ donation more or less, but these are not the deepest internal struggles. Chinese people influenced by traditional Confucian culture will make ethical value judgments different from other cultures when faced with individual choices. Potential donors and their families will inevitably think about this when faced with organ donation. For thousands of years, Confucianism has been influencing the minds of Chinese people. According to Confucianism, a person should love his/her relatives first, and then those less familiar people around him. If it is necessary to sacrifice individual benefits to satisfy group interests, this is contrary to the theory. At the same time, the strong emotional requisition of families for their members will also affect society's recognition of individual values. On the major issue of organ donation after death, it is inevitable that there will be a conflict between individual values and family ethics as well as emotional necessity.

1.5.1 Family-Based Ethics Has Become an Obstacle for Individual's Donation

Today, family relations are moving forward from traditional to modern status. But this does not mean that the individual is completely independent from the family. In most cases, individual choices are determined by family opinions. Individuals will compromise in the face of family benefits. This concession is not forced and authoritarian, but is taken for granted. Therefore, individuals often consider the value orientation of the whole family before deciding, thus lead to the non-self-inclination tendency of individuals [18]. The right of family members to give informed consent in medical care further illustrates that the individual's right to make health decisions is no longer limited to the individual himself, but is more "regulated" by the family. This "regulation" extends from the cradle to the grave, and even after death. This is why some young people with modern ideas have to stop after applying for organ donation because of the opposition of their elders or other members. Correspondingly, some elders have the willingness to donate but cannot withstand the opposition of their children; or when performing donations, the children refuse to donate on the grounds of "unfilial piety, great injustice." These family "regulations" restrict the development of organ donation.

1.5.2 The Emotional Necessity of Family Ethics Have Weakened Individual Willingness of Donation

Under the influence of our traditional Confucian ideology "benevolence," love is equally divided. It can be seen from "If one loves his family, he loves other people eventually," "Charity begins at home, but should not end there." In Confucianism, one should love one's own relatives first, and then love others, and finally one can attain the realm of "love the whole world." According to the distance of consanguinity, the interpersonal relationship established in this way must be an arithmetic sequence relationship [19]. People subconsciously distinguish the relationship of consanguinity and establish a strong emotional support for family members. The strong emotional needs of the family dilute the individual's value pursuit, and then the needs of social benefits are easily overlooked. Furthermore, when faced with the special donation model of controllable DCD, each potential donor and his/her family may have deeper concerns.

1.5.3 DCD's Technical Risks Make Donation Hover

The biggest difference between controllable DCD and other types of organ donation is that "the organ acquisition team systematically withdraws life support equipment, and organs are acquired after donor's circulation stops [20]. The warm ischemia time affect the donor organ quality, and the donor also has an adverse effect [21]. Therefore, there is a conflict between protecting the interests of donors and obtaining more high-quality organs. Faced with the medical and ethical debates between "rescue and abandonment," higher requirements have been put forward for the maturity of medical technology, the clarity of medical standards, the certainty of relevant policies, and the rigor of operational implementation. Imagine that when an individual donates, he/she realizes that his/her own life and body will be controlled by others in the future, and there are still various insecure factors in reality, how will you sacrifice yourself to help others? Donors' families cannot bear their relatives to endure more pain and take risks at the end of their lives. At this time, the technical management norms for DCD operations have created a gap among the interests of individuals, families, and the needs of society.

1.6 The Ethical Principles Adopted by DCD at Present

China currently regard DCD as the focus of organ donation and transplantation. In the "Guide," Chinese experts have drawn on the international DCD technical experience and basic ethical principles to establish the current DCD workflow, including procedures for death determination, medical intervention, persuasion, and organ harvesting. The experts put forward that in controllable DCD, the patient's family should be fully informed of the patient's condition, donation process, potential risks, etc., giving priority to the protection of the donor's interests, and not making unrealistic death judgments in pursuit of organ quality [22]. This involves informed consent and the principle of no harm in ethics.

1.6.1 Principle of Informed Consent

The World Health Assembly in May 2010 adopted and issued a new version of the "WHO Guidelines for Human Cell, Tissue and Organ Transplantation," which emphasizes that the principle of "voluntary-informed consent" is the primary principle of organ transplantation [23]. The guideline of China is based on the informed consent model of the "Human Organ Transplant Regulations" and other relevant regulations, emphasizing that "the problem of donation should be raised to all patients and/or family members who may be suitable for donation, and the meaning and specific implementation process of DCD should be explained in detail. The organ donation coordinator should discuss all issues related to DCD with the donor's family members in depth after their agreement and sign a formal informed consent form. The details of the procedure are reflected in full notification of the condition, voluntary choice to give up treatment, free choice of donation, and minute notification of donation details. The whole process is supervised by the hospital donation committee or ethics committee. The establishment of the operation of informed consent not only respect for the patient's autonomy, but also reflect the autonomy of the patient's family. So, usage of the patient's organs has the meaning of the subjective desire to rescue others. At a higher level, organ donation is raised to realize the value of human life, so that the donor's disposal of his/her own organs is ethically protected.

The principle of informed consent considers the independent decision-making power of patients and their families, and also raises the donation of organs to the height of realizing the value of life. According to Confucianism, the value of a person after death is based on the value of life, and it is possible to transcend death to make life eternal. DCD is not only a dedication act, donors save others' lives by donating their organs in a subjective behavior, which has gone beyond death. Therefore, all potential donors and their families should make their own choices after fully weighing the relationship between individuals, family, and social interests, and at the same time, those activities must accept ethical, regulatory, and policy restrictions in the practice of DCD.

1.6.2 No Harm Principle

The "Guide" in China emphasizes that "it is necessary to consider the interests of donors and avoid harming donors. Measures that can alleviate the suffering of donors should not be restricted or reduced, and measures that accelerate the death of donors should not be applied." At the same time, medical interventions related to transplantation can only be carried out after the death of the patient. This is particularly important in the process of donation of controllable DCD and is also the ethical bottom line of DCD. Do not hurt the interests of donors in order to improve the quality of organs, including the removal of donors' circulation support and medical intervention and other medical behaviors. In the process of organ transplantation, the donor's interest should take priority over the recipient's. Under certain circumstances, after obtaining the consent of the patient's family, the necessary minor harm to obtain greater benefits is allowed, although all emphasize the protection of the donor's interests. Each country sets different levels of donor-related medical intervention before transplantation. In the "Guideline," China particularly emphasizes the principle of harmlessness, stipulating the transparency of the evaluation and intervention process; not restricting or reducing measures that can alleviate the suffering of patients; no drugs that accelerate patient death; medical interventions should show clear evidence or effect. Physicians are required to be cautious and take everything for the benefit of patients to avoid harming patients. Any medical behavior that accelerates the death of the patient is absolutely prohibited.

1.6.3 Principle of Donation After Death

The transplant can only be carried out if the patient is determined to be dead. This principle is an important principle emphasized by international DCD transplantation. Because in the controllable DCD donation process, special operations for removing the circulatory system are required. Organ donation could be performed after the patient's death has been confirmed, determining whether DCD donation crosses the ethical bottom line. The "Guideline," specifies the details of confirming death: confirm that the circulation stop is irreversible or permanent, and should be observed for 2–5 min; two or more attending doctors declare the death, accurately record the time and record the video; emphasize that it cannot be taken any measures to restore the circulation; within a certain time after the removal of cardiopulmonary support, the circulation has not stopped irreversibly, then the patient should be sent back to the ward and continue to carry out hospice care. Because our country has always adopted the death judgment standard for cardiac arrest, the norm of confirming death is relatively general and simple compared to some countries with brain death standards. Compared with the regulations of some technologically developed countries, China's practical application of the principle of donation after death is relatively cautious, and these regulations basically conform to the technical level of our country at the beginning. At the same time, it also conforms to the legal regulations of our country.

1.7 Strategy of Sustainable Development for DCD

1.7.1 Establish a Fair, Equitable, and Open Organ Allocation and Sharing Mechanism

In China, the number of organs available for transplantation is much lower than the number of patients who need organ transplantation. It is a worldwide question. The huge demand for human organs, a scarce resource, has also caused serious problems related to organ transplantation, including organ trading, organ transplant tourism, and even murder. Although DCD can alleviate the contradiction of organ shortage to a certain extent, what is more important is how to ensure the fair and open distribution of this public resource of organs, which is not only respect for donors and their families, but also the fundamental guarantee for long-term health promotion of DCD work.

According to news from the National Health and Family Planning Commission, China has established an organ allocation and sharing system, including an organ transplant waiting list system, organ donor registration, and organ allocation and/or matching system. The system automatically ranks patients waiting for organ transplantation by computer, and assigns organs based on objective factors such as the severity of the disease, postoperative expectations, blood type, age, organ anastomosis, and region. This network system will be promoted nationwide to make organ distribution open and transparent. In addition, China has established organ acquisition organizations, which are specifically responsible for transplant coordination and organ acquisition.

1.7.2 Give Reasonable Compensation to Donors

China's "Human Organ Transplant Regulations" explicitly forbid any form of organ sales, emphasizing the "volunteer" principle of organ donation. A purely unpaid donation is a donation that does not have any strings attached, but if the donor's family not only suffers from the loss of a loved one, but may also have to pay additional costs, then this purely unpaid donation is not conducive to the sustainable promotion of the DCD. On the contrary, if properly handled, the nonutilitarian compensation given to the donor's family does not violate the medical ethical principle of "harmless, beneficial, respectful, mutual aid and justice," but also reflects the humanistic care given to the donor by society.

Many countries increase the number of bodies and live organs donation by means of economic measures. At the current stage, China needs to improve the organ transplant management system and related laws and regulations as soon as possible. At the same time, the country should give relevant provisions in the ethical norms and medical system, to prevent DCD to become a disguised way of buying and selling organs. On the other hand, the establishment and improvement of the reasonable compensation mechanism in DCD, both materially and spiritually, can reflect the social recognition and affirmation of the selfless dedication of organ donors, to help solve the problems of individuals and families after death. Not only can this effectively increase the number of transplanted organ donors without contrary to the ethical principles, but also more moral and practical. In the specific implementation, the compensation content may include reducing the cost of treatment after the donor family agrees to donate. The reduction amount should vary according to the actual situation. Partial compensation is not paid immediately, and families may apply for relief after the donation. The Red Cross shall give priority compensation on the basis of the assessment results. For now, it is feasible and a compensation mechanism with Chinese characteristics to be provided by the Red Cross, a third-party, independent of physicians and donors.

1.7.3 Improvement of DCD Utilization and Organ Quality

The scarcity of transplanted organ resources determines the necessity of making the best use of the organ available for transplantation. We should not only expand the organ resources available for transplantation as far as possible, but also strive to improve the utilization rate and the success rate of the existing organ transplant, in which Chinese scholars have made an active and effective exploration. Social surveys have found that many people have the idea of donating organs after death, but the proportion of people who can actually implement them is very low. If the donated organs are in short supply and low quality, the prognosis of transplant is not good, and the recipient even needs to be transplanted again, this will lead to more demand for organs.

1.8 Conclusion

Although China's DCD work was carried out late, the proposed solution of DCD in line with China's national conditions is put forward, based on foreign experience and in compliance with China's laws and regulations. The current DCD donation is basically adapted to the current stage of China's technical level. The pilot work has also achieved exciting results in recent years. Either way, organ donation begins with a range of social, ethical, legal, and human rights issues. Therefore, it is necessary to strengthen the management of laws and regulations, adhere to a rigorous, fair, and scientific attitude in organ acquisition and distribution, in order to ensure the healthy and orderly development of DCD organ donation. In the long run, we believe that

China's DCD organ donation will certainly be able to get more support and trust from the whole society. China's organ transplant work has also been more recognized and praised by the international community.

References

1. Zheng S. Organ transplantation in China is approaching to the world. Chin J Digest Surg. 2015;14(1):5–6. https://doi.org/10.3760/j.issn.1673-9752.2015.01.023.
2. Zhu Y, Cai C, Guan X. Donor management for organ donation in ICU. Chin J Crit Care Med (Electr Ed). 2017;3(2):85–90. https://doi.org/10.3877/j.issn.2096-1537.2017.02.002.
3. Gao T, Tian H. Evaluation, maintenance and care of organ donation donors after the death of citizens. Pract J Organ Transplant (Electr Vers). 2017;5(1):31–3. https://doi.org/10.3969/j.issn.2095-5332.2017.01.011.
4. Agopian VG. Liver transplantation with donation after cardiac death donors as a strategy for recipients with model for end-stage liver disease score > 15: Has the die been cast? Liver Transplant. 2017;23(5):579–80. https://doi.org/10.1002/lt.24756.
5. Katsaros GD, Schucht J, Jones CM, Cannon RM. Nationwide outcomes after renal transplantation from kidney-only versus multiple-organ deceased donors. Am Surgeon. 2019;85(9):1066–72.
6. Kootstra G, Daemen JHC, Oomen APA. Categories on non-heart-beating donors. Transplant Proc. 1995;27(5):2893–4.
7. Ridley S, Bonner S, Bray K, Falvey S, Mackay J, Manara A. UK guidance for non-heart-beating donation. Br J Anaesth. 2005;95(5):592–5. https://doi.org/10.1093/bja/aei235.
8. The Organ Transplantation Branch of the Chinese Medical Association. Guidelines for Organ Donation from Donors after Cardiac Dearh in China (2nd ed.). Chin J Organ Transplant. 2011;32(12):756–8. https://doi.org/10.3760/cma.j.issn.0254-1785.2011.12.014.
9. Xiaoliang Wu, Donghua Zheng, Zhiming Ding, Wenshi Jiang. Development trends and main points of clinical practice in global DCD. Organ Transplant. 2020(Issue 1):93–7.
10. Manning J. Changing to deemed consent for deceased organ donation in the United Kingdom: should Australia and New Zealand follow? J Law Med. 2020;27(3):513–26.
11. Reiling J, Forrest E, Bridle KR, Britton LJ, Santrampurwala N, Crawford D, et al. The implications of the shift toward donation after circulatory death in Australia. Transplant Direct. 2017;3(12):e226. https://doi.org/10.1097/TXD.0000000000000743.
12. Israni AK, Zaun D, Hadley N, Rosendale JD, Schaffhausen C, McKinney W, et al. OPTN/SRTR 2018 annual data report: deceased organ donation. Am J Transplant. 2020;(20 Suppl s1):509–41. https://doi.org/10.1111/ajt.15678.
13. Rudge C, Matesanz R, Delmonico FL, Chapman J. International practices of organ donation. Br J Anaesth. 2012;108(Suppl 1):i48–55. https://doi.org/10.1093/bja/aer399.
14. Wijdicks EF. Brain death worldwide: accepted fact but no global consensus in diagnostic criteria. Neurology. 2002;58(1):20–5. https://doi.org/10.1212/wnl.58.1.20.
15. Draft for Evaluation of Brain Death (adults). Natl Med J China. 2003;83(3):262. https://doi.org/10.3760/j:issn:0376-2491.2003.03.028.
16. Jiang W, Gomez MP, Paez G, Manyalich M. The beauty of data-focusing on the development trend of global organ donation. Chin J Transplant (Electr Vers). 2019;13(1):28–33. https://doi.org/10.3877/cma.j.issn.1674-3903.2019.01.007.
17. The Organ Transplantation Branch of the Chinese Medical Association. The process and norms of organ donation after death of Chinese citizens (2019 edition). Organ Transplant. 2019;10(2):122–7. https://doi.org/10.3969/j.issn.1674-7445.2019.02.003.
18. Xu W. Ethical research on the problem of brain death. Southeast University; 2005.
19. APing Zheng. Re-understanding of Confucian ethical culture. Sun Yat-sen University Forum 2000;20(2):212–217.
20. Yongfeng Liu. The ethics of organ acquisition from DCD and clinical application of liver transplantation. Chin J Transplant (Electr Vers). 2009;3(4):268–72. https://doi.org/10.3969/j.issn.1674-3903.2009.04.002.
21. Youhua Zhu. Application and results of non-heartbeat donors. In: Key Laboratory of Organ Transplantation, Ministry of Education, Wuhan Branch of Organ Transplantation 'editor'. The 2nd national symposium on organ donation and transplantation; 2009, Wuhan. p. 131–40.
22. Obermann K, Nagel E, Pichlmayr R. Ethical considerations in procuring organs from non-heart-beating donors after sudden cardiac death. Transplant Proc. 1995;27(5):2924–5.
23. WHO Guidelines for transplantation of human cells, tissues and organs. Chin J Transplant (Electr Vers) 2010;4(02):152–5.

Current Situation of Organ Donation After Cardiac Death in China

2

Xiaoshun He and Maogen Chen

Abstract

Organ transplantation and related medical products had developed rapidly and saved lots of patients with end-stage disease in the 1990s. However, organ shortage, placing restrictions on the development of organ transplantation, is a severe problem facing all over the world. The beneficiary of organ transplant has been up to 50–90 per million in Europe and American countries. But the number of people dying at end stage of organ disease has not decreased. On the contrary, due to awareness of the effect of organ transplantation by dying patients, the number in the waiting list is growing daily. The ratio of organ requirements to organ supply is 5:1 in the United States, other than 150:1 in China. Facing the large demand, there is an utterly inadequate amount of organs from donation after brain death (DBD). Based on the traditional culture and recognition to death in China, donation after cardiac death (DCD) becomes the best choice of donation type to expand the donor pool. Here, we will discuss the current situation of DCD development in China.

X. He (✉) · M. Chen
The First Affiliated Hospital of Sun Yat-sen University, Guangzhou, China

2.1 Preclinical Research on Non-Heart-Beating Donor

A paucity of donor organs is the principal limitation in human solid organ transplantation. As early as in the 1990s, the Western countries have tried to use non-heart-beating donor hearts in the animal models first. Since 1985 Loma Linda University Medical Center reported a successful case of using pediatric donor hearts that had been resuscitated after cardiac arrest up to 1 h, which prompted researchers to study how ischemia-reperfusion injured hearts can be used as donor organs [1–3]. After that, there was another case reported that a patient survived to use pediatric donor hearts that had periods of arrest and cardiopulmonary resuscitation for up to 2 h in 1993. Then, Dr. Gundry began a laboratory investigation into the feasibility of "reanimating" dead pulseless donor hearts in lambs. Lamb's hearts were successfully used for orthotopic heart transplantation after 1/2 h of cardiac electric standstill caused by either anoxia or exsanguination. The short-term anoxic and exsanguination models' experiments in lambs demonstrated that reperfusion modification could produce "normal" donor hearts reliably and consistently even after 30 min of warm ischemia, whether or not there is donor pretreatment. We can make these "dead" hearts produce short-term successful orthotopic transplantation and reanimation by pretreating the recipient with sublingual nifedipine; infusing

X. He (ed.), *Organ Donation and Transplantation after Cardiac Death in China*,
https://doi.org/10.1007/978-981-16-0815-5_2

prostaglandin E_1; reperfusing with a low hematocrit value (3–5%), low ionized calcium (0.3–0.5 mg/dl), low pressure (mean arterial pressure 20 mmHg), and low flow blood (25 ml/m^2) [4].

Because tolerance to ischemia varies widely among species, we suggest that these results must be replicated in a long-term subhuman primate model. Then the same reperfusion modifications in juvenile baboons were applied by these researchers to determine the human applications in an anoxic arrest model in 1995. In this experiment, donors were pretreated with prostaglandin, steroids, nifedipine, and dextrose. As described for the lamb model, recipients received the same reperfusion modifications. In addition, a leukocyte- depleting filter was added to the terminal blood cardioplegic solution for its successful intervention in hearts preserved for more than 24 h. After electric cardiac arrest 15, 22, 30, 30, and 31 min, the donors' hearts were harvested. And animals survived 1 day with the death caused by a stroke. Some survived 9 days with the death caused by dehydration. Others survived 13, 16, and 34 days with the death due to rejection [3]. In conclusion, with the use of clinically applicable methods, baboon hearts can be transplanted, reperfused, and reanimated successfully if they recovered 15–31 min after cardiac standstill caused by anoxia. These data suggest that it is feasible to use these techniques in human beings.

2.2 Current Situation of DCD Organ Transplantation Out of China

Joseph Murray and David Hume finished the first case of DCD renal transplantation in 1962 [5]. One year later, the first case of lung transplantation and liver transplantation using DCD donor has been completed by James Hardy and Thomas Starzl, respectively [6]. Then, Starzl completed the first case of liver transplantation which survived more than 1 year [7]. The first case of combined pancreas and kidney transplantation with DCD donation was performed by William Kelly and Richard Lillihei in 1967 [8]. Christian Barnard completed the first case of DCD heart transplantation in 1967, and another case of DCD heart recipient survived more than 1 year in 1968 [9, 10]. In 1968, Richard Lillihei finished the first case of DCD pancreas transplantation [11].

Transplanted organs were mainly from DCD (donation after cardiac death) or non-heart-beating donation with unsatisfactory survival until the 1960s. In 1968, the brain death concept was defined and accepted by clinical hospital and the independent legal committee of Harvard medical school. Then DCD was gradually replaced by DBD (donation of brain death) donation in the United States [7]. The clinical usage of cyclosporine since 1978 greatly improved the long-term survival of solid organ transplants and recipients, but it also increased the discrepancy between organ supply and demand of transplantation. The number of DBD could not be enough to satisfy the clinical needs. After the 1980s, transplant centers in Europe and the United States started to refocus on DCD donation to amplify the number of organ donors, which unlocked a new chapter for DCD organ transplantation.

The development of international DCD organ transplantation is unbalanced. Lots of factors are involved in the restriction of DCD implementation, including the legislation, ethics, cultural background, and different levels of social civilization in various countries. This difference is the most striking in Europe, such as in the United Kingdom, Holland, and Switzerland, where DCD has been supported by the government legislation. However, Germany has legislated to prohibit all organ acquisition behavior except for the DBD. And French and Spanish legislations prohibit controlled DCD organ transplantation. After the 1980s, many transplant centers in the United States have started to popularize the DCD organ transplantation derived from controllable Massachusetts III donation. In Japan, DBD donation was legislated in 1997. Due to the conceptual differences of culture, ethics, and legislation to the West, the main source of transplant organs is still mainly dependent on living donors and controlled Massachusetts IV DCD donation.

DCD organ transplantation has been accepted by more and more countries in recent years. They promote DCD popularization via legislation to achieve their clinical rational usage, and the number of DCD transplants increased rapidly in the past 10 years. The number of DBD derived transplantation decreased by 10%, while DCD increased by 280% from 2001 to 2005 data in the United Kingdom. Eleven percent of the kidney came from DCD donation by 2005. In a Belgian, DCD donor organs accounts for 11.38% of all transplanted organs, while 38%, 47% in Spain and Holland separately. In Europe, 6% of the kidneys came from DCD in 2005. The DCD transplantation has increased by 726% in the past 10 years in the United States, and DCD has accounted for 11% of all organ donors in 2008. In February 2005, the Canadian Medical Association organized a nationwide seminar on DCD, which consequently issued the national guidelines for non-heart-beating organ donation in 2006. DCD is becoming one of the solutions to alleviate the shortage of transplanted organs in the world [12, 13].

The rate of organ donation in China is extremely low. To improve this situation, Chinese government has started reformation with big strides to increase the donation. Since March 2010, China has officially launched DCD organ donation in 10 provinces and cities, including Tianjin, Shanghai, and Guangdong. In the first 2 years of innovation, the 11 pilot provinces and cities only finished about 130 cases of donation case which is equal to 0.34 per million donation rate. However, the organ donation rate was up to 24.1 per million population in the united states, and even in Japan it has reached 4.27 per million population [14]. The gap is obviously huge. It is Chinese feudal superstition and imperfect legal system construction that resulted in this phenomenon. But in the current situation, DCD is easier to get recognition and promotion, since it is fitful for the existing laws and regulations. It is a key strategy to resolve the problem of organ shortage. According to the China liver transplant registry (CLTR) data report, the total number of liver transplantation was 2025 cases in 2012, including 322 cases of DCD donation accounting for 15.9% of total liver donors.

2.3 Discussion of Death Criteria and the Origination of Brain Death

The death criteria are always a focal issue of medicine, law, philosophy, and ethics research. Medicine has proved that people's death was not a sudden event but a course. Not all organs end up together, but from the dysfunction of one or some important organs, the other important organs gradually cease to work eventually die. A dysfunctional cadaver has no value for transplantation. Those unaffected organs will be able be transplanted if death has confirmed before all organ dysfunction.

The standard of death definition was terrific before people recognized the human physical system very well. In 1740, Jacques Benigne Winslow thought the only mark of death was body rottenness in the united states. As time passes, cardiac arrest and pulseless was the major standard of death judge. The death idea of cardiac arrest was formulated from high antiquity via daily view and hunting activity by primitive human beings. But the heart arrest was officially defined as a death symbol until the invention of stethoscope in 1819. For a long time, the cease of heart, pulse, and breath became the prevailing criterion of death judgment almost in all countries, without argument. Then, with the invention of heart pacemaker and artificial ventilator, some patients were able to wake up and breathe for several hours after their heart palpitations stopped and cardiopulmonary dysfunction. People can sustain life with help of a heart pacemaker and artificial ventilator, which brings serious challenges for the death criteria. However, this kind of death criteria was still the only benchmark of decease till the emergence of organ transplant technology.

In the 1960s, with gradual improvement of kidney, liver, and heart transplantation, it appears to a huge demand for organs. But those organs in the body of heart arrest mean functional failure. How to obtain live organs for transplantation after death is a key issue. In 1968, Dr. Henry Beecher, chairman of the death review special committee in the Harvard University School of medicine, presides over the meeting discussing the criteria of death ascertainment. In the subsequent meeting report, it put forward a new concept of the definition that the standard of death is "irreversible coma or brain death." They proposed the new criteria for the diagnosis of death which has attracted worldwide attention. According to its definition, brain death is the decease of whole central nervous system, which is an irreversible state with functional incapacitation of the whole brain including the brainstem. Brain death manifested in the following four aspects: (1) There was no clinical evidence of brain function upon physical examination with completely unconscious; (2) There were no spontaneous respiration; (3) There was no physiological reflex reaction, including no response to pain and no cranial nerve reflexes, such as pupillary response (fixed pupils), oculocephalic reflex, corneal reflex, and caloric reflex test; (4) The EEG was flat. In 1973, the Eighth International Congress of clinical neurophysiology presented a more detailed definition: "brain death is an irreversible loss of the whole brain function, including the cerebellum, the brainstem till to the first cervical cord" [15].

Although the definition of brain death has been proposed for a half century, the acceptance of brain death was different in each country. Brain death was legislated by some countries including the United States, Germany, Japan, France, Finland, and so on; but brain death was only recognized in clinical practice without formally legal provision in Britain, Switzerland, South Korea, Austria, and so on; however, the standard of brain death was not approved by most of the developing countries. Many countries recognize both cardiac death and brain death as the death judgment standard, especially the United States, Japan, Austria, Switzerland, Finland, etc.

At present, there are no laws and legislations about brain death definition in China. Only some death-related academic discussions have been carried out. Representative academic activities were a cerebral resuscitation forum held in June 1986 in Nanjing, in which experts drafted the first Chinese consensus of diagnostic criteria of brain death. In 1988, experts from related disciplines conducted a discussion on the proposed diagnostic criteria for brain death in Shanghai. In 1989, the first draft of diagnostic criteria for brain death in children was drawn up in China. In October 2002, "China brain death criteria (adult) (third drafts)" was first published in the annual meeting of Chinese organ transplantation in Wuhan [16]. Then, the drafting group for brain death criteria of the Ministry of Health of the People's Republic of China has officially published the judgement standard of brain death for adults in 2003 [17]. In March 2012, Xuanwu Hospital Capital Medical University was authorized by the National Health and Family Planning Commission as a quality evaluation center for brain injury. After 10 years of clinical practice and research, this center optimized a new version of adult and children quality control version "brain death criterion and technical specification" [18, 19]. The publication of this medical professional standard would promote brain death criterion work effectively and development of organ donation.

In medical practice, cardiac death and brain death are affecting each other and reciprocal causation. When the heart and lung function are a failure, the blood circulation will stop and the brain cells will certainly die. On the other hand, the control center of respiratory and circulatory function is in the brainstem, and the brainstem failure will eventually lead to the stop of the heart stroke and the respiratory function. As far as the world is concerned, due to the profound influence of the traditional concept of heart and lung death, the concept of cardiopulmonary death is still taken into account when accepting the criteria of brain death. Judging from the basic national conditions of China, Chinese traditional culture attaches importance to humanistic care, and views about life and death has always been one of the important connotations and manifestations of culture. In a certain sense, this traditional concept of death organically unifies both standards of heart death and brain death and provides the traditional humanistic and theoretical basis for the establishment of death standards in China.

2.4 Impact of Brain Death Criterion on Transplant Development

Since the late 1970s, the research of organ transplantation technology has reached an advanced level in the world, but the source of organ is seriously lacking. A series of medical difficulties have been gradually overcome, organ transplantation confronted with legal dilemma without legislation of "brain death." Since only donor organs procured within brain death status were the most optimizing organ with viability and function. The lagging legislation of brain death has become the bottleneck of this life reengineering project, but also caused great waste of medical resources, which brings endless pain and annoyance to the patients and families. According to the survey, about one million patients in our country need organ transplants, but only 13,000 cases can acquire organ transplantation every year. Only 10% of the transplant recipients on the waiting list survive, and many critical patients die due to shortage of organs. On the other hand, a large number of people died in accidents such as traffic accidents, who could become organ donors. Due to the current brain death was not legislated in China, no doctor dared to make a decision of procurement. So there is isolation between organ needs and lacks. Under such circumstances, our country had put forward the work of organ donation and taken donation after cardiac death (DCD) as the dominant donor type, which would solve the dilemma of organ transplantation development [20].

2.5 Classification of DCD Donation

The first International Symposium on non-heart-beating donors published the DCD Maastricht classification criteria of organ donation in 1995 [21]. The standard DCD will be divided into 4 categories: Type I is prehospital death. There is a clear record of the time of death, cardiopulmonary resuscitation process before admission. Type II is cardiopulmonary resuscitation failure patients in the emergency ward. The majority of patients are wounded ones in trauma, with detailed records of the cardiopulmonary resuscitation process. Type III is a patient waiting for cardiac arrest or close to dying without reaching the standard of brainstem death. Type IV is cardiac arrest after brain death or accident cardiac arrest after definite brainstem death. Among them, the majority of type III and type IV patients are in intensive care units. In accordance with China's existing national conditions and international classifications, the Ministry of Health proclaimed three categories of citizen organ donation after death in China: China one category (C-I): the international standard of brain death organ donation (DBD). A rigorous medical examination is necessary, and the indicators are in line with the international brain death standards and the latest domestic standard of brain death. It is further acquired clear brain death from brain death diagnosis expert approved by the Ministry of Health commissioned institutions. The donor family fully accept and choose to stop treatment and agree to procure organ within brain death criteria. At the same time, the consent of the relevant department of the donating hospital should be obtained before procurement. China two category (C-II): International standardized cardiac death organ donation (DCD), including types I–IV of the Maastricht Standard Classification. China three category (C-III): donation after brain death plus cardiac death (DBCD). The donor has already fully met the DBD standard. But in view of the absence of legal support for brain death, it is implemented according to strict procedures of DCD. At present, C-III is the main mode of organ donation after the death of Chinese citizens.

Cardiac death organ donation is divided into uncontrolled and controlled types. Due to the randomness of cardiac arrest time, the uncontrolled DCD patients often have warm ischemia injury when organ procurement organization got intervention, resulting in poor organ quality. The precondition of control type DCD is that patient exists irreversible brain death, ventilator dependence, and informed consent about removal of all treatment. After the withdrawal of life support measures including ventilator and 3–5 min after cardiac arrest to declare donor death, the organ procurement staff waiting in another room then will start organ resection [22]. The controlled DCD refers to the planned removal of the life support equipment by the organ acquisition group. Family consent and the medical team and other works initiation can be completed before the removal of life support therapy. Therefore, the donor organs have short warm ischemia time and can be safely used for transplantation. There was no difference in long-term prognosis between controlled DCD donors and brain death donors. Uncontrollable DCD refers to the failure of cardiopulmonary resuscitation or cardiac arrest, or death on the way to hospital. Such donors are generally emergency patients who can seek organ donation after the patient has died of cardiac arrest or death. Because the donor-related procedures launched by the declaration of death, the donor organs experienced a longer duration of warm ischemia. Most uncontrolled DCD organs are not available for transplant.

2.6 Clinical Application and Prognosis of DCD Organ Transplantation

The donor liver pool was extended by application of cardiac death donor, and more and more patients with end-stage liver disease were saved and survived well. According to the 2007 annual report of American Organ Procurement and Transplantation Network (OPTN) and Scientific Registry of Transplant Recipient (SRTR), the total number of liver transplant in the United States was 35,598 cases by the end of 2006, of which DCD liver transplantation was 1007, accounting for only 2.8% of the total [23].

However, unlike the brain dead organ donor, the DCD donor proceeded in cardiac arrest. Before organ perfusion, the tissue experienced a process of ischemia and hypoxia. Ischemia-reperfusion injury of donor organs caused by cardiac arrest has a great influence on graft function and prognosis. And the effect of DCD transplantation varies greatly.

Kidney transplantation is the earliest clinical application and research using DCD donors. Most clinical reports came from one single transplant center, and the results were not entirely consistent. In the long-term follow-up, the prognosis of the recipients are affected by many factors, such as changes in immunosuppressive agents and updates in matching techniques. Kidney transplantation appeared to the best effect among different DCD-derived organ transplants. The short- and long-term outcomes of controlled and uncontrolled DCD renal transplantation are close to other types of donated organ transplants. The 6 years graft survival was 73.2% [24]. Multivariate analysis found that the incidence of delayed graft function dialysis after renal transplantation increased by two times, such that 50% of PRA, glucocorticoid resistance, rejection, re-transplantation, nontraumatic caused deceased donor and donor over 35 [25]. University of Wisconsin experience showed that there were 382 transplants from DCD donors and 1089 cases from DBD donors from January 1984 to August 2000. There was no statistical difference in cold ischemic time, rate of primary nonfunction, or graft loss in the first 30 days after transplantation. The rate of delayed graft function (DGF) was higher for DCD donors (27.5% vs. 21.3%; $p = 0.016$). There was no statistical difference in 5-, 10-, or 15-year allograft survival when DCD donors were compared with DBD donors (64.8%, 44.8%, 27.8% vs. 71.3%, 48.3%, 33.8%; $p = 0.054$), which indicated that the results of renal transplantation from DCD donors are equivalent to long-term allograft survival from DBD donors despite an increase at the rate of DGF [26].

The overall effect of DCD liver transplantation is inferior to that of renal transplantation. Noncontrolled DCD liver transplantation is very limited in clinical application. Before 2006, a few centers reported the therapeutic effects of DCD and DBD liver transplantation were relative. There is a significant difference between the large sample of controlled DCD and DBD liver transplantation.

A study by the Wisconsin University showed 1- and 3-year survival rates for recipients as 80% and 68% respectively in DCD, while 91% and

84% in DBD. The graft 1- and 3-year survival rates were 67% and 56% in DCD, while 86% and 80% in DBD, respectively. All of them were significantly less in the DCD group. The 1- (33% vs. 10%) and 3-year (37% vs. 12%) overall rate of biliary strictures were greater in the DCD group. There was no difference in the incidence of primary non-function, hepatic artery thrombosis, ischemic-type biliary stricture (ITBS), and portal vein stenosis/thrombosis. However, the incidence of biloma formation, hepatic abscess, and hepatic artery stenosis in DBD group were always higher than DCD group [27]. In recent years, the latest clinical data has brought more confidence in DCD liver transplantation. Nguyen [28] reported that the survival rates of grafts and recipients in DCD 1, 3, 5 years were 73.7%, 68.4%, 63.2% and 89.5%, 89.5%, 89.5%, respectively. Mateo et al. [29] reported 226 cases of DCD liver transplant recipients with warm ischemia time less than 30 min and cold ischemia time less than 10 h. The survival rates of 1 and 3 years were 81% and 67%, respectively, compared to 80% and 72% years after DBD liver transplantation, which was no significant difference. Lee et al. [30] reported that the survival rates of liver transplant recipients at 1 and 5 years were 84.9% and 69.4%, respectively, which were not different from those of DBD liver transplantation recipients. This happened only with strictly controlled donor parameters, including those aged less than 45 years, without fatty liver, warm ischemia time less than 15 min, and cold ischemia time less than 10 h. At present, most scholars believe that DCD donor liver quality could be improved by appropriate screening of donors, including the limitation of warm ischemia time and reasonable matching donor recipient.

The clinical experience of DCD pancreas and islet transplantation is very limited. A group of studies at the University of Wisconsin reported that there was no significant difference in graft and recipient survival between DCD and DBD [31]. The graft survival rates at 1 and 3 years were 55% and 36%, respectively, but the incidence of hemodialysis after transplantation was higher in the DCD group [32]. In 2003, Markmann et al. [33] reported that DCD-derived islet transplantation could be successfully used in patients with type 1 diabetes mellitus, but lack of large sample of clinical experience.

DCD lung transplantation experience is also limited. A large study of international, multicenter experience demonstrates excellent survival after lung transplantation using DCD donors. In a retrospective study, there were 306 lung transplants performed using DCD donors and 3992 transplants using DBD donors during January 2003 and June 2013 data from the International Society for Heart and Lung Transplantation (ISHLT) DCD Registry. Thirty-day survival was 96% in the DCD group and 97% in the DBD group. One-year survival was 89% in the DCD group and 88% in the DBD group. Five-year survival was 61% in both groups [34]. The incidence of early acute lung injury was not different from that of other donor organs. Uncontrolled DCD lung transplantation has also been reported sporadically, but the overall therapeutic effect is not ideal. Because of persistent ischemic injury during organ donation, it is generally accepted that DCD is not suitable for lung transplantation [35–37].

Clinically, the source of DCD organs is increasing year by year. The long-term outcome of DCD renal transplantation has been close to that of other standard donors. In recent years, the effect of DCD liver transplantation has gradually been recognized by many transplant centers. With the accumulation and promotion of related experience, DCD has become one of the most important donor sources for organ transplantation. At present, the research on the factors affecting lung, pancreas, and heart transplantation from DCD is in the beginning, but some early experience reports are very encouraging.

2.7 The Development of Organ Donation After the Death of Domestic Citizens in China

China had made a pioneering achievement in organ transplantation legislation and management system construction. China's liver transplantation registration project was initiated in February 2005. In March 2007, the State Council promulgated and implemented management file "the regulations on human organ transplantation." In order to promote organ donation move forward, the Ministry of Health (now named as the National Health and Family Planning Commission) commissioned the Red Cross Society of China to launch human organ donation-related work in January 2010. In March of the same year, the Ministry of Health and the Red Cross Society of China jointly issued the "China human organ donation pilot work program," which wanted to establish the organ donation system in 10 provinces first. Ten provinces including Guangdong, Wuhan, Tianjin, Liaoning etc. have gradually carried out human organ donation work and achieved some experience in the promotion and establishment of organ donation system. Based on the experience of the pilot work program, the National Health and Family Planning Commission issued "the management of the procurement and distribution of human organs (Trial Implementation)" in 2013, which was promulgated on September 1, 2013.

According to the rule, our country established the leadership of the Administrative Department of Health (Health and Family Planning Commission) as the policy and guidance department. And the organ procurement organization (OPO) is dependent on the transplant hospital. At the same time, it stipulate the principle that donated organ must be distributed and shared through the "China Organ Transplant Response System". The social forces are also fully involved in the donation scheme. Because of the huge contribution in organ donation and system construction, the Red Cross participates in the process of organ donation as a third party. The implementation of the rule is a sign that our country has initially explored and established the "China organ donation model." This model is similar to the Spanish model and has made great achievements in the actual work.

OPO, which worked on the frontline of organ donation, plays an important role in every successful donation case. OPO personnel were mainly composed of organ transplantation center, department of neurology and neurosurgery, ICU, physicians and nurses, etc. Transplantation hospitals, as the support unit of OPO, should play a role in the aspect of organization, management, and construction, including performing strictly the death judgment process and standardization, financial management, and standardization of organ donation procedures.

Since the rule was published, the provinces and municipalities have promulgated the implementation details. Taking Guangdong Province as an example, the Guangdong provincial health and Family Planning Commission issued a letter on September 29, 2013, on human organ donation acquisition and distribution management work notice. According to the notice, Guangdong province will set up 6 OPO base on the transplant hospital. In order to ensure the orderly development of organ donation, the administrative department has stated that Guangdong would be divided into 6 regions correlated to the 6 OPO service range, and each OPO should work in its designated region. Then on June 17, 2014, the health and Family Planning Commission of Guangdong provincial issued a file on "notice about establishment of Guangdong Province organ donation death evaluation expert group." The expert group composed of neurology and neurosurgery experts was established to standardize the death judgment of organ donors.

References

1. de Begona JA, Gundry SR, Razzouk AJ, Boucek MM, Kawauchi M, Bailey LL. Transplantation of hearts after arrest and resuscitation. Early and long-term results. J Thorac Cardiovasc Surg. 1993;106(6):1196–201. 1200-1
2. Kawauchi M, Gundry SR, de Begona JA, Razzouk AJ, Bailey LL. Utilization of pediatric donors salvaged by cardiopulmonary resuscitation. J Heart Lung Transplant. 1993;12(2):185–8.
3. Gundry SR, Fukushima N, Eke CC, Hill AC, Zuppan C, Bailey LL. Successful survival of primates receiving transplantation with "dead," nonbeating donor hearts. J Thorac Cardiovasc Surg. 1995;109(6):1010–97., 1101–2. https://doi.org/10.1016/S0022-5223(95)70193-1.
4. Gundry SR, Alonso DBJ, Kawauchi M, Liu H, Razzouk AJ, Bailey LL. Transplantation and reanimation of hearts removed from donors 30 minutes after warm, asystolic 'death'. Arch Surg. 1993;128(9):989–91. 992–3

5. Murray JE, Merrill JP, Harrison JH, Wilson RE, Dammin GJ. Prolonged survival of human-kidney homografts by immunosuppressive drug therapy. N Engl J Med. 1963;268:1315–23. https://doi.org/10.1056/NEJM196306132682401.
6. Starzl TE, Marchioro TL, Vonkaulla KN, Hermann G, Brittain RS, Waddell WR. Homotransplantation of the liver in humans. Surg Gynecol Obstet. 1963;117:659–76.
7. Starzl TE, Porter KA, Brettschneider L, Penn I, Bell P, Putnam CW, et al. Clinical and pathologic observations after orthotopic transplantation of the human liver. Surg Gynecol Obstet. 1969;128(2):327–39.
8. Kelly WD, Lillehei RC, Merkel FK, Idezuki Y, Goetz FC. Allotransplantation of the pancreas and duodenum along with the kidney in diabetic nephropathy. Surgery. 1967;61(6):827–37.
9. Barnard CN. The operation. A human cardiac transplant: an interim report of a successful operation performed at Groote Schuur Hospital, Cape Town. S Afr Med J. 1967;41(48):1271–4.
10. Barnard CN. Human cardiac transplantation. An evaluation of the first two operations performed at the Groote Schuur Hospital, Cape Town. Am J Cardiol. 1968;22(4):584–96.
11. Lillehei RC, Simmons RL, Najarian JS, Weil R, Uchida H, Ruiz JO, et al. Pancreatico-duodenal allotransplantation: experimental and clinical experience. Ann Surg. 1970;172(3):405–36.
12. Qian J, Ma Z. The history and current situation of donors after cardiac death. Chin J Transplant (Electronic Version). 2009;3(4):273–6. https://doi.org/10.3969/j.issn.1674-3903.2009.04.003.
13. Dominguez-Gil B, Haase-Kromwijk B, Van Leiden H, Neuberger J, Coene L, Morel P, et al. Current situation of donation after circulatory death in European countries. Transpl Int. 2011;24(7):676–86. https://doi.org/10.1111/j.1432-2277.2011.01257.x.
14. Huang J. A key measure to promote the healthy development of organ transplantation in China—Principle thinking on the pilot work of DCD. Chin J Organ Transplant. 2011;32(1):1–4. https://doi.org/10.3760/cma.j.issn.0254-1785.2011.01.001.
15. Dai Q. The ethical pain and legal helplessness in death criterion and organ transplantation. Med Philos. 2006;27(13):42–4.
16. Liu M, Sui S. Discussion on ethical and legal issues of brain death criterion. Chin Hospitals. 2016;20(2):62–4. https://doi.org/10.3969/j.issn.1671-0592.2016.02.025.
17. Draft for criterion of brain death (adults). Natl Med J China. 2003;83(3). https://doi.org/10.3760/j:issn:0376-2491.2003.03.028.
18. Brain Injury Quality Control Evaluation Center of National Health and Family Planning Commission. Criterion and technical specifications for brain death (Adult's Quality Control Version). Chin J Neurol. 2013;46(9):637–40. https://doi.org/10.3760/cma.j.issn.1006-7876.2013.09.015.
19. Brain Injury Quality Control Evaluation Center of National Health and Family Planning Commission. Criterion and technical specifications for brain death (Children's Quality Control Version). Chin J Pediatr. 2014;52(10):756–9. https://doi.org/10.3760/cma.j.issn.0578-1310.2014.10.008.
20. Wang L. Ethical Research on Death Criteria. Med Soc. 2003;16(2):24–5., 29. https://doi.org/10.3870/j.issn.1006-5563.2003.02.010.
21. Kootstra G, Daemen JH, Oomen AP. Categories of non-heart-beating donors. Transplant Proc. 1995;27(5):2893–4.
22. Chen Z. The development history of the source of human organ transplantation donors. Chin J Transplant (Electronic Version). 2009;3(4):264–7. https://doi.org/10.3969/j.issn.1674-3903.2009.04.001.
23. Liu Y. The ethics of organ acquisition from DCD and clinical application of liver transplantation. Chin J Transplant (Electronic Version). 2009;3(4):268–72. https://doi.org/10.3969/j.issn.1674-3903.2009.04.002.
24. Rudich SM, Kaplan B, Magee JC, Arenas JD, Punch JD, Kayler LK, et al. Renal transplantations performed using non-heart-beating organ donors: going back to the future? Transplantation. 2002;74(12):1715–20. https://doi.org/10.1097/01.TP.0000039165.58547.87.
25. Weber M, Dindo D, Demartines N, Ambuhl PM, Clavien PA. Kidney transplantation from donors without a heartbeat. N Engl J Med. 2002;347(4):248–55. https://doi.org/10.1056/NEJMoa020274.
26. Cooper JT, Chin LT, Krieger NR, Fernandez LA, Foley DP, Becker YT, et al. Donation after cardiac death: the university of wisconsin experience with renal transplantation. Am J Transplant. 2004;4(9):1490–4. https://doi.org/10.1111/j.1600-6143.2004.00531.x.
27. Foley DP, Fernandez LA, Leverson G, Chin LT, Krieger N, Cooper JT, et al. Donation after cardiac death: the University of Wisconsin experience with liver transplantation. Ann Surg. 2005;242(5):724–31.
28. Nguyen JH, Bonatti H, Dickson RC, Hewitt WR, Grewal HP, Willingham DL, et al. Long-term outcomes of donation after cardiac death liver allografts from a single center. Clin Transpl. 2009;23(2):168–73. https://doi.org/10.1111/j.1399-0012.2009.00968.x.
29. Mateo R, Cho Y, Singh G, Stapfer M, Donovan J, Kahn J, et al. Risk factors for graft survival after liver transplantation from donation after cardiac death donors: an analysis of OPTN/UNOS data. Am J Transplant. 2006;6(4):791–6. https://doi.org/10.1111/j.1600-6143.2006.01243.x.
30. Lee KW, Simpkins CE, Montgomery RA, Locke JE, Segev DL, Maley WR. Factors affecting graft survival after liver transplantation from donation after cardiac death donors. Transplantation. 2006;82(12):1683–8. https://doi.org/10.1097/01.tp.0000250936.73034.98.
31. D'Alessandro AM, Fernandez LA, Chin LT, Shames BD, Turgeon NA, Scott DL, et al. Donation after cardiac death: the University of Wisconsin experience. Ann Transplant. 2004;9(1):68–71.

32. D'Alessandro AM, Odorico JS, Knechtle SJ, Becker YT, Hoffmann RM, Kalayoglu M, et al. Simultaneous pancreas-kidney (SPK) transplantation from controlled non-heart-beating donors (NHBDs). Cell Transplant. 2000;9(6):889–93.
33. Markmann JF, Deng S, Desai NM, Huang X, Velidedeoglu E, Frank A, et al. The use of non-heart-beating donors for isolated pancreatic islet transplantation. Transplantation. 2003;75(9):1423–9. https://doi.org/10.1097/01.TP.0000061119.32575.F4.
34. Oto T. Lung transplantation from donation after cardiac death (non-heart-beating) donors. Gen Thorac Cardiovasc Surg. 2008;56(11):533–8. https://doi.org/10.1007/s11748-008-0315-y.
35. Cypel M, Levvey B, Van Raemdonck D, Erasmus M, Dark J, Love R, et al. International Society for Heart and Lung Transplantation donation after circulatory death registry report. J Heart Lung Transplant. 2015;34(10):1278–82. https://doi.org/10.1016/j.healun.2015.08.015.
36. Del RGF, Nunez PJ, Soria GA, Moreno RM, Varela A, Calatayud J. Non heart beating donors. Successfully expanding the donor's pool. Ann Transplant. 2004;9(2):19–20.
37. Martin J, Lutter G, Ihling C, Siepe M, Wagner S, Hilberath J, et al. Myocardial viability twenty-four hours after orthotopic heart transplantation from non-heart-beating donors. J Thorac Cardiovasc Surg. 2003;125(6):1217–28.

3 Cardiac Death Donor Evaluation and Management

Guixing Xu and Zimeng Liu

Abstract

Donation after cardiac death (DCD) describes the retrieval of organs for the purposes of transplantation that follows death confirmed using circulatory criteria (the cessation of the heart beat). The persisting shortfall in the availability of organs for transplantation has prompted many countries to reintroduce DCD schemes not only for kidney procurement but increasingly for other organs with a lower tolerance for warm ischemia such as the liver, pancreas, and lungs. Compared with donation after brain death, the challenge in the practice of DCD includes how to identify patients as suitable potential DCD donors, and how to manage the consequences of warm ischemia in a fashion that is professionally, ethically, and legally acceptable. Since the organ procurement from the uncontrolled DCD is hard to practice, this chapter mainly focuses on the practice of controlled DCD. DCD after the withdrawal of life-sustaining treatment accounts for a substantial proportion of deceased organ donors overall. Generally speaking, after the withdrawal of life-sustaining treatment, DCD accounts for a substantial proportion of deceased organ donors. Where this occurs, there is an increasing consensus that organ and tissue donation might be considered a alternative part of end-of-life care in intensive care unit.

3.1 The Evaluation of Cardiac Death Donor

For patients with end-stage failure of different vital organs, organ transplantation is often the only therapeutic option. However, there is a worrisome disproportion between the demand for organ transplants and the number of transplants. Donation after cardiac death (DCD), the process of organ procurement after withdrawal of life-sustaining treatment (WLST) and cardiac death in the operating room, is an increasing practice. The challenge that is faced by today's organ procurement organization (OPO) is how to evaluate patients as potential DCD donors. Potential DCD donors are mainly divided into two groups: Group1—A person whose circulatory and respiratory functions have ceased and resuscitative measures are not to be attempted or continued; Group2—A person in whom the cessation of circulatory and respiratory functions is anticipated to occur within a time frame that will enable organ recovery [1].

G. Xu (✉)
The Neurosurgery Department, The First Affiliated Hospital of Sun Yat-sen University, Guangzhou, China

Z. Liu
The Intensive Care Unit, The First Affiliated Hospital of Sun Yat-sen University, Guangzhou, China

X. He (ed.), *Organ Donation and Transplantation after Cardiac Death in China*,
https://doi.org/10.1007/978-981-16-0815-5_3

Because the number of people who are waiting for organ transplants is far greater than the rate of organ donation, medical professionals, especially in the ICU, should continue to capture potential organ donors as clinically indicated. Critical care professionals must manage not only anxious patients and family members during stressful situations but also often have to work through "difficult end-of-life decisions, evaluating when to call the OPO, caring for brain death patients, managing a potential DCD candidate" within institutional and standard of care guidelines.

Since patients with catastrophic, irreversible brain injury who do not meet the criteria for brain death, also named as neurocritical patients, are the most frequent candidates for DCD. Currently, the prediction of brain death in these neurocritical patients is based on neurological examination, neuroimaging, controlled ventilation, vasopressor use, GCS, and brain stem reflexes. Recently, these variables are used to predict cardiac death in neurocritical patients, so they can also be used to evaluate the potential DCD donor in neurocritical patients [2]. It is an encouraging step to identify the potential DCD donors on the basis of neurologic lesions and the organ transplantation enters into the neurological era.

3.1.1 The Classification of DCD

The modified Maastricht classification is widely used to categorize DCD, and there are five categories in this classification (Table 3.1). Categories II, V, and I describe organ retrieval that follows unexpected and irreversible cardiac arrest (uncontrolled DCD), so they were hard to be evaluated as a potential DCD donor. While categories III and IV refer to retrieval that follows death resulting from the planned WLST (controlled DCD), so the evaluation of potential DCD donors focuses on these two controlled categories [3]. The evaluation of potential DCD donors in category III is based on the prediction of cardiac death, while category IV is based on the prediction of progress to brain death.

The vast majority of DCD donors are controlled donors, patients who die after WLST. The quality of organs of DCD donors is highly dependent on the time between WLST and cardiac death. Cardiac death beyond 60 min can result in donor ineligibility because of inferior quality of organs as a result of suboptimal oxygen levels. Therefore, for practical and ethical reasons, the ability to predict whether a patient will die within 60 min after WLST is of interest for the transplantation.

3.2 Cardiac Death Prediction

Based on a cardiac death criterion, the potential DCD donor turns to an actual DCD donor when respiration and circulation have ceased and cardiopulmonary function will not resume spontaneously. The current predictive scores that can be used to evaluate the potential DCD donor are as follows.

3.2.1 The UW Criteria

The University of Wisconsin is unique because it has continuously performed DCD since 1974. About 10–15% of the donors obtained by them are DCD donors. The University of Wisconsin has developed an algorithm—the UW criteria—for the evaluation of the potential DCD donor. The UW criteria are calculated based on the six parameters of patients and composed of a numeric scale from 7 to 21 (Table 3.2) [4].

Table 3.1 The modified Maastricht classification of DCD

Classification	Description	Type
I	Dead on arrival	Uncontrolled
II	Unsuccessful resuscitation	Uncontrolled
III	Anticipated cardiac arrest	Controlled
IV	Cardiac arrest in a brain-dead donor	Controlled
V	Unexpected arrest in ICU patient	Uncontrolled

Table 3.2 The UW criteria for predicting cardiac death after WLST

Variables	Subcategory	Scale
Spontaneous respirations after 10 min (WLST)	Rate > 12	1
	Rate < 12	3
	Tidal volume > 200 ml	1
	Tidal volume < 200 mL	3
	Negative inspiratory force >20	1
	Negative inspiratory force <20	3
	No spontaneous respirations	9
Body mass index	<25	1
	25–29	2
	>30	3
Vasopressors	No vasopressors	1
	Single vasopressor	2
	Multiple vasopressors	3
Age	0–30	1
	31–50	2
	>51	3
Intubation	Endotracheal tube	3
	Tracheostomy	1
Oxygenation after 10 min (WLST)	O_2 saturation > 90%	1
	O_2 saturation 80–89%	2
	O_2 saturation < 79%	3

Table 3.3 The likelihood of cardiac death according to the UW criteria

	Cardiac death	
Score	Within 60 min (%)	With 120 min (%)
10	8	26
11	13	34
12	20	42
13	28	51
14	38	59
15	50	68
16	62	75
17	72	81
18	81	86
19	87	90
20	92	92
21	95	95
22	97	96
23	98	97

The University of Wisconsin Donation After Cardiac Death Evaluation Tool is derived from standard weaning protocols utilized in hospitals for patients with withdrawn life support treatment. Respiratory rate and tidal volume (VT) predict whether a patient can breathe without the assistance of a ventilator. An increased respiratory rate in combination with a decreasing VT may indicate that the respiratory of a patient will arrest without the aid of a ventilator. Vasopressors and inotropes increase systolic blood pressure output and contracts peripheral vessels thereby shunting blood to important organs. When vasopressors and inotropes are removed, the heart function begins to fail. The secondary effect of heart failure is a decrease in the amount of oxygen delivered to the organ. Arterial oxygen saturation of less than 90% caused hypoxemia. The UW criterion gives points for either an endotracheal (ET) tube or a tracheostomy. When the ET tube is withdrawn, these structures resume their anatomical position and may occlude the airway.

The UW criteria are originally designed to predict cardiac death after WLST, and now it also can be used to evaluate the potential DCD donor by anticipating cardiac arrest in patients. The expiration likelihood of cardiac death with 60 and 120 min with the UW criteria is shown in Table 3.3. A score between 10 and 23 is assigned based on these variables, with a higher score presumed to be associated with a higher probability of death. As shown in Table 3.3, the patients with a score of more than 17 can be treated as potential DCD donors, since the expiration likelihood of cardiac death after WLST within 60 min is more than 80%.

3.2.2 The UNOS Criteria

The United Network for Organ Sharing (UNOS) also developed criteria that can be helpful in evaluating potential DCD candidates (Table 3.4) [5]. Based upon the number of UNOS criteria present, a score is assigned between 0 and 5, with 5 presumed to be associated with a higher likelihood of death within 60 min. The criteria will be helpful for clinicians in determining an individual's potential for DCD.

The number of UNOS evaluation criteria has a "dose-response curve." Compared with the UW criteria, the UNOS criteria are simpler and easier to utility in clinical experience, but less precise. There are five categories of variables in the UNOS criteria, it just needs to calculate the number of variables (Table 3.5). According to the Table 3.5, patients with number of UNOS criteria present more than 2 are more likely to be a potential DCD donor, since the percent of cardiac death after WLST is more than 60% among them.

3.2.3 The DCD-N Score

The most frequent candidates for DCD are patients with catastrophic, irreversible brain injury who do not meet the criteria for brain death, but about half of these patients continue to breathe and maintain circulation for more than 60 min after WLST. Prolongation of the withdrawal phase of warm ischemia time (i.e., the time between WLST and end of cardiopulmonary function) beyond 60 min can compromise organ function. The success of DCD relies on the evaluation of patients who are most likely to die within 60 min. Available variables to estimate the time to cardiac death after WLST, such as the UW criteria or the UNOS criteria, include little information about the neurological status of the patient, so they have less prognostic value in patients with catastrophic brain injury who have not progressed to brain death. Meanwhile, patients with catastrophic, irreversible brain injury who do not meet the criteria for brain death, also named as neurocritical patients, are the most frequent candidates for DCD, therefore methods used to evaluate the potential DCD donor should be especially applicable to patients in neurocritical state.

Some scoring system has been specifically designed to be used in neurological patients with severe, irreversible brain injury and it can be fully assessed while the potential donor remains supported by mechanical ventilation. The most representative one is the DCD-N score reported by Rabinstein (Table 3.6) [2]; there are 3 neurological variables and 1 no-neurological variable in this score. The information about brain injury included in the score can improve the accuracy of cardiac death prediction within 60 min after WLST in neurocritical patients. The DCD-N score can be useful to evaluate the best candidates for donation among patients in a neurocritical state, thus reducing the chances of unsuccessful activation of retrieval teams and improved allocation of resources.

The probabilities of death within 60 min according to the DCD-N score are shown in the Table 3.7, according to it, scores more than 3 are most likely to occur cardiac death within 60 min.

Table 3.4 The UNOS criteria for evaluating potential DCD patients

Variables	Subcategory
Breath	Apnea
	RR < 8
	RR > 30 during trial off mechanical ventilation
Cardiac assist	LVAD
	RVAD
	V-A ECMO
	Pacemaker unassisted heart rate < 30
Oxygenation	PEEP ≥10 and SaO2 ≤ 92%
	FiO2 ≥ 0.5 and SaO2 ≤ 92%
	V-V ECMO
Vasoactive agents	Norepinephrine, epinephrine, or phenylephrine ≥0.2 μg/kg/min
	Dopamine ≥15 μg/kg/min
IABP	IABP 1:1 or Dobutamine or dopamine ≥10 μg/kg/min CI ≤ 2.2 L/min/m^2
	IABP 1:1 and CI ≤1.5 L/min/m^2

RR respiratory rate, *LVAD* left ventricular assist device, *RVAD* right ventricular assist device, *V-A ECMO* venoarterial extracorporeal membrane oxygenation, *PEEP* positive end-expiratory pressure, SaO_2 arterial oxygen saturation, FiO_2 fraction of inspired oxygen, *V-V ECMO* venovenous extracorporeal membrane oxygenation, *IABP* intra-aortic balloon pump, *CI* cardiac index

Table 3.5 The likelihood of cardiac death within 60 min among potential DCD donor with the UNOS criteria

Group	Number of UNOS criteria present	Death percent within 60 min
1	0	33%
2	1	41%
3	2	67%
4	3	88%

Table 3.6 The DCD-N score for evaluation of cardiac death in neurocritical patients

Variables	Subcategory	Score
Corneal reflex	Present	0
	Absent	1
Cough reflex	Present	0
	Absent	2
Extensor or absent motor response to pain	Present	0
	Absent	1
Oxygenation index	<3	0
	>3	1

Table 3.7 Probabilities of death within 60 min according to the DCD-N score

Corneal reflex	Cough reflex	Extensor or absent motor response	Oxygenation index > 3	Score	Probability (%)
+	+	–	No	0	8
+	+	–	Yes	1	16
–	+	–	No	1	18
+	+	+	No	1	20
+	–	–	No	2	26
–	+	–	Yes	2	34
+	+	+	Yes	2	37
–	–	+	No	2	40
+	–	–	Yes	3	45
–	–	–	No	3	48
+	–	+	No	3	51
–	+	+	Yes	3	61
–	–	–	Yes	4	68
+	–	+	Yes	4	71
–	–	+	No	4	74
–	–	+	Yes	5	87

Contrarily, scores more than 3 can be used to identify the potential DCD donors among neurocritical patients. Unlike the UW criteria and the UNOS criteria, the DCD-N score mainly focuses on the neurocritical patients treated as potential DCD donors, so the applications are limited.

3.2.4 The C-DCD-Nomogram

As a simple graphical representation of a statistical predictive model, the nomogram creates a numerical probability of a clinical event. Compared with traditional staging systems, nomogram has higher predictive accuracy and discrimination. Thus, nomograms have been proposed as an alternative or even as a new standard for providing prognostic information.

A nomogram called the Chinese Donation after Circulatory Death Nomogram (C-DCD-Nomogram) was established and validated by Xiaoshun He et al. for predicting death within 60 min after WLST [6]. There were 10 predictors were incorporated into the C-DCD-Nomogram. These predictors included five neurological examination variables and four neuroimaging variables (Fig. 3.1). They are:

1. Hospitalization days: <30 days or>30 days
2. Pupil size: Normal, anisocoric, or bilaterally dilated
3. Pupil light reflex: Brisk, sluggish, or fixed
4. Corneal reflex: Present or absent
5. Cough reflex: Present or absent
6. Motor response to pain: Normal, extensor, or absent

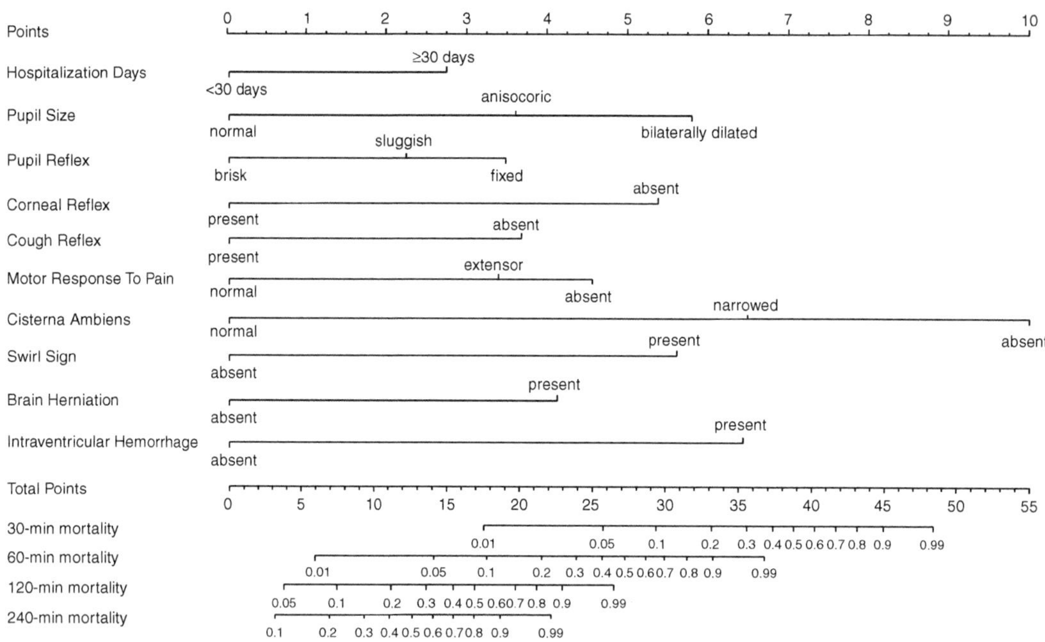

Fig. 3.1 The C-DCD-nomogram

7. Cisterna ambiens: A sheet-like curved layer of subarachnoid space extending from the cisterna quadrigeminalis and partially encircling the midbrain on each side, connecting with the cisterna interpeduncularis) (normal, narrowed, or absent)
8. Swirl sign: Noncontrast CT appearance of low attenuation or radiolucency inside intracranial hyperattenuated hematomas, absent, or present.
9. Brain herniation: Absent or present
10. Intraventricular hemorrhage: Absent or present

According to Fig. 3.1, each predictor was divided into different levels, each level is pointed. Further, in order to use it easily, four different risk groups were created according to the total points:<22, 22–25.9, 26–36.9, ≥37. Concordant with the nomogram prediction, the actual proportion of deaths among patients who scored >22 at 240 min, scored >26 at 120 min, or scored >37 points at 60 min were 94.7%, 97.0%, and 99.0%, respectively (Table 3.8).

In 2018, the C-DCD-Nomogram was further validated with much better performance than the UWDCD evaluation tool, the UNOS criteria, and the DCD-N score [7]. The C-DCD-Nomogram is superior to the other 3 tools in predicting death within a limited duration after WLST in Chinese neurocritical patients, suggesting it is a reliable tool for identifying potential donors after cardiac death. Having not been validated in a non-Chinese population, the C-DCD-Nomogram in the intensive care unit varies in centers in the same country, let alone centers in different countries. Moreover, the C-DCD-Nomogram was developed using data from a neurocritical patient cohort, which limits its application in other potential DCD donors.

Table 3.8 Proportion of cardiac deaths at each time point stratified by different risk groups with Nomogram

	Cardiac deaths (%)		
Risk groups	60 min	120 min	240 min
<22	4.1	49.3	84.9
22–25.9	5.3	68.4	94.7
26–37	67.9	97.0	97.8
>37	99.0	100	100

3.3 Prediction of Progress to Brain Death

Before the development of tracheal positive-pressure ventilators, clinicians determined death by showing the prolonged absence of respiratory and cardiocirculatory functions since the brain functions also ceased at this time. However, once mechanical ventilation could sustain respiratory functions, it became possible for a brain dead patient to have respiration and ventilation supported mechanically. The critical functions of the brain include consciousness, control of circulation, respiration and temperature, and control of homeostasis (fluid, electrolytes, neuroendocrine). Loss of all brain functions whose respiratory and circulatory functions are maintained by life-sustaining therapy including mechanical ventilation with endotracheal intubation [8].

Brain death is defined as the irreversible loss of brain functions (including the brainstem) manifested by unresponsive coma, absence of brainstem reflexes, and apnea. Traumatic brain injury (TBI) and stroke are the most common causes of brain death, which account for more than 90% of potential organ donors. Before progressing to brain death, many patients exhibit a state known as "imminent brain death" [9] from which they might pass to the status of possible organ donors. This condition should be clearly defined and recognized in neurocritical patients, and it should be emphasized that these patients are not brain dead and thus must receive the required intensive care until brain death is confirmed. Based on the above, a patient with a devastating brain injury sustained with mechanical ventilation may be a possible donor, a person who is suspected to fulfill the clinical brain death criteria can be identified as a potential donor. Therefore, a systematic search of possible donors with progress to brain death utilizing clinical routine parameters (mainly included neurological examination, neuroimaging, and spontaneous respiration evaluation), was crucial to identify the potential organ donors.

3.3.1 Neurological Examination

All possible donors need to meet the following criteria: under mechanical ventilation, with devastating irreversible brain injury of known origin, deep coma (score of 3 on the Glasgow Coma Scale, Table 3.9) [10] and absence of one or more brainstem reflexes.

Prior to the assessment of coma, some prerequisites should be fulfilled to rule out coma by reversible causes: (A) presence of irreversible brain injury of known etiology able to cause the condition; (B) absence of evidence of exogenous intoxication or use of central nervous system depressants; (C) absence of severe hydro-electrolytic or acid–base abnormalities; (D) core temperature ideally ≥36.5 °C (core blood, rectal, bladder, or esophageal temperature); and (E) mean arterial pressure (MAP) ≥ 60 mmHg or systolic arterial pressure (SAP) ≥ 90 mmHg. Deep coma patients must lack all evidence of responsiveness. Eye movement or motor response to noxious stimuli is absent. Standard noxious stimuli should be exerted on the head and face, which can avoid confusion with spinal responses, including compression of the supraorbital nerves and bilateral temporomandibular joint compression with deep pressure [11].

Table 3.9 The Glasgow Coma Scale

Score	Eye	Verbal	Motor
6			Obeys commands
5		Oriented	Responds to pain with purposeful movement
4	Open spontaneously	Disoriented, but able to answer questions	Withdraws from pain stimuli
3	Open to verbal command	Inappropriate answers to questions; words discernible	Responds to pain with abnormal flexion (decorticate posture)
2	Open in response to pain applied to the limbs or sternum	Incomprehensible speech	Responds to pain with abnormal (rigid) extension (decerebrate posture)
1	None	None	None

Combined scores < 8 are typically regarded as coma

The Glasgow Coma Scale (GCS) plays an important role in evaluating patients with acute neurological injury and in their management. Reported as a predictive factor of poor outcome in stroke patients, the impact of a low initial GCS score may reflect severe brain injury and hydrocephalus due to high stroke volume and herniation. GCS score ≤ 6 without sedation is a simple score usable at the patient's bedside to help physicians evaluate patients likely to progress to

Table 3.10 The corresponding location of brainstem reflex

No.	Brainstem reflexes	Corresponding location	
1	Pupillary light reflex	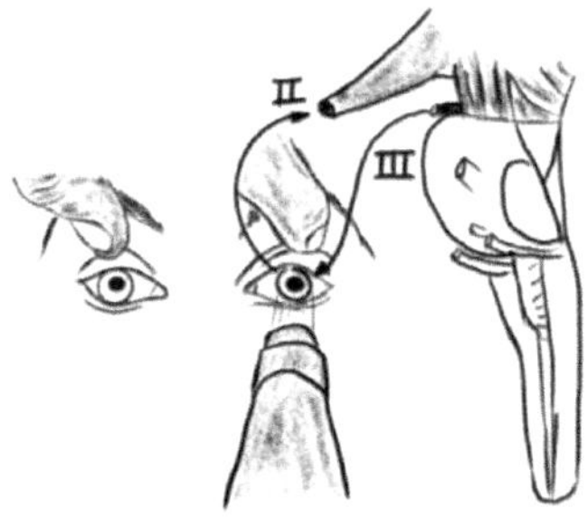	Midbrain
2	Corneal reflex	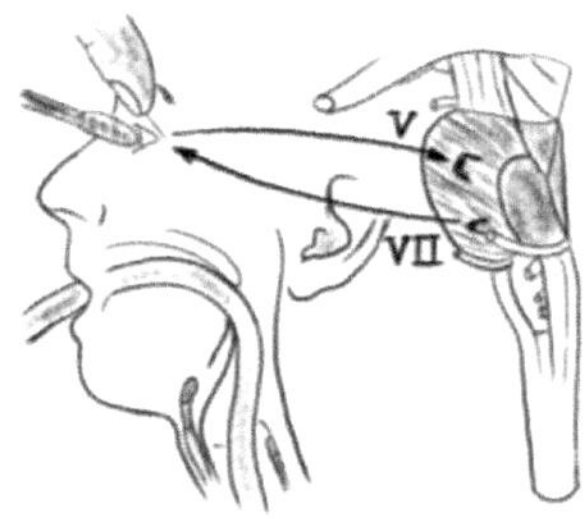	Pons
3	Oculocephalogyric reflex	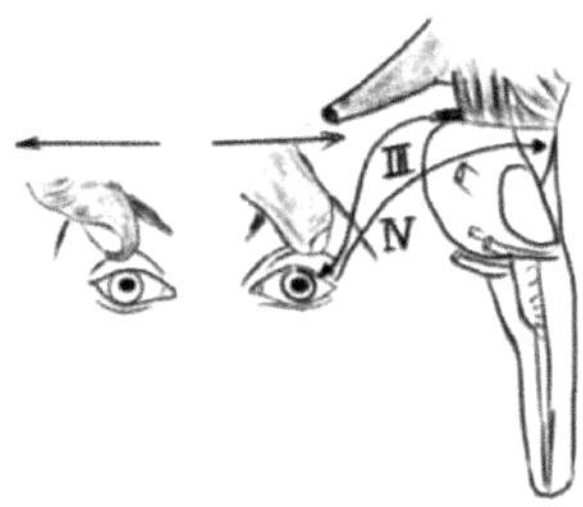	Midbrain Pons
4	Oculovestibular reflex	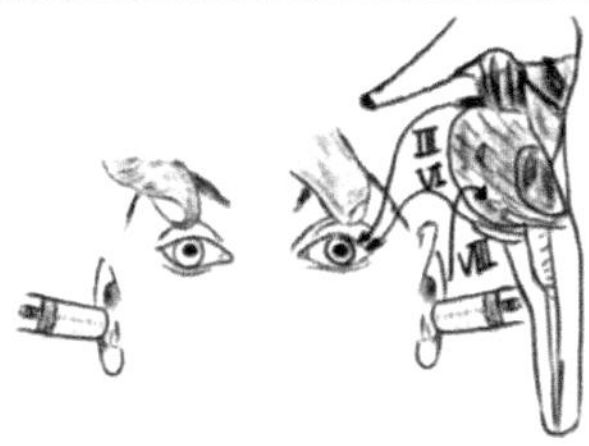	Pons
5	Cough reflex	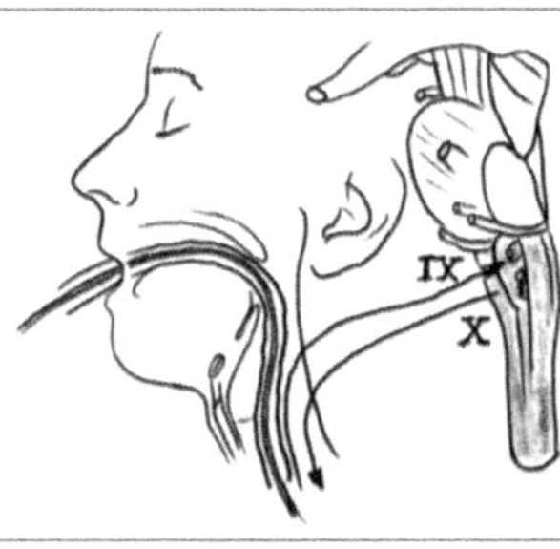	Medulla

brain death. Once the presence of deep coma is established, 5 brainstem reflexes should be tested (pupillary, corneal, oculocephalogyric, oculovestibular, and cough reflex, Table 3.10), and the cessation of respiration should be assessed according to a standardized technique (Apnea test).

3.3.2 Neuroimaging

Neuroimaging, especially the brain Computed Tomography (CT) scan, is the direct and important method to conform the original brain injury. Evidence shows that radiological data along with neurological examination findings can better reflect the severity of brain injury and provide useful information for determining outcomes in neurocritical patients. Brain CT imaging findings can provide important prognostic information of neurocritical patients; brain CT scan for initial evaluation of traumatic brain injury (TBI) had been well established. Brain CT scans produce clear, high-quality images in short time and the analysis of data has been further enhanced by the use of various graphics workstation programs that have produced detailed images and 3D reconstructions of specific areas of interest, allow radiologists to make accurate diagnoses [6].

3.3.2.1 Swirl Sign [12]

The swirl sign described as non-contrast CT scans appearance of low attenuation or radiolucency inside intracranial hyperattenuated hematomas (Fig. 3.2a). The swirl sign seen on non-enhanced CT scans represents active bleed-

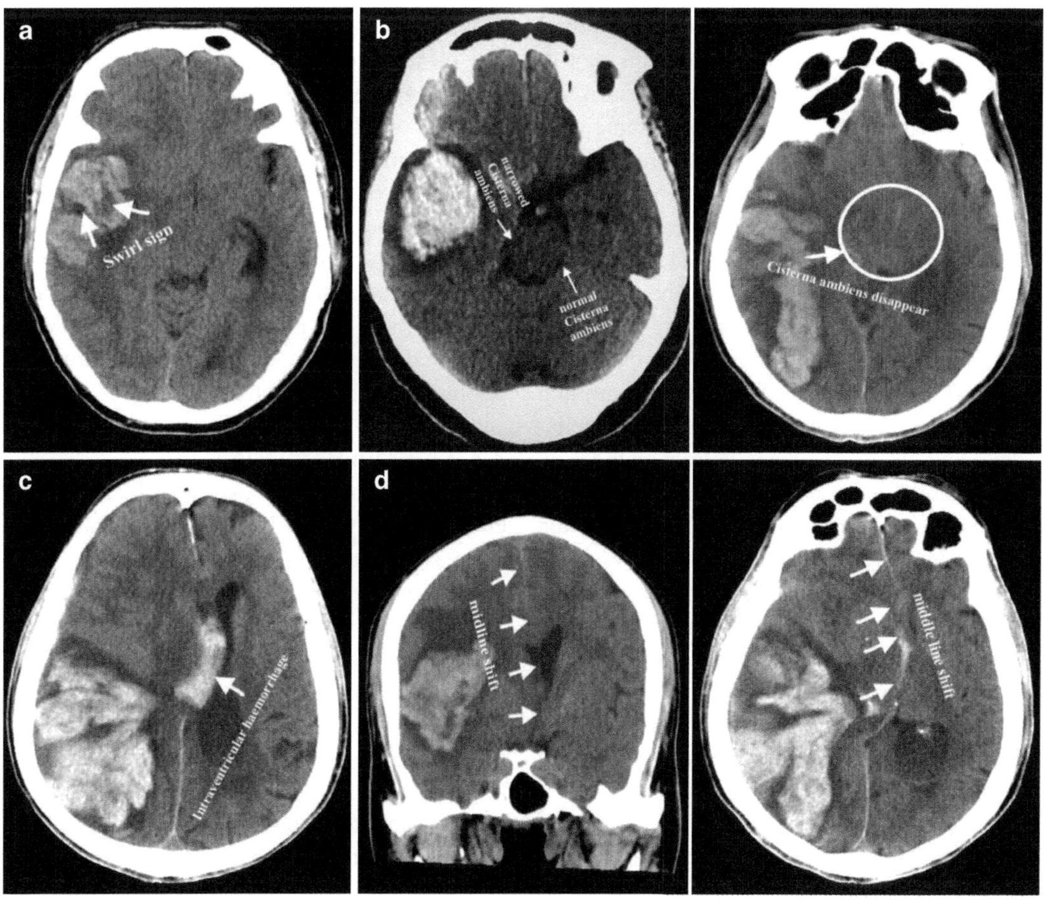

Fig. 3.2 The serious manifestation of brain injury in brain CT scan. (**a**) Swirl sign. (**b**) Cisterna ambiens. (**c**) IVH. (**d**) The midline shift

ing in the hematoma, it represents actively extravasating non-coagulated fresh blood which is of low attenuation with clotted blood (50–70 HU) surrounds it. Studies showed that the volume growth at 24 h was higher in the heterogeneous hematoma (with swirl sign) than in the homogeneous hematoma (without swirl sign). The growth leading to increasing intracranial pressure (ICP), decreasing cerebral perfusion pressure, and brain death, is highly predictive of neurological deterioration and is an independent predictor of mortality.

3.3.2.2 Cisterna Ambiens [13]

The ambient cistern is a thin, sheet-like extension of the quadrigeminal cistern that extends laterally around the midbrain and posterior to the thalami. It acts as the connection between the quadrigeminal cistern and the interpeduncular cistern (Fig. 3.2b). Cisterna ambiens are cerebrospinal fluid circulation path with posterior cerebral artery, superior cerebellar artery, anterior choroidal artery, posterior choroidal artery, basal veins and the fourth cranial nerve through. Acute traumatic brain injury causes high intracranial pressure (ICP), because the pressure of lesion is higher than other parts of the cerebral, this hemicerebrum will shift to the contralateral first but restricted by the falx cerebri, and the bottom of the hemicerebrum near the midline structures such as uncinate gyrus, parahippocampal gyrus will shift downward also blocked by tentorium cerebelli and more apparent, cause suprasellar cistern and cisterna ambiens narrow or blocked. When these happen, cerebrospinal fluid circulation disorder continues to develop compression of the brainstem, the aqueduct of sylvius obstruction in whole or in part to form the hydrocephalus, lead to increased ICP finally. Whether brainstem damage or not is an important factor to decide the prognosis of patients. The blocking of cisterna ambiens is one of the important signs of cerebral compression, is reliable evidence of brainstem injury.

3.3.2.3 Intraventricular Hemorrhage [14]

IVH (Intraventricular Hemorrhage) causes blockage of ventricular conduits leading to hydrocephalus, increased ICP, and a reduced level of consciousness. IVH is a common neurosurgical emergency usually seen in cases of hypertensive intracerebral hemorrhage with the extension into the ventricular system, termed as secondary IVH (Fig. 3.2c). Many studies previously showed that the volume of IVH, presence of hydrocephalus, patient's age, and admitting GCS score are among the predictors for mortality and functional outcome. IVH contributes to morbidity in three main ways. First, hemorrhage in the ventricular system leads to blockage of ventricular conduits, producing acute hydrocephalus. If left untreated, acute hydrocephalus leads to elevation of ICP and progression to death. Besides raised ICP, the direct mass effect from the IVH may be another contributing pathophysiologic event that determines prognosis independent of ICP elevation. The prolonged presence of clots deep within the brain is related to ventriculomegaly, brain edema, and inflammatory responses. Communicating and obstructive hydrocephalus is another common complication of IVH. Blood degradation products of IVH will flow via CSF pathways to the cisterns and arachnoid granulations. Prolonged contact of the blood breakdown products with the pathways, cisternal surfaces, and arachnoid granulations leads to an inflammatory response that permanently scars the granulations and pathways and may alter the cisterns, which leads to delayed development of communicating or obstructive hydrocephalus.

3.3.2.4 Brain Herniation [15]

Brain herniation is a deadly side effect of a mass effect and very high ICP that occurs when the brain shifts across structures within the skull. Herniation can also occur in the absence of high ICP when mass lesions such as hematomas occur at the borders of brain compartments. Brain herniation usually presents with abnormal posturing a characteristic positioning of the limbs indicative of severe brain damage. Traumatic brain injury can cause brain herniation. The brain can shift by such structures as the tentorium cerebelli, the falx cerebri, and the foramen magnum. The shift of midline across the falx cerebri was the typical manifestation (Fig. 3.2d). Supratentorial and infratentorial are two major classes of herniation. A supratentorial herniation is of structures normally above the tentorial notch and infratentorial is of structures normally below it. Supratentorial herniation includes uncal herniation, central herniation, cingulate herniation, and transcalvarial herniation. Infratentorial herniation includes upward herniation and tonsillar herniation. It is often fatal when herniation occur, because herniation puts extreme pressure on parts of the brain and thereby cuts off the blood supply to various parts of the brain. When herniation is visible on a CT scan, the prognosis for a meaningful recovery of neurological function is poor. Respiratory arrest and cardiac arrest will be caused by damage to the cardiorespiratory centers in the medulla oblongata. Damage to the midbrain, which contains the reticular activating network regulating consciousness, will result in coma.

3.3.3 Spontaneous Respiratory Arrest Prediction

Respiratory-related risk factors, such as controlled mode of ventilation and a higher level of oxygen support, are also strongly correlated with the time progressing to brain death. The etiology of spontaneous respiration arrest is often linked to catastrophic brainstem injury, and withdrawal of ventilator support may often lead to a rapid cardiac death associated with rapid development of respiratory acidosis. In a subset of studies, the withdrawal of high levels of oxygen support (FiO_2 or PEEP) has also been associated with a shorter time to cardiac death. Hypoxemia will cause anaerobic metabolism, severe lactic acidosis, and electrolyte and hemodynamic instability, eventually leading to cardiac death; the higher the oxygen support, presumably the more rapid the progression to cardiac death.

Assessment of respiration patterns is a core skill for clinicians to identify the potential DCD donor, since the irregular respiratory pattern or need for ventilation could demonstrate the severity of brain injury. The traditional DCD tool evaluates the patient's ability to breathe without the assistance of the ventilator. The patient is disconnected from the ventilator for 10 min; similar to the Apnea Test for brain death determination. Each minute of apnea causes the carbon dioxide level in the blood to increase by 3–6 mmHg [4]. A patient begins to develop hemodynamic instability when the pH of the blood drops below 7.17 ± 0.02, therefore, the evaluation for spontaneous respiratory should not exceed 10 min of apnea. If, during the 10-min period of observation, the patient becomes unstable (systolic blood pressure < 80 mm Hg; oxygen saturation < 70%), the test is immediately stopped. Thus, the respiratory pattern is evaluated to assess their ability to support life. If the respiratory is ineffective or no spontaneous respiratory, cardiac arrest is predicted to occur within a short period after withdrawal of ventilator support.

The other traditional methods for evaluation of respiration, such as arterial blood gas analysis (ABG), have less value to identify the potential DCD donor. Though, Wijdicks EF and his partner introduced a new coma scale: the FOUR score [16], this score includes a breathing patterns grade, and it can be easily mastered by physicians and interpreted satisfactorily by nurses (Table 3.11). The most important one of the breathing patterns is conducive to predict early mortality in neurocritical patients. In this score, breathing patterns are graded into 5 levels on the basis of respiratory drive: level 1-not intubated, regular breathing pattern, level 2-not intubated,

Table 3.11 The respiratory pattern in FOUR score for probability of progress to cardiac death

Level	Respiratory pattern	Probability
1	No-intubated, regular respiratory pattern	0
2	No-intubated, Cheyne-Stokes respiratory pattern	53.3%
3	No-intubated, irregular respiratory	53.3%
4	Respiratory above ventilator rate	81.8%
5	Respiratory at ventilator rate or respiratory arrest	>90%

Cheyne-Stokes breathing pattern, level 3-not intubated, irregular breathing, level 4-breathes above ventilator rate, level 5-breathes at ventilator rate or apnea. Regular breathing pattern (level 1) means the normal function of respiratory centers located in the brainstem, patients with this breathing pattern nearly cannot be treated as potential DCD donors. In no-intubated patients, the Cheyne-Stokes respiration (level 2) and irregular breathing (level3) can represent bihemispheric or lower brainstem dysfunction of respiratory control; patients with these two breathing patterns have a chance of 53.3% to become potential DCD donor. In intubated patients, overbreathing the mechanical ventilator (level4) represents the impairment of respiratory centers, patients with this level have a chance of 81.8% to become potential DCD donors. Patients who breathe at ventilator rate or apnea (level 5) are progressing to brain death, mostly can become the candidate of brain death donor; however, the brain death precipitates a massive adrenergic release (catecholamine storm) leading to cardiovascular collapse (cardiac death) without advanced management, so when the diagnosis of brain death is not available, this group of patients can be treated as potential DCD donor [17].

A lower GCS, absence of cough reflex, absence of corneal reflexes, extensor motor reflexes were associated with faster time to death in neurocritical patients. These variables lead to cardiac death is associated with the loss of effective respiratory due to brainstem injury. Thus, a patient clinically manifested with low GCS or loss of brainstem reflexes, may develop hemodynamic instability as a result of a cascade of inflammatory mediator release associated with cellular necrosis (Fig. 3.3). In summary, patients with these risk factors could be treated as potential cardiac death donors, because they have a catastrophic and irreversible brain injury (do not meet the brain death standard).

3.4 Donor Management in ICU

Mortality on the waiting list for transplantation remains high [18]. The role of intensive care medicine should focus on the protection and optimization of organ functions. The time between donor diagnosis and operation provides an opportunity to apply interventions to protect or even improve organ function. The intensivists are quite important in this process. The purpose of this chapter is to provide a practical and critical summary of general interventions and specific measures of organ protection, so as to maximize the chance of successful transplantation.

3.4.1 Goal-Directed Protocols

The use of bedside checklists to maintain cardiovascular, respiratory, and endocrine-metabolic stabilization has increased the chance of transplanted organs and decreased DCD losses in cardiac arrest [19]. In shock states, the "VIP" rules named for the Ventilation, Infusion, and Pumping/Pressure approach are the key aspects of the management [20]. Providing a systematic sequence of procedures aimed at restoring DO_2 by adjusting mechanical ventilation, fluid and drug Infusions, and maintaining heart function (pumping/pressure), an adapted version of the VIP approach was proposed to simplify and improve management standards of PBDD [21]. Twenty-seven hospitals used the bedside checklist based on the VIP approach as a quality intervention in over 24 months. Implementation of the checklist reduced the chance of cardiac arrest and increased the number of actual donors and organs recovered per donor [22]. The management of DCD is a complex process. In order to improve the effectiveness of management, clinical guidelines and warning tools can be used to control the quality. The process needs the close cooperation of medical staff, effective implementation, and monitoring. In addition, interaction between the intensive care team, operating room professionals, and transplant teams is required.

3.4.2 Ventilation

The neurogenic pulmonary edema (NPE) is common in the DCD donor due to the raised hydrostatic pressures and capillary damage in the pulmonary vascular, which leads to the leakage of plasma into pulmonary interstitial and alveolar

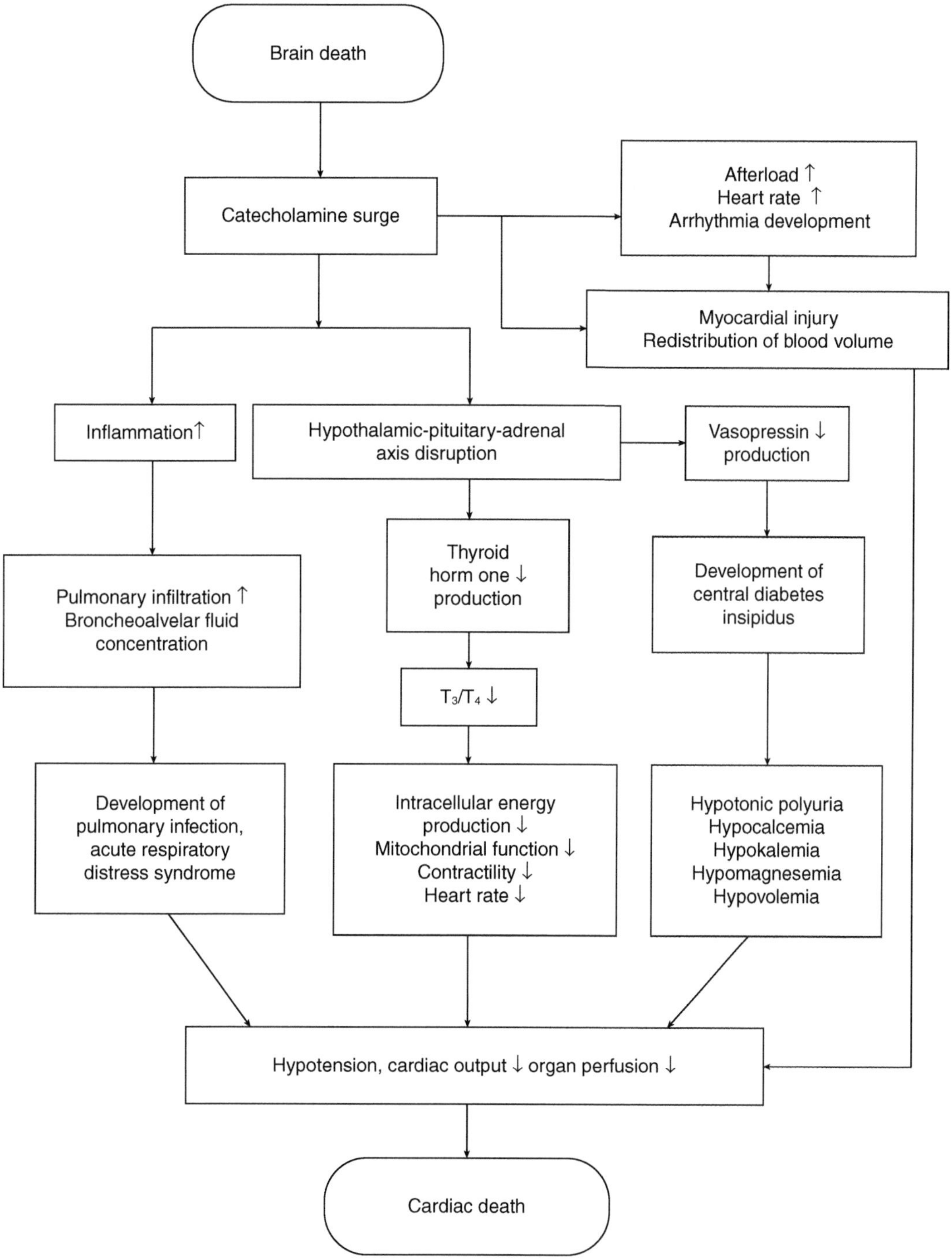

Fig. 3.3 Brain death leads to cardiac death

space [23]. Severe brain injury increases the response of the lungs [24] to mechanical or ischemia/reperfusion injury. The expression of inflammatory mediators increased, neutrophil infiltration and activate macrophages gathered in the alveolar space, membrane lipid peroxidation and even alveolar hemorrhage happened. These hemodynamic and inflammatory changes are similar to the manifestation of acute respiratory distress syndrome (ARDS). These changes not only hinder the potential of lung donation but also damage the function of other organs. Therefore, ventilation management aims to maintain adequate oxygenation and gas exchange, avoid further lung injury, and protect other organs [25].

The objectives of respiratory management include maintaining a reasonable range of pH, achieving a proper oxygen pressure (PaO_2) at the lowest fraction of inhaled oxygen (FiO_2), oxygen saturation (SpO_2) above 95%, and partial pressure of carbon dioxide ($PaCO_2$). Previous guidelines suggested that NPE should be treated with a higher tidal volume [10–15 mL/kg predicted body weight (PBW)] [26] and a positive end-expiratory pressure (PEEP) of at least 5 cmh2o. However, more and more studies have confirmed that ventilator-associated lung injury is common in organ donors [27]. Lung protective ventilation strategy can better protect the lung and reduce the incidence of ventilator-associated lung injury [28]. A multicenter randomized controlled trial confirmed that the protective ventilator strategy (using 6–8 mL/kg of PBW, PEEP equal to 8–10 cmH_2O, a closed circuit for tracheal suction, alveolar recruitment maneuvers after any disconnection, and the use of continuous positive airway pressure during apnea test) was better than the conventional strategy [29]. The protective ventilator strategy increased the number of eligible and transplanted lungs, while the number of other transplanted organs was not influenced. Current guidelines recommend using lower tidal volumes of 6 mL/kg PBW, plateau pressures <30 cmH_2O, proper PEEP, and measures to recruit the atelectatic lung [25], which are similar to the management of ARDS.

3.4.3 Hemodynamic management

Hemodynamic instability is often the primary and prominent challenge in the management of circulating dead donors. The hemodynamic response after brain death has been well described [30]. Primary damage to the brain and/or brainstem immediately activates the sympathetic nervous system greatly. This "autonomic storm" may lead to arrhythmia, myocardial ischemia, and myocardial dysfunction. Systemic and local ischemia caused by circulatory instability can further trigger a strong systemic inflammatory response, which leads to the deterioration of hemodynamics.

3.4.3.1 Infusion/Fluid

Hypovolemia is a common cause of hemodynamic disorders in organ donors. Massive peripheral vasodilation and central diabetes insipidus aggravate hypovolemia. Therefore, prevention and immediate correction of hypovolemia are essential for maintaining hemodynamic stability and protecting the perfusion of potential transplantable organs. The pathophysiological changes of donors make it more difficult to evaluate the volume status of organ donors [25]. Appropriate monitoring is essential to guide fluid treatment. The guideline of the Society of Critical Care Medicine/American College of Chest Physicians recommended the following [25]:

1. Hemodynamic monitoring tools help to assess volume status and response to fluid. A central venous catheter can ensure fluid infusion and monitor CVP. Invasive monitoring techniques, such as SWAN-GANZ catheter, PiCCO or pulse profile analysis, or noninvasive monitoring techniques, can be established to continuously measure stroke volume, CO, cardiac index, vascular resistance, and mixed venous oxygen saturation.
2. General guidelines for adequate IV fluid resuscitation are as follows:
   (a) Mean arterial pressure at least 60 mmHg.
   (b) Urine output at least 1 mL/kg/h.
   (c) Left ventricle ejection fraction at least 45%.
   (d) Lower vasopressor dose (e.g., dopamine ≤10 μg/kg/min).
3. In the whole stage of donor management nursing, it is recommended to use hemodynamic parameters to maintain the normal blood volume of the donor for fluid replacement.

Isotonic crystalloid is the first choice for fluid resuscitation. In case of hyperchloremic metabolic acidosis, the use of 0.9% normal saline should be limited. Similarly, lactate Ringer solution may not be suitable for some donors due to its hypotonic effect and insufficient electrolyte content. In these cases, pH neutral isotonic solution can be considered. If the volume state is stable, but hypernatremia needs to be corrected, hypotonic fluid can be used. Patients with metabolic acidosis may benefit from solutions containing sodium bicarbonate. 0.45% saline with or without sodium bicarbonate can be used in hypernatremic donors. Colloidal solution is commonly used in severe intravascular insufficiency. 5% albumin and hydroxyethyl starch (HES) are the most commonly used colloidal solutions in ICU. However, it should be noted that the use of HES is associated with acute kidney injury, coagulation disorders, and hepatic reticuloendothelial system involvement. It can also lead to acute hypervolemia, which may adversely affect the impaired right ventricular function. Delayed graft function and graft failure have been associated with the use of HES in donor management [31]. One study compared 130 kDa HES with 200 kDa HES, and showed a delay of the decline of graft function in 130 kDa HES group [32]. The results suggest that the low molecular weight HES solution with rapid degradation may have better side effects. According to the existing data, conventional use of HES is not recommended, but if it is used, the injection volume should be limited to 500–1000 mL.

In summary, crystal or colloid can be used as the choice of fluid resuscitation. The preferred isotonic crystals are 0.9% normal saline and lactate Ringer solution. HES should not be routinely used for colloidal resuscitation of organ donors [25].

3.4.3.2 Vasoactive Drugs

For donors, the discussion of these vasoactive drugs is not limited to vasopressors and inotropic drugs alone, but also HRT (vasopressin, steroid, and thyroid hormone). Once hemodynamics are unstable, vasopressors should be used to maintain perfusion pressure when volume resuscitation cannot reach the threshold hemodynamic target. The use of vasoactive drugs should be based on hemodynamic monitoring, and evaluate hemodynamic conditions at any time, such as cardiac function, volume, and vascular resistance.

In the past, it was demonstrated that norepinephrine might increase pulmonary capillary permeability, leading to excessive contraction of mesentery or coronary artery, or increase left ventricular afterload [25]. Therefore, dopamine was recommended as a catecholamine choice in donor management guidelines. Norepinephrine and phenylephrine were rarely used. However, recent sepsis guidelines pointed out that dopamine might bring more adverse reactions and increase mortality than NE. Now, NE is recommended as the first choice of vasopressors. Dopamine was only used in patients with low risk of arrhythmia. Dobutamine may be used in conditions of cardiac pump dysfunction. Vasopressin can improve the vascular tone in the state of vasodilative shock related to brain death [33], effectively fight against diabetes insipidus (DI), and reduce the dosage of catecholamine. A combination of thyroid hormones and hormones that make up HRT is usually given at the beginning of donor management, rather than hemodynamically, or reserved for unstable donors, rather than responding to fluid and/or vasoactive support.

3.4.4 Endocrine Management

In severe brain injury and brain death donors, endocrine abnormalities occur frequently. Massive cerebral injury leads to brain edema and ischemia, which increases ICP. When the elevation in ICP forces the brainstem to herniate through the foramen magnum, brain death occurs causing additional ischemic injury and ultimately brainstem infarction [30]. The hypothalamic–pituitary axis is particularly sensitive to ischemic injury. Vasopressin production reduced which led to DI [30]. Anterior pituitary hormone deficits, resulting in hypothyroidism and hypocortisolism, have also been reported, although at relatively lower rates [34]. Pharmacologic replacement of these hormones may be a benefit to hemodynamic stability, organ function, and the likelihood of multiple organ retrieval.

3.4.4.1 Vasopressin Deficiency

Decreased or undetectable levels of arginine vasopressin (AVP or antidiuretic hormone) are common in donors. The reason is mainly the damage of the structure of posterior pituitary, supraoptic nucleus of hypothalamus, and paraventricular nucleus. AVP deficiency is associated with hypovolemia, hypertonic pressure and hypernatremia, and may lead to inappropriate diuresis. According to guideline [25], when continuous hypotension still occurs in the presence of active fluid resuscitation or DI, the treatment of AVP dysfunction should be considered. DI should be diagnosed if one or more of the following criteria are confirmed after excluding other causes:

(a) Urine output greater than 3–4 L/day or 2.5–3.0 mL/kg/h
(b) Normal or increased serum osmolality
(c) Hypotonic urine (urine osmolality <200 mOsm/kg H_2O, specific gravity <1.005)
(d) Hypernatremia ($Na^+ > 145$ mmol/L)

3.4.4.2 Hypothyroidism

After brain death with usually low levels of the biologically active triiodothyronine (T_3), alterations in the thyroid axis are common. However, several studies of brain dead organ donors demonstrated normal to elevated thyroid-stimulating hormone levels due to the residual pituitary function in the majority of patients and internal carotids supply. Evidences were confused on whether thyroid replacement should be routinely used in DCD donors. Guidelines recommended to consider thyroid hormone replacement in hemodynamically unstable donors [25]. Both T_4 and T_3 substitutions have been used for this purpose, although T_4 is increasingly degraded to inactive reverse-T_3.

3.4.4.3 Corticosteroid

The prevalence of corticosteroid deficiency after brain death is different among reports. Therefore, the indications for corticosteroid therapy in brain dead organ donors remain unclear. However, in the case of hemodynamic instability, corticosteroid deficiency and corticosteroid treatment should be considered. Importantly, since corticosteroids may reduce the expression of HLA [35], the use of corticosteroids should be used after donor tissue typing and sampling.

3.4.5 Nutrition and Glycemia

The optimal feeding strategy of brain dead organ donors is lack of effective clinical research. At present, the guidelines recommend continued nutritional support for donors [25]. Enteral nutrition is the first choice for critically ill patients. Potential adverse effects of parenteral nutrition on critically ill patients include increased risk of infection and prolonged organ failure. Therefore, it is not recommended to start early parenteral nutrition in potential donors [36].

Due to insulin resistance and unsuppressed gluconeogenesis hyperglycemia was so common in donors as in critically ill patients. It has been reported that hyperglycemia was associated with reduction of donor renal function and with pancreas allograft loss [25, 36]. What is more, severe hyperglycemia may induce osmotic diuresis leading to fluid and electrolyte disturbances, and is associated with a higher risk of infections in critically ill patients [37]. The ideal blood glucose target for potential donors remains unclear, due to the lack of evidences in this population. Consensus guidelines recommend to treat at least severe hyperglycemia (>180 mg/dL) [25].

3.4.6 Temperature Management

Temperature dysregulation following death by neurologic criteria is inevitable [30], which might imply a poor prognosis, unless temperature is actively corrected. Temperature dysregulation is induced by the integration of loss of hypothalamic control, reduction in metabolic rate, absence of muscular activity, and increased heat loss because of profound vasoplegia. Because hypothermia can activate intravascular coagulation and produce organ damage, it may have negative consequences [38]. Initial measures for reaching the temperature target include thermal blankets reducing passive heat loss, hot air devices, and warmed fluid infusions. In a recent RCT [39], the requirement for early dialysis after kidney transplantation was significantly reduced by mild hypothermia in the organ donor (34 °C–35 °C), compared with normothermia (36.5 °C–37.5 °C). The current target to keep the body temperature above 35 °C seems reasonable [18], although a higher target may be warranted in the presence of severe cardiovascular instability requiring high doses of vasopressors or inotropes.

3.4.7 Transfusion

To address severe anemia that could potentially compromise oxygen delivery to vital organs, packed RBCs may be required. The optimal hemoglobin in this population is unknown, but a target above 7 g/dL has been recommended in other critically ill populations. Other blood products (fresh-frozen plasma, cryoprecipitate, and platelets) may be required to manage associated hematologic problems or bleeding.

3.4.8 Infection Management

Infections in the donor might complicate organ donation. The reported rate of unexpected infection transmission from donor to receptor was low, which was less than 1% of solid organ transplant recipients [40]. However, the consequences may be devastating, and sometimes even fatal. The infective assessment of the donor should include previous infections, travels, contact with animals, other environmental exposures, sexual history, and intravenous drug abuse [40].

In the ICU, the incidence of infection (mainly hospital acquired Infections such as pneumonia or catheter-related bloodstream infections) can reach up to 40%, especially in patients with longer length of stay [41]. Infections usually are not contraindications to donation, in those cases patients were treated with appropriate antibiotics for at least 48 h prior to procurement [25], and without shock, multiorgan failure, or poor response to antibiotic treatment. If infections are diagnosed after transplantation, it is very important to communicate with the coordinating transplant organization to prescribe treatment of the recipient [41].

For many of the management strategies in circulatory-dead donors, the evidences were still too weak to demonstrate an effect on receptor outcomes. Hence, some of the elements in circulatory-dead donor management protocols are based on pathophysiological reasoning, epidemiological observations, or extrapolations from general ICU management strategies.

References

1. Manara AR, Murphy PG, O'Callaghan G. Donation after circulatory death. Br J Anaesth. 2012;108:108–21.
2. Rabinstein AA, Yee AH, Mandrekar J, Fugate JE. Prediction of potential for organ donation after cardiac death in patients in neurocritical state: a prospective observational study. Lancet Neurol. 2012;11(5):414–9.
3. Kootstra G, Daemen JH, Oomen AP. Categories of non-heart beating organ donors. Transplant Proc. 1995;27:2893–4.
4. Lewis J, Peltier J, Nelson H, et al. Development of the University of Wisconsin donation after cardiac death evaluation tool. Prog Transplant. 2003;13:265–73.
5. De Vita MA, Mori Brooks M, Zawistowski C, Rudich S, Daly B, Chaitin E. Donors after cardiac death: validation of identification criteria (DVIC) study for predictors of rapid death. Am J Transplant. 2008;8:432–41.
6. He X, Xu G, Liang W, et al. Nomogram for predicting time to death after withdrawal of life-sustaining treatment in patients with devastating neurological injury. Am J Transplant. 2015;15(8):2136–42.
7. Xu G, Guo Z, Liang W, et al. Prediction of potential for organ donation after circulatory death in neurocritical patients. J Heart Lung Transplant. 2018;37(3):358–64.
8. Dalle Ave AL, Bernat JL. Using the brain criterion in organ donation after the circulatory determination of death. J Crit Care. 2016;33:114–8.
9. de Groot YJ, Jansen NE, Bakker J, Kuiper MA. Imminent brain death: point of departure for potential heart-beating organ donor recognition. Intensive Care Med. 2010;36(9):1488–94.

10. Teasdale G, Jennett B. Assessment of coma and impaired consciousness. A practical scale. Lancet. 1974;2:81–4.
11. Brain Injury Evaluation Quality Control Centre of National Heath, Neurocritical Care Committee of Chinese Society of Neurology, Neurocritical Care Committee of Chinese Neurologist Association. China criteria and practical guidance for determination of brain death in adults(second edition). Natl Med J China. 2019;99(17):1288–92.
12. Wagemans BA, Klinkenberg S, Postma AA. Teaching NeuroImages: Swirl sign and spot sign in intraparenchymal hematoma. Neurology. 2016;87(18):225–6.
13. Adelson PD, Bratton SL, Carney NA, Chesnut RM, du Coudray HE, Goldstein B, et al. Guidelines for the acute medical management of severe traumatic brain injury in infants, children, and adolescents. Chapter 5. Indications for intracranial pressure monitoring in pediatric patients with severe traumatic brain injury. Pediatr Crit Care Med. 2003;4(3 Suppl):S19–24.
14. Tuhrim S, Horowitz DR, Sacher M, Godbold JH. Volume of ventricular blood is an important determinant of outcome in supratentorial intracerebral hemorrhage. Crit Care Med. 1999;27:617–21.
15. Barras CD, Tress BM, Christensen S, et al. Density and shape as CT predictors of intracerebral hemorrhage growth. Stroke. 2009;40:1325.
16. Wijdicks EF, Bamlet WR, Maramattom BV, Manno EM, McClelland RL. Validation of a new coma scale: the FOUR score. Ann Neurol. 2005;58(4):585–93.
17. Nyam TE, Ao KH, Hung SY, Shen ML, Yu TC, Kuo JR. FOUR score predicts early outcome in patients after traumatic brain injury. Neurocrit Care. 2017;26(2):225–31.
18. Citerio G, Cypel M, Dobb GJ, et al. Organ donation in adults: a critical care perspective. Intensive Care Med. 2016;42:305–15.
19. Martin-Loeches I, Sandiumenge A, et al. Management of donation after brain death (DBD) in the ICU: the potential donor is identified, what's next? Intensive Care Med. 2019;45(3):322–30.
20. Weil MH, Shubin H, et al. The "VIP" approach to the bedside management of shock. JAMA. 1969;207:337–40.
21. Westphal GA. A simple bedside approach to therapeutic goals achievement during the management of deceased organ donors an adapted version of the "VIP" approach. Clin Transpl. 2016;30:138–44.
22. Hunter JP, Ploeg RJ. An exciting new era in donor organ preservation and transplantation: assess, condition, and repair! Transplantation. 2016;100:1801–2.
23. Busl KM, Bleck TP. Neurogenic pulmonary edema. Crit Care Med. 2015;43:1710–5.
24. Mascia L, Sakr Y, Pasero D, et al. Extracranial complications in patients with acute brain injury: a post-hoc analysis of the SOAP study. Intensive Care Med. 2008;34:720–7.
25. Kotlof RM, Blosser S, Fulda GJ, et al. Management of the potential organ donor in the ICU: society of critical care medicine/American college of chest physicians/association of organ procurement organizations consensus statement. Crit Care Med. 2015;43:1291–325.
26. MacLean A, Dunning J. The retrieval of thoracic organs: donor assessment and management. Br Med Bull. 1997;53:829–43.
27. Wheeler AP, Bernard GR. Acute lung injury and the acute respiratory distress syndrome: a clinical review. Lancet. 2007;369:1553–64.
28. Krebs J, Tsagogiorgas C, Pelosi P, et al. Open lung approach with low tidal volume mechanical ventilation attenuates lung injury in rats with massive brain damage. Crit Care. 2014;18:R59.
29. Mascia L, Pasero D, Slutsky AS, et al. Effect of a lung protective strategy for organ donors on eligibility and availability of lungs for transplantation. JAMA. 2010;304:2620.
30. Smith M. Physiologic changes during brain stem death lessons for management of the organ donor. J Heart Lung Transplant. 2004;23:S217–22.
31. Cittanova ML, Leblanc I, Legendre C, et al. Effect of hydroxyethyl starch in brain-dead kidney donors on renal function in kidney-transplant recipients. Lancet. 1996;348:1620–2.
32. Blasco V, Leone M, Antonini F, et al. Comparison of the novel hydroxyethyl starch 130/0.4 and hydroxyethyl starch 200/0.6 in braindead donor resuscitation on renal function after transplantation. Br J Anaesth. 2008;100:504–8.
33. Pennefather SH, Bullock RE, Mantle D, et al. Use of low dose arginine vasopressin to support brain-dead organ donors. Transplantation. 1995;59:58–62.
34. Dimopoulou I, Tsagarakis S, Anthi A, et al. High prevalence of decreased cortisol reserve in brain-dead potential organ donors. Crit Care Med. 2003;31:1113–7.
35. Meyfroidt G, Gunst J, et al. Management of the brain-dead donor in the ICU: general and specific therapy to improve transplantable organ quality. Intensive Care Med. 2019;45(3):343–53.
36. Casaer MP, Van den Berghe G. Nutrition in the acute phase of critical illness. N Engl J Med. 2014;370:1227–36.
37. Marvin MR, Morton V. Glycemic control and organ transplantation. J Diabetes Sci Technol. 2009;3:1365–72.
38. Weiss S, Kotsch K, Francuski M, et al. Brain death activates donor organs and is associated with a worse I/R injury after liver transplantation. Am J Transplant. 2007;7:1584–93.
39. Niemann CU, Feiner J, Swain S, et al. Therapeutic hypothermia in deceased organ donors and kidney-graft function. N Engl J Med. 2015;373:405–14.
40. Fishman JA, Greenwald MA, Grossi PA. Transmission of infection with human allografts: essential considerations in donor screening. Clin Infect Dis. 2012;55:720–7.
41. Vincent J-L, Marshall JC, Namendys-Silva SA, et al. Assessment of the worldwide burden of critical illness: the intensive care over nations (ICON) audit. Lancet Respir Med. 2014;2:380–6.

4 Organ Procurement, Quality Evaluation, and Perfusion

ZhiYong Guo

Abstract

Graft quality is directly related to the clinical prognosis of recipients. Organ procurement, organ function evaluation, and organ preservation are the main contents in the process of deceased donation (DD), which determine the efficacy and safety of clinical organ transplantation. Optimizing these three steps is the main method to improve the quality of grafts.

4.1 Organ Procurement

4.1.1 Liver Acquisition Technology

In February 2011, the Chinese Citizens' Organ Donation Standards, referred to as "Chinese Standards," were formulated by the Chinese Committee for Clinical Application of Human Organ Transplant Technology, which are divided into three categories, namely: China Class I (C-1): International Standardization Donation after Brain Death (DBD) is a case of brain death. After rigorous medical examinations, all indicators meet the international standards for brain death and the latest domestic brain death standards. Brain death experts trained and certified by the former Ministry of Health have clearly determined China Class II (C-II): International Standardized Cardiac Death Organ Donation (DCD), which includes cases of Class I to IV in the Maastricht Standard Classification. China Class III (C-III): Brain-heart death. Standard organ donation (donation after brain death waiting for death, DBCD), similar to the Maastricht standard IV, meets the diagnostic criteria for brain death. Because the brain death law has not yet been established, and family members cannot accept organ donation under a beating heart state, for this type of accumulation in Europe and the United States, the source of organ donation is mostly brain death donors, the proportion is as high as 95% or more [1, 2]; In this case, the donor should perform the donation according to the DCD procedure, that is, remove the life support, and implement the donation after the heart stops beating. As the laws related to brain death have not yet been implemented, heart-dead organ donation (China Class II, III) has become the main source of liver donors [3].

4.1.1.1 Rapid DCD Donor Organ Procurement Technology

For DCD donors or fresh donors without heartbeat or brain dead donors but with hemodynamic mutations, rapid donor organism procurement technology should be used. Based on the experience of obtaining a large number of donors, the

Z. Guo (✉)
Organ Transplant Center, The First Affiliated Hospital of Sun Yat-sen University, Guangzhou, China

X. He (ed.), *Organ Donation and Transplantation after Cardiac Death in China*,
https://doi.org/10.1007/978-981-16-0815-5_4

center has formed a complete set of rapid donor liver acquisition strategies, which are briefly described as follows.

Position: supine with a pillow on the waist and back. Disinfection drapes: 0.1% iodophor, rapid disinfection of the chest and abdomen, regular drapes.

The procedure is as follows:

Vertical selection: The abdomen is a large "ten" long, lengthwise up to under the xiphoid process, down to the top of the pubic symphysis, crossing the meridian level to the coaxial midline at both ends.

Donor liver graft: After entering the abdomen, push the small intestine to the upper right side, cut the posterior peritoneum before the sacrum, separate, expose the lower part of the abdominal aorta and ligate the distal end, cut the abdominal abdomen above the ligature, insert the modified 22-gauge Foley catheter with 3–4 side holes into the artery. The insertion depth is from the bladder to the level of the celiac artery opening (about 20 cm). The balloon is quickly injected with 30 ml of saline to intervene the thoracic aorta and avoid perfusion. The urinary catheter was ligated and fixed, and 4 °C kidney transplant solution (HCA) was implanted at a pressure of about 100 cm H_2O. It is required that the implant fluid must be implanted quickly in a line.

Free the inferior hepatic inferior vena cava, intubate the inferior vena cava under the kidney, insert a large silicone tube to drain the perfusate, and drain the perfusate out of the abdominal cavity to avoid interference with the surgical field.

The second assistant lifts up the transverse colon, and then separates the superior mesenteric vein 2–3 cm below the peritoneal reflex of the transverse colon. After ligating the distal end of the superior mesenteric vein, incise the proximal end and insert an 18-gauge silicone tube with an anti-dropping ring. The insertion depth is 6–8 cm. Be careful not to insert too deep, and fix it with silk thread. Immediately connect the perfusion tube to the HCA perfusion solution for gravity perfusion. The abdominal aorta and superior mesenteric vein were perfused with a total of 3000 ml of HCA (about 1500 ml each).

Use gauze to protect the gallbladder and cut the bottom of the gallbladder to drain the bile in the gallbladder. The intubation is continued to flush the biliary tract with about 500 ml of 0–4 °C HCA solution to minimize the residual bile components in the biliary tract and ensure that the biliary tract is effectively lavaged (if the lavage is unsatisfactory, after the donor liver is cut out, the biliary tract is flushed again through the common bile duct).

Preliminary assessment of the quality of the donor liver: While performing low-temperature lavage, the round ligament and the falciform ligament of the liver are cut, and the donor organs are quickly evaluated to determine whether they are suitable for transplantation. At the same time, put crushed ice on the surface of liver, kidney, pancreas, etc. Open both sides of the perirenal fat sacs, spread ice debris on both sides of the kidneys, and check that the kidneys are well perfused. If the perfusion of one pole of the kidney is not good, be careful that the accessory renal artery is sent out from the distal end of the abdominal aortic cannulation ligature.

Dissociation and extraction of the donor liver: After the portal vein and abdominal aorta are perfused with HCA solution, the portal vein and abdominal aorta are reperfused with 1000–1500 ml UW solution, respectively. Cut the hepatic round ligament, falciform ligament, and left and right triangular ligaments, and then explore the liver for disease again, and further judge whether the quality of the donor liver and the effect of lavage are satisfactory, whether the perfusion pipeline is unobstructed and whether the perfusion speed meets the requirements. The liver and kidney ligaments are incised, and the duodenum is freed downward. Cut the liver and kidney ligaments to expose the inferior inferior vena cava, and free the inferior vena cava above the kidney veins. Cut off all ligaments around the liver, and be careful not to damage the upper and lower inferior vena cava. After the color of the donor liver turns white, the temperature drops, and the drainage fluid is clear, the inferior inferior vena cava is transected above the left renal vein. Make a Kocher incision, free the pancreas and duodenum, and transcribe the pancreas from the middle of the head of the pancreas approximately 2–3 cm from the upper edge of the pancreas. The surgeon held the celiac artery with his left hand and cut the abdominal aorta about 0.5 cm below the opening of the celiac artery (be careful not to damage the bilateral renal arteries), and then remove the liver. After the removal of the donor liver, 4 °C UW solution was given through the choled end of the common bile duct, and the intrahepatic and extrahepatic biliary tracts were repeatedly washed again. Finally, the donor liver was placed in 4 °C UW solution for storage. During the extraction process, surgeons need to pay special attention to the length and resection position of the hepatic artery, portal vein, suprahepatic, inferior vena cava, and common bile duct, which must meet the needs of liver transplantation. Lift the abdominal aorta and the distal end of the inferior vena cava, and cut the bilateral iliac vessels and femoral arteries and veins. Store the donor liver and spare blood vessels in a 0–4 °C preservation solution, wrap them in four layers of sterile intestinal bags, and store them in a 0–4 °C refrigerator.

4.1.1.2 Collect DCD in Whole to Donate Liver, Pancreas, Spleen, Duodenum, Part of Jejunum, and Bilateral Kidneys

In the current DCD organ donation process, some donors need to cut abdominal organ clusters for transplantation, or if small bowel transplantation is required, then obtain organs in one piece. As early as 2003, the center carried out the first successful upper abdominal organ cluster transplantation in Asia, and gradually developed improved organ cluster transplantation strategies for the treatment of liver cirrhosis or liver cancer with type 2 diabetes, and the results were gratifying. At present, more than 20 cases of organ cluster transplantation have been completed.

As with the rapid donor organ procurement technique for intubation and perfusion, the abdominal aorta, inferior vena cava, portal vein, and gallbladder can be intubated and perfused. Then cut off the round ligament of the liver, falciform ligament, coronary ligament, left and right triangular ligaments, cut the diaphragm to the left and right to the diaphragm foot. Free the ascending colon, ileocecal area, and small mesenteric; incise the outer peritoneum of the ascending colon to the ileocecal area, turn the large and small intestines to the upper left to expose the roots of the mesentery, and cut off the transverse mesentery and small intestine. After double ligation at the pylorus of the stomach, it was severed. After double ligation of the jejunum 15 cm below the ligament of flexion, it was transected. Proximal jejunum iodophor disinfection: Lift the large intestine and small intestine out of the abdominal cavity. Free bilateral kidneys outside the fat sac. The superior and inferior hepatic vena cava near the atrium, the thoracic aorta above the diaphragm, and the distal end of the thoracic aorta fracture are lifted. The assistant holds up the abdominal organs and bilateral kidneys, close to the front of the spine, and sharply separate from top to bottom. Abdominal organs, kidneys, ureters, abdominal aorta, and inferior vena cava were taken out together and placed in a UW liquid ice basin at 4 °C. Check the organs for damage. Store the donor organs and spare blood vessels at 0–4 °C. Stored in liquid, wrapped in four layers of sterile intestinal bags, and stored in a constant temperature refrigerator at 0–4 °C.

If multiple organ transplantation or combined pancreas-kidney transplantation is performed, sequential intestinal lavage is required after biliary lavage. Method: The gastric antrum was ligated at the distal end of the gastric antrum, an lavage tube (made by trimming the end of the gastric tube) was inserted into the gastric antrum at the distal end of the ligation line, and the distal gastric antrum was ligated and the lavage tube was fixed. Inject 150 ml of renal perfusion solution, 100 ml of 0.5% metronidazole, and 100 ml of UW solution through the lavage tube with a 50 ml syringe. During each flush, the duodenum and jejunum perfusion solution are pushed distally and in the Treitz ligament. Block the jejunum at the end 20 cm to prevent reflux. The Treitz ligament was ligated 2 cm away from the UW fluid injection site. The jejunum 10 cm distal to the Treitz ligament is ready to be cut. Note that the amount of UW fluid should be appropriate so as not to cause pressure in the duodenum.

4.1.1.3 Precautions in the Process of Donating Liver

1. Ensure that the temperature of the perfusate and preservation solution is 0–4 °C.
2. Ensure that the perfusion tube is fully exhausted.
3. Ensure that the arterial cannula is above the opening of the abdominal trunk, and the portal vein cannula is next to the main portal vein.
4. Pay attention to observe the hepatic artery variation and take some necessary protection.
5. The perihepatic ligament should be separated sharply, and the assistant's exposure should be gentle to avoid damage to the liver capsule.
6. Pay special attention to the length and resection position of the hepatic artery, portal vein, suprahepatic, inferior vena cava, and common bile duct during the cutting process. They should meet the needs of implantation and reconstruction, while avoiding damage to renal arteries, veins, and ureters.
7. The air in the four-layer intestinal bag should be emptied, and the crushed ice in the heat preservation refrigerator should be sufficient and completely cover the intestine bag. For long-distance transportation, attention should be paid to check whether the ice in the heat preservation refrigerator is sufficient.
8. The heat preservation refrigerator is labeled with donor information.

4.1.2 Kidney Acquisition Technology

4.1.2.1 Preoperative Preparation

For controllable DCD donors (Maastricht Class III and IV, Class III in China), before organ procurement, the donor can be injected intramuscularly with 10 mg of phentolamine, intravenous injection of 200 mg of heparin and 300,000 U of urokinase. Thereby expanding the donor's renal artery, preventing blood clotting in the kidney and dissolving possible thrombi, which improves the perfusion effect. For uncontrollable DCD donors (Maastricht Class I, II and V), 200 mg of heparin and 300,000 U of urokinase can be added to the perfusion solution (3000 ml of HCA solution). It has been reported that injecting phentolamine (10 mg/50 kg) before kidney extraction can improve the indicators of machine perfusion of the kidney (the flow rate increases by 23%, and the resistance decreases by 30%), and can reduce the incidence of delayed recovery of graft function after kidney transplantation [4]. In the rat model without a heartbeat donor, injecting heparin and phentolamine before organ procurement can improve the perfusion effect of the donor liver, and phentolamine can improve the uniformity of perfusion [5].

4.1.2.2 Entire Kidney Removal Method (Fig. 4.1)

All content is presented in the form content is shown in Fig. 4.1 to improve visualization.

4.1.3 Heart and Lung Acquisition Technology

4.1.3.1 Acquisition Technology of Donor Heart

Protection of donor heart: At all stages of heart transplantation, there are factors that cause donor heart injury: before transplantation, the pathophysiological changes of the brain dead or the hemodynamic instability, hypothermia, electrolyte abnormalities, and metabolic disorders caused by improper treatment during the maintenance treatment stage can lead to myocardial ischemia, and these are important reasons for the hypofunction of the donor heart after surgery; Inappropriate operation in the process of obtaining the donor heart and long-term exposure of the donor heart to a dry environment can also cause significant damage; Ischemia-reperfusion injury when the aorta is open after donor heart transplantation [6, 7]. Therefore, the protection of the donor heart should run through the entire process of heart transplantation, which can be divided into three stages: preoperative, intraoperative, and postoperative (Fig. 4.2).

Acquisition surgery of donor heart: The surgical position of the donor is the same as that of conventional heart surgery. Routinely perform the following inspections after pericardiotomy:

Surgical incision:
1. The donor is placed in a supine position, and a sterile towel is placed on the 12th rib of the back to raise it.
2. Lodophor disinfection, spread surgical towels.
3. A large "ten" incision in the abdomen: the longitudinal incision starts from the xiphoid process and reaches above the pubic symphysis; the transverse incision is at the level of the umbilicus to the posterior axilla lines on both sides.

In situ perfusion:
After entering the abdomen, push the small intestine to the head, cut the posterior peritoneum before the sacrum, find and separate the abdominal aorta, and ligate the distal end with a 7 -gauge silk thread. After the abdominal aorta at the level of the inferior mesenteric artery, thread a 7-gauge silk thread. Cut the anterior wall of the abdominal aorta, insert a modified balloon catheter about 15 cm, inflate about 20 ml of the balloon to block the proximal end of the abdominal aorta, and ligate the abdominal aorta at the catheterization site. Quickly turn on the perfusion fluid switch and quickly perfuse 3000ml HCA solution and 1000ml UW solution. Separate the inferior vena cava on the right side of the abdominal aorta cannulation, and insert a drainage tube to drain blood and erfusion fluid.

Free the left kidney and ureter:
Push the intestine to the right and pull the splenic flexure of the colon and descending colon inward. After incising the peritoneum on the lateral side of the descending colon, incise the mesangium of colon splenic flexure and diaphragmatic colon ligament upward to expose the left kidney. Lift part of the left renal fascial sac, incise the fascia and push the tail of the pancreas to the right. The surgeon uses his left hand to protect the kidney, and his right hand cuts open the left pararenal fascia and tissues on the head of the left kidney to free the left kidney. Cut the descending mesocolon downward and push open the intestine to the inside to expose the left ureter. Clamp the ureter with mid-curved forceps below the iliac blood vessel, cut the distal end, lift the ureter, cut it sharply toward the medial and lateral mesangium, and try to preserve the surrounding tissues of the ureter.

Free the right kidney and ureter:
The Cattel-Braasch manoeuvre (Cattel-Braasch manoeuvre) was used to free the duodenum, the right colon and the mesenteric root of the small intestine and push the intestinal tube to the left. Cut the peritoneum on the outside of the ascending colon, and cut upward to the liver flexure of the colon, exposing the right kidney. Use the Kocher manoeuvre to free the duodenum and the head of the pancreas, lift the duodenum, cut the right posterior peritoneum of the duodenum, and expose the inferior vena cava, abdominal aorta, right renal hilum and left Renal vein. The surgeon uses his left hand to protect the kidney, and his right hand cuts the right pararenal fascia and posterior renal tissue, as well as the liver and kidney ligaments. Push open the intestine to the left and cephalic side to expose and free the right ureter. The right ureter is adjacent to the inferior vena cava. When freeing the right ureter, be careful not to damage the inferior vena cava to avoid blood outflow and unclear vision.

Resection of the gastrointestinal tract and cut out both kedneys:
Lay both kidneys flat and lift up the intestine. Cut the root tissue of the small mesenteric (including Treitz ligament, abdominal trunk and superior mesenteric artery), and turn the small intestine and colon out of the abdominal cavity. Turn the ureter to the side of the head, and the assistant gently supports the kidneys. The surgeon clamped the abdominal aorta and inferior vena cava with curved forceps and cut them off. Lift the proximal end and sharply free the abdominal aorta and inferior vena cava in the anterior spine. Turn the ureter down, the surgeon grasps both kidneys with his left hand, cuts off the abdominal aorta and inferior vena cava as close to the heart as possible, and removes the kidneys in one piece.

Fig. 4.1 Entire kidney

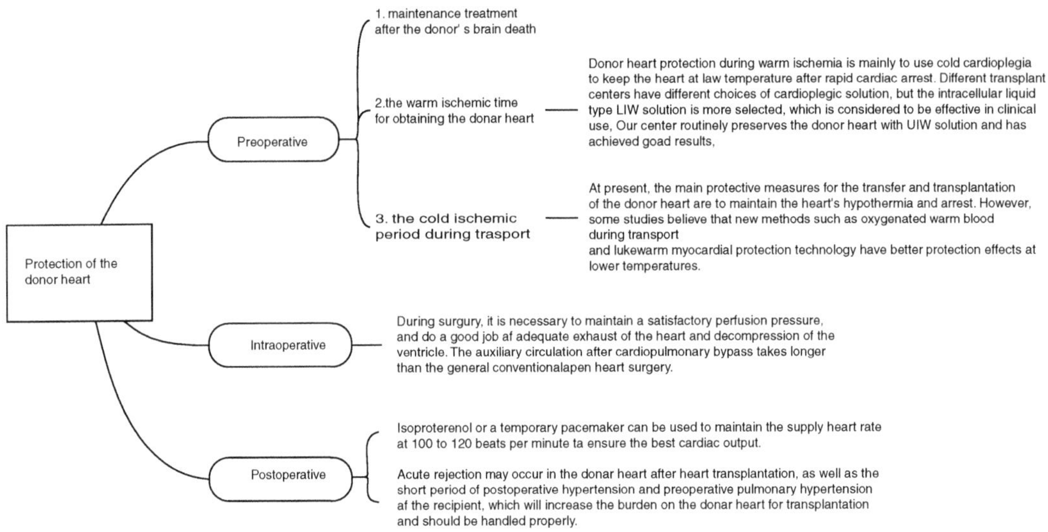

Fig. 4.2 Three stages of donor heart protection

(1) Stroke each chamber and blood vessels on the surface of the heart for tremor; (2) Check whether there are traumas, scars on the surface of the heart, and whether the contractile force is strong; (3) Palpate whether the main coronary artery and main branches have arteriosclerosis Plaque.

A midline sternum incision is routinely used to make a longitudinal incision to explore the heart to determine whether there is any trauma or obvious damage to the outside of the heart caused by chest compression. Free the superior and inferior vena cava. The donor is fully heparinized (3 mg/kg), then the ascending aorta is blocked at the level of the brachial trunk, and the aortic root is perfused with 4 °C cold cardioplegia (10 ml/kg), and sufficient perfusion pressure is ensured. At the same time, the inferior vena cava and the right upper pulmonary vein were cut to decompress the left and right ventricles, and the icy debris in the pericardial cavity was locally cooled. Cut the ascending aorta with the distal end of the aortic clamp, and cut the pulmonary artery at the branches of the left and right pulmonary arteries. Cut the inferior vena cava near the diaphragm level. When cutting the superior vena cava, try to keep some superior vena cava. Cut off four pulmonary veins at the left and right pericardial reflexes. Lift the apex of the heart, separate the mediastinal tissue behind the atria and great vessels, and take out the donor heart completely. Put it in a double-layer sterilization bag containing 4 °C preservation solution or ice salt water for further cooling. The double bag is also filled with ice salt water, and it is transported in a container with ice chips. For long-distance transportation, intermittent perfusion or continuous low-flow perfusion (3–6 ml/kg) can be used.

Pruning of donor heart: The trimming of the donor core should be completely immersed in the cold storage solution. The bottom of the container is cushioned with gauze so that the donor core does not collide with the container wall. Different methods are used for pruning according to different surgical procedures of heart transplantation. In standard orthotopic heart transplantation, 1/3 to 1/2 of the full length of the right atrium wall should be cut along the right side of the entrance of the inferior vena cava and the right atrial appendage. Remove the membranous tissue around the aorta and pulmonary artery to completely separate the two. Make an “X” cross incision along the entrance of the four pulmonary veins left atrium; or along the entrance of the superior inferior pulmonary vein on the same side, posterior wall of the left atrium, and then cut atrium horizontally. In orthotopic whole-heart transplantation, the trimming method of the aorta and pulmonary artery is the same as the trimming method of the standard orthotopic heart transplantation, but the right atrium wall is not cut, and the superior and inferior vena cava are kept as long as possible; The left upper and lower lung veins and the right upper and lower lung veins of the donor heart are, respectively, trimmed into two common openings. When the double vena cava orthotopic heart transplantation trims the donor heart, the treatment of the pulmonary vein is the same as the standard orthotopic transplantation, and the treatment of the upper and inferior vena cava is the same as the whole-heart orthotopic transplantation. In the process of donor heart implantation, the aorta and pulmonary artery can be trimmed to the appropriate length after the atrial anastomosis is completed. Some simple defects, such as patent foramen ovale, can be trimmed before implanting the donor heart.

4.1.3.2 Combined Acquisition Technology of Donor Heart and Lung

A median sternum incision was used to cut the donor heart and lungs. The retractor is opened to the maximum, the pleural cavity is opened, and both lungs are explored to determine whether there are adhesions, nodules, or trauma. Lightly press the lungs and cut the lower lung ligaments with an electric knife. The thymus is removed, the pericardial cavity is opened, and the aorta, pulmonary artery, and superior and inferior vena cava are freed. The ascending aorta and the superior and inferior vena cava cross bands. Free the trachea between the superior vena cava and the ascending aorta and pass the band. The free range exceeds the four cartilage rings on the carina. Extensively remove the pericardium up to both hilar. Continuous mechanical ventilation, FiO_2 is 40%, and PEEP is 3–5 cm H_2O. After the donor was fully heparinized (3 mg/kg), the ascending aorta and main pulmonary artery were cannulated. Ligate the superior and inferior vena cava. After the heart is empty, the ascending aorta is blocked, cardioplegia is perfused, and lung protection fluid is perfused through the pulmonary artery. The lung protection solution contains prostaglandin, a powerful vasodilator. After blocking the ascending aorta, immediately cut off the inferior vena cava and quickly open the left atrial appendage. The perfusion time is 10 min. Ice salt water was poured into the chest cavity to cool down, and the tidal volume remained at about half of the normal value. After the perfusion, the lungs are completely collapsed, and the ice saline in the chest cavity and pericardium is sucked out.

Push the heart to the left, open the posterior mediastinum, and bluntly separate the esophagus and descending aorta. The aorta can be cut off at the descending aortic segment or arch. Avoid damaging the lungs, trachea, heart, and large blood vessels during the whole process. To avoid contamination, the esophagus should not be damaged. Check again the hilar tissues that has been separated. After the lungs are inflated normally, the trachea is cut off at least 4 cartilage rings on the carina with a closure device, and the heart and lungs are completely removed. Immediately wrap it with sterile gauze and put it into ice salt water packed in a 3-layer sterile plastic bag. Pour the cardioprotective liquid or lung protective liquid into the innermost bag containing the heart and lungs, and transport it in a container with ice debris [9, 10].

Attachment: Preparation and surgical procedures for donors of combined heart-lung transplantation in the First Affiliated Hospital of Sun Yat-sen University

1. Tracheal intubation, FiO_2 is 40%, PEEP 3–5 cm H_2O;
2. Fiberoptic bronchoscopy and sputum suction test;
3. After making a median incision and loosening the adhesion, separate the lower lung ligament, Shupu 2 g + normal saline 20 ml iv (when cutting the skin);
4. The fluid supplement rate is 45–100 ml/h;
5. Mean arterial pressure 70–80 mmHg, CVP 5–8 cm H_2O;
6. Open the pericardium, heparin 3 mg/kg;
7. Methylprednisolone 30 mg/kg or 1 g (when the heart is free), carefully check the heart condition, explore the lungs, free the ascend-

ing aorta, innominate vein, superior and inferior vena cava;

8. Resection of the pericardium to the hilum of both lungs, including the phrenic nerve and thymus;
9. Cardioplegia: After blocking the aorta, infuse 1000 ml of 4 °CUW solution at the root of the aorta at a pressure of 60–80 mmHg;
10. Lung protection solution (EC 4000 ml + Tris 0.8 ml + PGI 100 μg): After blocking the pulmonary artery, the pulmonary artery is perfused with 4000 ml, and the perfusion pressure is 20-30 mmHg;
11. Cut off the vena cava and aorta, separate the esophagus and other attachments behind the heart and lungs, block the trachea from the clamp, cut off the trachea at the far side of the clamp, and cut the heart and lungs in one piece.
12. Other precautions for donor protection:
    (a) After lung resection, try to minimize touching and squeezing the lungs, and the lungs continue to expand slightly to prevent prolonged atelectasis;
    (b) The heart and lungs are placed in a protective solution at 4 °C, and a sterile bag is placed outside it, and then transferred to the refrigerator. Avoid volume overload and prevent pulmonary edema.

4.1.3.3 Acquisition Technology of Donor Lung

Cut the open heart bag and both pleural cavities to observe the expansion of both lungs. Exploring the lungs to find out whether there are adhesions, masses, nodules, and trauma. The main pulmonary artery was sutured and intubated (14Fr.). The depth of the intubation should be at the bifurcation of the left and right pulmonary arteries. Infuse 4 l of 6 °C lung protection solution, the perfusion pressure is 15–20 mmHg, and the perfusion time is 10 min. At the same time, open the left atrial appendage to drain the lung lavage fluid. Continue to ventilate during lavage to avoid atelectasis and facilitate the uniform distribution of the protective fluid. During perfusion, FiO_2 should be around 50%, breathing rate 12 beats/min, tidal volume 15 ml/kg, and PEEP of 6–8 cm H_2O should be used to fully inflate the lungs and clamp the trachea at the end of inhalation. After the lavage was completed, the pulmonary artery cannula was pulled out and the organs were beginning to be procured.

The heart should be removed first, and the inferior vena cava and right atrium should be cut off at the proximal end of the inferior vena cava. Ligate and cut the superior vena cava 1 cm above the junction of the superior vena cava and the right atrium. Cut the ascending aorta at the distal end of the ascending aorta, and cut the main pulmonary artery at the beginning of the left and right pulmonary arteries. Cut the root pulmonary vein where the pulmonary vein enters the left atrium, and remove the heart. Immediately perform retrograde implantation at each pulmonary vein opening to ensure that bronchial and lung blood vessels are lavaged, which is beneficial to reduce the contraction of the pulmonary artery and the removal of clots in the distal pulmonary artery bed, and improve the function of the transplanted lung. The specific method is as follows: a urinary catheter with a balloon is inserted through the pulmonary vein, the blood vessel is filled with water to expand to block the backflow of the lavage fluid, and then the lung protection fluid is implanted retrogradely. Each pulmonary vein was perfused with 500 ml protective solution. It takes about 2 and a half minutes to fill, and it takes 10 min in total. The donor lung can be obtained from the right side. The lower pulmonary ligaments on both sides are cut off, and the posterior pulmonary vein is closely attached to the posterior mediastinum along the posterior edge of the hilum. The upper pulmonary vein, bronchi, carina, and trachea are sharply separated. Separate the left hilum to the trachea in the same way. When the lungs are inflated, use a closure device to cut off the trachea to remove both lungs. A section of the aortic wall can be attached to the arterial duct ligament junction. After taking out the donor lung, immediately put it into ice saline packed in 3 layers of sterile plastic bags. Put 1000 ml of 4 °C lung protection solution upside down in the innermost bag for lungs, and transport it in a container with crushed ice.

4.1.4 Special Organ Acquisition Technology

4.1.4.1 In Vivo Split Liver Transplantation Technology

Introduction to split liver transplantation: Split liver transplantation (SLT) refers to splitting a complete donor liver into two independent anatomical and functional grafts, which are transplanted to two recipients, respectively, a kind of liver transplantation technology, as an important transplantation technology to increase the source of donor liver. It avoids the shortcomings of living donor liver transplantation (living-related donor liver transplantation, LDLT), such as donor risk, and has become a recognized new transplant technology and research hotspot today.

Introduction to the methods of in vivo *split liver transplantation:* SLT includes two methods: in vitro SLT (Ex situ split liver transplantation, ESSLT) and in vivo SLT (In situ split liver transplantation, ISLT). The latter is developed on the basis of the former. The first SLT implemented by Pichlmayr [8] in Germany in 1988 was ESSLT—on the donor liver dressing table, they split a complete donor liver into left and right donor livers. The left and right donor livers were transplanted into a 63-year-old woman with biliary cirrhosis and a child with congenital biliary atresia. The first ISSLT in my country was completed in 2012 by the Organ Transplant Center of the First Affiliated Hospital of Sun Yat-sen University.

In vivo *split liver transplantation indications:* Busuttil [9] and others believe that if the donor liver is grossly observed for signs of congestion, swelling, hardening, etc., ISSLT should be excluded first without the need for more specific inspections to determine whether it is appropriate to discard. In addition to the general observation of the quality of the donated liver, the following needs to be met: (1) Stable hemodynamics; (2) No need for high-dose booster drugs to maintain (dopamine <15 mg/kg·min); (3) age 10–40 years old; (4) ICU Hospital stay <5 days; (5) Liver function <3 times the normal value; (6) Blood Na + <160 mg/dl.

Donor-recipient matching is the key to the selection of split liver transplantation recipients. Recently, the graft-to-recipient weight ratio (GRWR) and the recipient standard liver volume ratio (SLV) are commonly used in clinical practice to assess the minimum donor liver volume. If the donor liver is too small, it can easily lead to severe small liver syndrome. In living donor liver transplantation, GRWR>0.8% is sufficient. Kilie [10] even thought that as long as the recipient does not have severe cirrhosis or portal hypertension, CRWR>0.7% is sufficient. For split liver transplantation, most scholars believe that GRWR>1% is essential to maintain normal postoperative graft function. In addition to GRWR, Urata [11] and others believe that SLV ≥ 40% can also achieve the minimum effective liver volume. Strasberg [12] found that nearly half of the graft's function was lost during the SLT process. Therefore, the concept of functional transplanted liver volume (FGS) has received increasing attention, that is, the actual function of the transplanted liver in the recipient.

In general, for ISSLT, adult segments II and III donor livers are suitable for children weighing 6–20 kg. However, for about 10–20% of young children, the sections II and III liver donation is too large for them, causing difficulty in closing the abdomen; adult sections II, III, and IV liver donation are suitable for patients weighing less than 60 kg; The adult segment I–IV donor liver is suitable for patients weighing about 65 kg; the adult segment V–VII donor liver is suitable for patients with the same weight as the donor; the adult segment I, IV–VII over the right hemiliver or the segment I, V–VII. The right hemiliver can be used for patients weighing less than 80 kg. If the recipient weighs more than 100 kg or a donor with a history of liver surgery, ISSLT should not be performed.

4.1.4.2 Technical Points of In Vivo Split Liver Transplantation

ISSLT of the left lateral lobe segments (II, III) and super right hemihepatic (I, IV, VI–VII): a median incision is made to separate the abdominal aorta and the inferior mesenteric vein. In this way, rapid intubation cold perfusion can be performed when the donor gives up ISSLT in emergency situations such as unstable hemodynamics. Disconnect the falciform ligament of the liver, expose the second hepatic hilum, carefully free the left hepatic vein and avoid damage to the middle hepatic vein to ensure smooth circulation. The left hepatic artery, the left branch of the portal vein, and the left hepatic duct were dissected at the first hepatic portal at the bottom of the hepatic round ligament. Along the left side of the liver falciform ligament 1.0 cm (the junction of II, III, and IV), the liver parenchyma was separated to 1.0 cm above the umbilical fissure with electric knife or bipolar electrocoagulation, ultrasonic surgical suction knife (CUSA). Ligate the perforating small blood vessels and small bile ducts in the liver section carefully. Close the left liver section and sharply cut the remaining liver parenchyma, expose the left liver duct section, press to stop bleeding, and try not to stitch. Perform in situ perfusion of the donor liver, sharply cut the left hepatic artery and the left branch of the portal vein, and lavage the biliary tract of segments II and III. The left lateral lobe donor liver was taken out and stored cold. Then cut the super right hemiliver, perform cold biliary lavage, and suture the left side cut ends of the inferior vena cava, proper hepatic artery, portal vein, and common hepatic duct, and preserved in UW liquid cold for later use.

ISSLT of the left liver (segments II, III, IV) and the right liver (segments I, V–VII): moderately free the extrahepatic segment of the left hepatic vein and the middle hepatic vein at the second hepatic portal. Dissect the left hepatic artery, left portal vein, and left hepatic duct to the level of the round ligament at the first hepatic portal, temporarily block the left hepatic artery and the left portal vein or the right hepatic artery and the right portal vein to determine the cut of the liver parenchyma Line (Cantlie line, the projection of the middle hepatic vein on the surface of the liver near the diaphragm). Using electrosurgical knife or bipolar coagulation, CUSA splits the liver parenchyma along the right side of the Cantlie line, ligating the intrahepatic blood vessels and small bile ducts in the liver section. The branch of the middle hepatic vein with a diameter greater than 5 mm on the right hepatic section is retained, and the cut end corresponding to the left hepatic section is sutured. Sharply cut the left hepatic duct at the first hepatic hilum. After in situ cold perfusion of the donor liver, the left branch of the portal vein was sharply cut at the bifurcation of the portal vein and the right hepatic artery was cut off at the beginning of the proper hepatic artery. The proper hepatic artery, common hepatic artery, and abdominal trunk are preserved in the left liver. The left hepatic vein and the middle hepatic vein are cut at the confluence of the inferior vena cava, and the inferior vena cava is reserved in the right hemiliver. The left liver was taken out and kept cold. The right liver was cut and trimmed with conventional liver transplantation. The left and right liver and biliary tracts were lavaged with cold UW fluid.

In order to ensure smooth circulation of the veins in the V–VII segment, the middle hepatic vein branch of the right hepatic section with a diameter greater than 5 mm can be interposed between the donor's saphenous vein or the inferior mesenteric vein and the recipient's inferior vena cava. Regarding the attribution of the inferior vena cava, Colledan [13] believed that it can be retained in the left hemiliver, but when the short hepatic vein is thick, it is best to retain it in the right hepatic. Gundlach et al. [14] suggested that the inferior vena cava should be cut longitudinally, and the left and right hemilivers should retain part of the venous cuff, which should be anastomosed with the recipient's inferior vena cava. However, if the recipient is two adults, in order to obtain a sufficient volume of the left liver, the middle hepatic vein is usually reserved in the left liver, and the inferior vena cava should be reserved in the right liver. Since the left hepatic artery is relatively thin, the proper hepatic artery and common hepatic artery are generally reserved in the left hemiliver. Rela [15], etc., reported 41 cases after applying this method, only 1 case had hepàtic artery embolism. However, it has also been reported that only the left vascular branch of the left liver is retained, and complications such as hepatic artery embolism are not increased after transplantation.

ISSLT of the left liver (segments I-IV) and the right liver (segments V-VII): free the right hemiliver and the extrahepatic part of the right hepatic vein, separate and ligate the short hepatic vein on the right side of the inferior vena cava. The left side of the vena cava was not dissected, and the short hepatic vein with a diameter of >5 mm was reserved for reconstruction. The antidote along the right side of the right hepatic artery at the first hepatic portal can protect segment IV hepatic artery from damage. Separate the right branch of the portal vein to its full length at the bifurcation of the portal vein. Using an electric knife or bipolar coagulation, CUSA splits the liver parenchyma along the right side of the Cantlie line to the right front of the inferior vena cava on the posterior side of the right liver, and ligate or suture the small blood vessels and bile ducts in the liver section. Cut the middle hepatic vein to segment V and segment VIII, and reserve the branch with a diameter of >5 mm in the right hemiliver. The donor liver needs to be reconstructed when implanted. Free the left hepatic duct to the median fissure, cut the left hepatic duct sharply at the first hepatic hilum, and use compression to stop bleeding when the cross-section is bleeding. Perform in situ cold perfusion of the donor liver, cut the right hepatic artery at the beginning of the right hepatic artery, and cut the right branch of the portal vein at the bifurcation of the portal vein. Cut the right hepatic vein where it joins the inferior vena cava, thus completing the right hemihepatic split. The right hemiliver was taken out and stored cold and the biliary tract was lavaged with cold UW solution. Obtaining the left hemiliver is the same as conventional donor liver procurement. The biliary tract is lavaged with cold UW fluid, the right hepatic vein entrance of the inferior vena cava and the corresponding cut ends of the proper hepatic artery and the main portal vein are closed. The donor liver is cold stored for future use.

4.1.5 Kidney Acquisition in Children

The cutting method of abdominal organs from pediatric donors is basically similar to that of adult donors. Due to the small diameter of the abdominal aorta, inferior vena cava, and superior mesenteric vein of pediatric donors, donors under 3 years of age still need to retain the intact abdominal aorta and inferior vena cava for double kidney transplantation, and organ procurement has its advantages, special aspects.

In situ *perfusion:* Due to the small diameter of the abdominal aorta, it is often impossible to use a balloon catheter to block it. In order to preserve the intact abdominal aorta for bilateral whole kidney transplantation, the arterial perfusion cannula (using a plastic gastric tube or a 16-gauge urinary catheter) can be inserted through the right common iliac artery or the distal end of the abdominal aorta, and the diaphragm is incised. Block the distal thoracic aorta in the chest cavity. Plastic gastric tube should be used for inferior vena cava drainage, and the intubation position should be at the distal end of the inferior vena cava or the right common iliac vein. The superior mesenteric vein is relatively thin, and the portal vein can be inserted with a ventricular drainage tube.

Reduce the amount of perfusion fluid: Compared with adult donors, the amount of perfusion fluid should be reduced, which can generally be adjusted according to the weight of the donor. Generally, donors under 5 years old can be perfused with 1500 ml of HCA solution and 1000 ml of UW solution through the abdominal aorta and 1000 ml of UW solution through the portal vein.

Excision of the great abdominal blood vessels: For donors less than 5 years old, the both kidneys should try to keep the abdominal aorta and inferior vena cava as long as possible. When the liver and kidney are separated after the whole organ is cut, the abdominal aorta should be cut along the opening of the superior mesenteric artery, and the abdominal aortic trunk should be preserved. Part of the anterior wall of the abdominal aorta was cut off and left for the donor liver, and the remaining arteries were left for the donor kidney. The thoracic aorta should be routinely cut for use.

Resection of bilateral ureters and bladder: The surrounding tissues of the ureters should be preserved as much as possible. If the donor is 1-year-old, both ureters and bladder should be removed. During the transplantation of the recipient's kidneys in a whole block, the bladder flap with the triangle of the donor bladder can be used to directly anastomize the recipient's bladder, which can simplify the operation and avoid ureteral obstruction and reflux; the bladder flap can obtain adequate blood supply through bilateral ureters. When cutting the double ureter and bladder, care should be taken to preserve enough tissue around the ureter.

Gentle operation to protect blood vessels: Due to the fragility of the pediatric donor's blood vessel, the damaging to the blood vessel can easily lead to thrombosis of the transplanted renal artery. The operation process should be careful and gentle to avoid violence.

4.1.6 Multiple Organ Procurement Technology

Abdominal multiple organ transplantation refers to the transplantation of more than three organs in the abdominal cavity that are related to each other in anatomy and function, such as hepatopancreaticoduodenal transplantation, which has the characteristics of comprehensive replacement of organ functions and maintenance of the normal anatomical and physiological structure of the transplanted organs. At present, the First Affiliated Hospital of Sun Yat-sen University has implemented eight cases of multiple organ transplants from DCD donors, all of which have achieved good results.

Selection of indications: To date, no comprehensive indication criteria have been formulated for multiple organ transplantation, which mainly include: (1) liver failure with diabetes; (2) liver tumor with diabetes; (3) extensive small bowel lesions leading to multiple organ failure; (4) extensive gastrointestinal tract polyposis or myopathy or nervous system adjustment disorder of all organs with cavity in the abdomina; (5) Severe abdominal trauma and abnormal development of the abdomen; (6) Pancreatic and duodenal sarcoma, carcinoid, pancreatic neuroendocrine tumors with liver metastases;

4.1.6.1 Multiple Organ Transplantation

At present, the trend of multiple organ transplantation is to reduce the number of transplanted organs as much as possible to reduce rejection and intestinal leakage. The earliest multiple organs were whole abdominal organ transplantation, including whole abdominal organs such as liver, pancreas, stomach, small intestine, and colon. Later, because of the many complications of whole abdominal organ transplantation, the types of transplanted organs gradually decreased, and only necessary vital organs were kept for transplantation. Now the most commonly used is the upper abdomen multiple organ transplant—hepatopancreaticoduodenal transplantation. In addition, if the patient has small bowel failure, hepatopancreas-duodenal small bowel transplantation should be performed, and hepatopancreaticoduodenal small bowel transplantation should be performed with total digestive tract disease. The following uses the commonly used hepato-pancreatic-duodenal transplantation as an example to introduce multiple organ transplantation methods.

4.1.6.2 Donor Surgery

For multiple organ procurement, in situ perfusion and en bloc resection are often used, which can simplify the procedure and avoid damage to ectopic blood vessels. According to the in situ perfusion method, the abdominal aorta and superior mesenteric vein were quickly perfused with UW solution at 4 °C. The multi-organ rapid extraction method completely cuts the donor liver, pancreas, duodenum, and part of the jejunum, and retains the bilateral iliac vessels for use. Understage multi-organ trimming: Trim the openings of the celiac trunk and superior mesenteric artery, and, respectively, anastomize them with the external iliac and internal iliac arteries taken from the donor, so that the first two are connected into one outlet, which is the common iliac artery outlet. The common iliac artery after the anastomosis is to be anastomosed with the recipient's abdominal aorta end-to-side. Finally, UW fluid was perfused through the superior mesenteric vein, and the small blood vessels around the pancreas were properly ligated. Store at 4 °C.

4.1.6.3 Recipient Surgery

Recipient surgery uses an inverted T-shaped incision on the upper abdomen. After the diseased liver is removed, the multiple organ donors are implanted in a modified piggyback method, and the pancreas graft is superimposed on the recipient's pancreas. The recipient's portal vein was anastomosed with the posterior wall of the graft's portal vein end-to-side, and the graft's common iliac artery was anastomosed with the recipient's common hepatic artery. After reflow, the biliary tract and external pancreas were drained by side-to-side anastomosis of the descending duodenum of the donor and the upper jejunum of the recipient. A drainage tube is placed near the opening of the donor's duodenum and pancreaticobiliary duct from the recipient's jejunum to facilitate postoperative intestinal anastomosis decompression and observation of pancreatic juice and bile secretion.

4.1.6.4 Treatment after Transplantation and Diagnosis and Treatment of Complications

Surgical technical complications: Common surgical complications include postoperative hemorrhage, leakage or stenosis of biliary tract and blood vessels, intestinal perforation, wound dehiscence, intra-abdominal abscess, and chylous ascites.

Diagnosis and treatment of internal environment disorders: Peripheral venous blood and arterial blood were drawn at different times during the operation for blood electrolyte, biochemical testing, and blood gas analysis, and comprehensive measures were taken for the internal environment changes at different stages of transplantation. Quickly correct acidosis, prevent and treat hyperkalemia, hypocalcemia, etc., adjust heart rate and vascular resistance with cardiovascular active drugs. After the inferior vena cava is blocked and the severe acidemia at the end of the visceral period, a large amount of alkali supplementation is given and bloodletting is performed after the anastomosis of the large vein to shorten the visceral period as much as possible. Venous bypass can also be used to reduce and correct acidemia.

Maintenance of pancreatic function: Take care to avoid pinching the pancreas during perfusion and transplantation to protect the pancreas and its blood supply. When the transplanted pancreas functions well, stop insulin as soon as possible to avoid severe hypoglycemia. According to the situation, measure C-peptide, blood insulin, blood sugar, blood amylase and lipase to monitor pancreatic function.

Treatment of immune rejection: Rejection after transplantation has always been an important link in restricting multiple organ transplantation. At present, the treatment of immune rejection is mainly the application of immunosuppressive agents, and the combination of drugs is often advocated to reduce the side effects of drugs. Monitoring graft rejection can be based on clinical observation, histopathological analysis of endoscopic-guided biopsy, and the treatment of rejection depends on the severity of rejection. In addition to immunosuppressive agents, RNAi currently serves as a new breakthrough point for alternative immune supplements to improve transplant prognosis [16].

Treatment of infection: After transplantation, immunosuppressive agents must be used for a long time to prevent rejection, which may cause local or systemic infections. Use ganciclovir and cytomegalovirus specific immune antibodies to prevent cytomegalovirus, fluconazole to prevent fungal infections, and determine whether to apply antibiotics systemically based on the results of rapid blood, urine, and exudate culture.

4.2 Quality Evaluation

DCD has been proposed as a means of increasing the pool of grafts. The poor graft quality of the DCD is a major cause of the inferior clinical outcome. Proper evaluation and maintenance of donor and graft function can effectively reduce postoperative complications.

4.2.1 Purpose of Evaluation

The purpose of donor evaluation includes: (1) defining the type of donation death (DD) and its reasonable donation process; (2) collecting all the medical information of the donor to facilitate the maintenance of donor and organ function; (3) evaluating the types and quantity of organs that can be donated; (4) eliminating donation contraindications, avoiding the occurrence of donor derived diseases and ensuring the safety of organ transplantation.

The absolute contraindications of organ donation include: (1) unexplained coma; invasive or hematological malignancies; (2) malignant infectious diseases, such as acquired immunodeficiency syndrome (AIDS), rabies, encephalitis B, etc.; (3) severe untreated or uncontrolled sepsis (especially sepsis caused by multidrug-resistant bacteria); (4) special types of infections, such as hematogenous disseminated tuberculosis, Mucor and cryptococcal infections, tetanus, etc.

4.2.2 Basic Evaluation

Information such as present medical history, previous medical history, personal history, and family history should be collected as far as possible. Medical providers should analyze carefully and fully find or exclude the contraindications of organ donation and transplantation, and provide comprehensive information support for the follow-up work of organ donation.

Basic information Including donor age, gender, ethnicity, height, weight, body temperature, heart rate, respiration rate, blood pressure, etc.

Present medical history (1) Etiology, diagnosis, and differential diagnosis; (2) medical examination results, including laboratory examination results and imaging data; (3) course of disease records, including donor treatment records, rescue records, nursing records, etc.; (4) treatment plan, including treatment for primary disease, anti-infection, or prevention of infection, etc.; (5) Donor life support measures, including start time, duration, drug type, and dosage.

Previous medical history Including hypertension, metabolic diseases, and other diseases that may affect organ function, infectious disease history, operation history, etc.

Personal history Including personal addiction, drug use history, adverse occupational environment exposure history, contact history in epidemic area, animal contact or bite history, vaccination history, sexual behavior, allergy history, etc.

Family history Including familial hereditary diseases, infectious diseases, etc.

4.2.3 Special Evaluation

Evaluation of organ donation type (1) Whether it meets the criteria of brain death (BD); (2) whether it meets the criteria of DCD; (3) the prediction of cardiac death after life support is withdrawn.

Characteristics of potential DCD donors: (1) To meet the medical conditions of organ donation; (2) Although it may become a donation after brain death (DBD), it does not meet the criteria of brain death; 3) catastrophic brain injury or other diseases; (4) the patient's attending physician determines that he has no survival expectation; (5) the family members who have the legal decision-making authority request to withdraw the respiratory support and organ perfusion support treatment; and; (6) before the removal of the life support treatment, it is possible to obtain the informed consent of family members [17].

Evaluation of donor derived infection (DDI) (1) Results of infection related tests; (2) The location and type of infection; (3) whether there are infection pathogen or the unclear type pathogen in the donor; (4) whether the risk of infection can be controlled by anti-infective drugs; (5) whether donor infection is a contraindication of organ donation and transplantation; (6) whether there is infection with unclear diagnosis or differential diagnosis; (7) whether they are high risk individuals of some infectious diseases; (8) the culture result of organ perfusate and preservation solution is also an important basis for infection evaluation, prevention, and treatment.

Organ donation is prohibited for patients with the following infectious diseases: (1) multi drug resistant bacteria, especially carbapenem resistant Enterobacteriaceae; (2) active tuberculosis; (3) untreated bacterial or fungal sepsis (e.g., Candida spp.); (4) active infection of endemic fungal diseases (e.g., Blastomyces, sporobacteria, histoplasmosis); (5) potential central nervous system (CNS) infections include unexplained CNS infections (encephalitis, meningitis), herpes simplex virus encephalitis, history of multiple tumor virus JC virus (JCV) infection, West Nile virus (WNV) infection, rabies, Creutzfeldt–Jakob disease, untreated cryptococcal infection, etc.; (6) Serological or molecular diagnosis of human T lymphotropic virus (HTLV)-1 or HTLV-2 infection; (7) serological or molecular diagnosis of human immunodeficiency virus (HIV) infection; (8) untreated parasite infection (Trypanosoma Kuwana, Leishmania donovani, Strongyloides faecalis), etc.

Evaluation of tumor donors (1) the diagnosis time, type, benign and malignant, differentiation degree and grade of tumor, pathological data, treatment plan, recurrence, etc.; (2) If it is CNS tumor, we should also consider whether the tumor is primary or metastatic, initial or recurrent, treatment plan, the possibility of extracranial metastasis, etc.; (3) based on the available clinical data, whether further screening is needed. In addition, attention should be paid to the exploration in the process of organ procurement [18].

Evaluation of encephalitis donors The evaluation includes: (1) whether the etiology or pathogen is clear; (2) the results of cerebrospinal fluid test; (3) whether the diagnosis and differential diagnosis are sufficient;(3) whether the donor has animal contact or bite history, vaccination or related treatment history; (4) whether the disease is a mass event, and the contact history of the donor in the epidemic area.

Evaluation of donors of intracranial hemorrhage (1) Whether the diagnosis and differential diagnosis of intracranial hemorrhage is clear; (2) whether there is the possibility of intracranial hemorrhage secondary to CNS tumor; (3) whether there is the possibility of intracranial hemorrhage secondary to infectious diseases.

4.2.4 Evaluation of Organ Function

Once it is confirmed that the donor meets the DCD criteria, the function evaluation of donor organs should be carried out in the process of donor evaluation and maintenance.

Various methods should also be used to evaluate organ function during and after organ procurement. The whole evaluation process is dynamic and continuous.

The contents of organ function evaluation should include: (1) which examination or evaluation contents need to be further improved; (2) which organs meet the donation conditions; (3) whether the donors are standard donors or extended criteria donor (ECD); (4) the functional status or damage severity of heart, lung, liver, kidney, pancreas, etc.; (5) Before the donor maintenance and procurement, whether there is the risk of injury aggravating.

4.2.4.1 Evaluation and Selection of Renal Function

Blood biochemical test: The baseline of Serum creatinine (Scr) is important, and SCR < 200 μmol/L at the time of procurement indicates better renal function. While the donor kidney with low Scr level may have poor recovery of renal function after transplantation or even primary non-function (PNF). Therefore, it is necessary to analyze the donor's actual situation in combination with the Scr in the early stage of the disease and the Scr before procurement. In the organ maintenance stage, Scr may rise sharply, and even need to be assisted with hemodialysis treatment. At this time, the causes for the increase of Scr should be carefully identified. If the increase of SCR is caused by irreversible renal injury, it is necessary to carefully consider whether the donor kidney is available; if the SCR increase is caused by reversible renal injury such as acute tubular necrosis, the donor kidney can be considered.

Ultrasound imaging examination: ultrasound is an essential means for the evaluation of donor kidney, which is helpful to judge the basic situation of donor kidney, such as the size, abnormal echo of parenchyma, calculus, tumor, hydrops, etc. color Doppler ultrasound can also observe the blood flow of donor kidney, so as to judge the function of donor kidney.

Appearance and texture of donor kidney: observing the appearance and texture of donor kidney during organ procurement is a very direct and practical way to evaluate the quality of donor kidney. Doctors can directly observe the size and texture of the donor kidney, the flow rate of perfusion fluid, and the color of the donor kidney after perfusion, whether there is tumor, cyst, vascular or anatomical malformation, thrombosis, infarction, and scar in the donor kidney. Further pathological evaluation or lifeport evaluation is feasible for the kidney in question.

Mechanical perfusion parameters: Mechanical perfusion parameters have been widely used in the evaluation of renal function in recent years. It is recommended that the reference index of lifeport for evaluation of donor kidney is resistance index <0.5 and flow rate >60 ml/min within 3 h of perfusion.

Pathological evaluation: Pathological evaluation has important clinical significance. Wedge biopsy or fine needle aspiration biopsy can be used for sampling. If the number of glomeruli to be biopsied reaches 20–25, it is conducive to accurate judgment. The indications include ECD, hypertension, diabetes, and kidney injury. Pathological sampling can be performed at three time points: the end of cold preservation, pre-reperfusion, and post revascularization. The pathological results were evaluated according to the Remuzzi score.

4.2.4.2 Evaluation and Selection of Hepatic Function

Fatty liver: The liver transplantation (LT) with mild bullous steatosis (<30%) is relatively safe, while the donor liver with moderate bullous steatosis (30–60%) can be selectively used in emergency; liver with severe bullous steatosis (>60%) is generally not recommended for transplantation. Since it is difficult to accurately determine the severity of steatosis by gross observation, pathological evaluation should be conducted and the degree of steatosis should be determined once obvious steatosis is suspected.

Warm ischemia time (WIT): After withdrawal of life support therapy, persistent severe hypotension (arterial systolic pressure less than 50 mmHg and lasting for more than 15 min) will increase the incidence of biliary ischemia and liver graft dysfunction after transplantation, as well as the mortality of recipients. Shortening the WIT can improve the quality of donor liver to a certain extent, so as to improve the effect of LT.

Cold preservation time: The cold preservation time of graft is generally less than 12 h. It has been found that the incidence of graft dysfunction increases by 6% every 1 h of cold ischemia time prolongation. Shortening the cold preservation time can promote the recovery of transplanted liver function and improve the effect of LT.

Protection and evaluation of donors with unplanned cardiac arrest: Donors are prone to unscheduled cardiac arrest, and prolonged cardiopulmonary resuscitation (CPR) can significantly damage organ function. Studies have shown that under the condition of chest compression, the oxygen transport capacity of patients is only 1/4 of physiological quantity, and the oxygen uptake rate is much higher than that of physiological state. On the basis of a comprehensive evaluation, the donor liver can be used for transplantation if the recovery time of the donor's autonomic circulation is less than 10 min and the liver function is basically normal.

Indocyanine Green Clearance (ICG) Test: The ICG retention rate at 15 min (ICGR15) of donors before procurement was independently associated with 3-month graft survival after

LT. A donor ICGR15 value of ≤11.0%/min could be used as an early assessment index of graft quality because it provides additional information to the transplant surgeon or organ procurement organization members who must maintain or improve organ function to adapt the LT [19].

4.2.4.3 Evaluation and Selection of Heart Function

Age: The donor's age is 45–55 years old, the donor heart can be considered to use when the cold ischemia time (CIT) is less than 6 h and the recipient has no complications. The donor age is more than 55 years old, so the donor heart is not recommended to use or only use it to save lives and other special circumstances.

Body weight: The matching of donor and recipient weight is the key to heart transplantation. It is safe to transplant if the donor's body weight is not less than 70% of recipient's. When the body weight of male donor is 70 kg, it is safe to transplant regardless of the recipient body weight. However, when the donor is female and the recipient is male, the donor body weight should not be less than 80% of the recipient body weight.

Cold ischemia time: The CIT of heart should be less than 6 h. Under the condition of normal cardiac function and no positive inotropic drug support, donor hearts with CIT > 6 h can be accepted.

Underlying cardiac diseases: It will not be considered for transplantation when any one of the main coronary arteries of the donor heart is found to be blocked. If there is no left ventricular hypertrophy according to electrocardiogram, the left ventricular wall thickness is less than 14 mm and only mild left ventricular hypertrophy is found, the donor can be considered for use.

Donor hearts that died of sepsis or central nervous system infection are not recommended for transplantation. The donor had uncontrollable ventricular arrhythmias, or the left ventricular ejection fraction (LVEF) is still less than 40% after hemodynamic stabilization under the application of positive inotropic drugs, it is not recommended to use this kind of heart.

The general criteria for cardiac donors are as follows: (1) age < 50 years old; (2) body mass difference < 20%; (3) no serious structural heart disease; (4) no persistent hypotension and hypoxemia; (5) stable hemodynamics, mean arterial pressure (MAP) > 60 mmHg, central venous pressure (CVP) 8–12 cm H_2O, dosage of vasoactive drugs (dopamine or dobutamine) < 10 μg/(kg min); (6) normal electrocardiogram; (7) normal echocardiography; (8) Normal coronary angiography (donors without coronary angiography need to been explored again during the operation to evaluate the coronary situation), myocardial enzymes were basically normal; (9) All blood transfusion items are negative (including HBsAg, HCV, and HIV).

4.2.4.4 Evaluation and Selection of Lung Function

The ideal donor lung criteria are as follows: (1) ABO blood type compatibility; (2) age < 60 years old; (3) smoking history <400 cigarettes/year; (4) continuous mechanical ventilation <1 week; (5) $PaO_2/FiO_2 > 300$ mmHg (PEEP = 5 cm H_2O); (6) Chest X-ray showed that the lung field was relatively clear; (7) Bronchoscopy showed that the lumen of each airway was relatively clean; (8) No special pathogenic bacteria were found in sputum.

The criteria of acceptable donor lung are as follows: (1) ABO blood type compatibility; (2) age < 70 years old; (3) smoking history <400 cigarettes/year; (4) ventilator time is not required; (5) $PaO_2/FiO_2 > 250$ mmHg (PEEP = 5 cm H_2O); (6) there is a small to moderate amount of exudation in the lung field of X-ray chest film; (7) donor lung volume reduction or lung transplantation can be carried out; (8) chest trauma is not considered as exclusion criteria; (9) slight aspiration or improved sepsis after treatment and maintenance was not considered as the exclusion criteria; (10) the purulent secretion in the airway of donor lung can be improved after treatment and maintenance, and can be used for transplantation; (11) the results of drug sensitivity test showed that Pan resistant or all resistant bacteria were excluded; (12) donor with underlying pulmonary diseases (such as active tuberculosis and lung cancer) should be excluded, but bronchial asthma is acceptable; (13) the unqualified donor lungs can be transplanted after repairing by perfusion in vitro and reach the donated criteria; (14) Cold ischemia time ≤12 h.

4.2.4.5 Evaluation and Selection of Pancreatic Function

The evaluation contents include: (1) the ideal age of pancreas donor is between 15 and 40 years old, which can be extended to 45 years old if the general condition is fine; (2) the donor body mass index (BMI) < 25 kg/m^2; (3) the primary disease is trauma; (4) no history of pancreatitis, hypertension, diabetes, or hyperlipidemia; (5) no pancreatic injury or trauma; (6) normal blood amylase and lipase; (7) The WIT of donor pancreas was less than 10 min and the CIT was less than 12 h; (8) glycosylated hemoglobin (HbA1c) was normal.

4.2.4.6 Evaluation and Selection of Small Bowel Function

Absolute contraindications: (1) patients with mesenteric vascular disease; (2) malignant tumors (except for skin basal cell carcinoma and glioma without metastasis); (3) severe abdominal trauma; (4) uncontrolled or untreated sepsis, sepsis of unknown infection source; (5) HIV antibody positive and high risk of HIV infection; (6) active syphilis; (7) Hepatitis B virus (HBV) negative recipients received HBV positive organs.

Relative contraindications: (1) age > 65 years old; (2) HBV and hepatitis C virus serological positive; (3) the result of cytomegalovirus polymerase chain reaction (PCR) is positive; (4) some serious medical diseases, such as diabetes, systemic lupus erythematosus, etc.; (5) serious macrovascular malformations or lesions.

4.3 Organ Perfusion in Donation After Cardiac Death

After the organ donated by qualified donors is procured, organ perfusion is required before transplantation, and its quality directly affects the functional recovery and the long-term efficacy of organ transplantation. Besides the inevitable cold preservation injury, organs donated from DCD are suffering from different degrees of warm ischemia injury. Therefore, for organs donated from DCD, we emphasize the use of machine perfusion to protect the organ function. Ex vivo machine perfusion has been proved to not only improve the quality of organs but also provide indicators for judging organ vitality, and provides a corresponding circulatory platform that approximates the physiological state of the isolated organs.

4.3.1 The History of Machine Perfusion and Preservation

The history of organ perfusion can be traced back to the nineteenth century. In 1849, *Loebel* reported the first case of Ex vivo organ perfusion [20]. In the 1930s, *Alex Carrel* began to try to use perfusion pumps to perfuse and preserve organs outside the body [21]. In 1960, *Folkert Belzer* began to use hypothermic perfusion to preserve the kidney, and plasma was used for hypothermic pulse perfusion in 1967. However, the huge and inconvenient transportation of perfusion equipment limited the development of this method at that time [22]. In 1971, a small portable perfusion pump for machine perfusion of kidneys was invented, which greatly promoted the clinical promotion of hypothermic machine perfusion of isolated organs. However, with the advancement of in vitro preservation solutions and postoperative anti-rejection drugs, the advantages of hypothermic machine perfusion were no longer obvious. Therefore, after the mid-1980s, static cold storage (SCS) has become the mainstream. The earliest isolated organ preservation solution was the Collins solution developed by the team led by Collins in 1969, and in 1976, the European Society of Transplantation improved it and developed the Euro-Collins (EC) solution. In the 1980s, *Belzer* developed University of Wisconsin (UW) solution, which can significantly extend the cold preservation time of solid organs such as kidney, liver, pancreas, etc., so it gradually replaced EC solution. At the same time, *Bretschneider* developed the histidine-tryptophan-ketoglutarate (HTK) solution, which was firstly used as a myocardial solution in heart transplantation operations. Later, HTK solution was discovered that it has a good effect on the preservation of other solid abdominal organs, so it is popularized and applied in the field of organ transplantation [23–25].

With the improvement of transplantation technology, the efficacy of transplantation has been steadily improved, and the shortage of organs has become the primary reason restricting the development of organ transplantation. The increasingly severe contradiction between supply and demand forces transplant experts to continuously expand the source of donor organs. Expanded criteria donors organs are thought to cause higher incidence of Primary Nonfunction (PNF) and Delayed Graft Function (DGF) [26–28]. The traditional static cold storage has been unable to meet the clinical needs, and machine perfusion has once again returned to the field of vision of transplant experts.

4.3.2 Machine Perfusion

4.3.2.1 Different Types of Machine Perfusion

According to the different perfusion temperature, machine perfusion (MP) can be divided into hypothermic machine perfusion (HMP), hypothermic machine perfusion (MTMP), subnormothermic machine perfusion (SNMP), and normothermic machine perfusion (NMP). According to whether it carries oxygen or not, it can be divided into oxygen-carrying and non-oxygen-carrying perfusion systems.

4.3.2.2 The Advantages of Machine Perfusion

The advantages of machine perfusion mainly include the following aspects: (1) Reduce the metabolic level of isolated organs, thereby reducing the consumption of oxygen and ATP by the tissue. (2) Make the solution circulate continuously in the blood vessels of the organs, provide nutrients, take away oxygen free radicals and toxic metabolites, and reduce cold ischemia damage. (3) Reduce vasospasm. (4) Detect indicators such as perfusion flow and resistance index to provide an important basis for evaluating donor kidneys. (5) Convenient to add drugs that help improve organ quality. (6) Preserve the hemodynamic stimulation in organ blood vessels during cold ischemia, which is of great significance to the recovery of organ blood vessel physiological functions after transplantation.

4.3.3 Machine Perfusion of Major Organs

4.3.3.1 Machine Perfusion of Kidney

Hypothermic machine perfusion of Kidney: Hypothermic machine perfusion refers to the application of centrifugal pumps or roller pumps to continuously perfuse organs with cold solution. After the organ is procured, the kidney is connected to the perfusion device through the renal artery to keep the vasculature sealed. The circulation of the perfusion solution is driven by a peristaltic pump to provide continuous or pulsed power, and the cold (0–4 °C) preservation solution is perfused through the renal artery.

The application of HMP in kidney transplantation has become increasingly mature, and there are currently many commercial kidney perfusion devices on the market. Including LifePort kidney perfusion device (Organ Recovery System, Chicago and Brussels), RM3 (Waters Medical System, Birmingham, USA), and Kidney Assist (Organ Assist, Groningen, Netherlands).

A large number of studies have reported that HMP has obvious advantages compared with static cold storage [26, 27]. According to a prospective, multi-center, randomized, controlled trial of Lifeport improving the quality of cadaveric kidney donors, LifePort can reduce the incidence of DGF and increase the survival rate of grafts [26]. However, in the three-year follow-up data published later, the HMP did not show obvious advantages in the DCD donor kidney subgroup analysis [29]. Another study analyzed the data of Scientific Registry of Transplant

Recipients, and MP did not reduce the DCD 0–1 year all-cause transplant failure rate [30].

The results of two large-sample, randomized, controlled trial comparing the efficacy of HMP and SCS in DCD donor kidneys showed that HMP cannot improve the 1-year survival rate of recipients and grafts [31, 32]. One of the studies confirmed that HMP can reduce the incidence of DGF and shorten the course of the disease [31], but another study did not [32]. Our research team conducted a meta-analysis of the relevant published literature, compared the clinical data of 175 machine perfusion and 176 static storage kidney transplants, and found that machine perfusion can reduce the incidence of DGF [33]. However, it is worth noting that the results of different studies are likely to be closely related to whether machine perfusion is performed immediately after procurement and whether the perfusion time is long enough. Therefore, we suggest that HMP in donor kidneys with high risk factors for DGF may be a more reasonable choice, and it is necessary to decide whether to use perfused organs based on the improvement of organ quality.

Normothermic machine perfusion of Kidney: Kidneys from DCD are less tolerant of low temperature, so improved machine perfusion technique is needed [34–36]. Improved HMP has been shown in animal experiments to reduce graft damage. For example, low-concentration oxygen supply [37] and therapeutic drugs [38] can be used in HMP. However, the efficacy of these treatments under low-temperature conditions is significantly inhibited.

Preserving the kidney at room temperature has many advantages. It is closer to its physiological state. It can observe and evaluate the quality of the transplanted kidney [39], and it can help the recovery of kidney function. There is a case report that a kidney which was originally rejected for transplantation due to insufficient perfusion has reached the standard for transplantation after NMP [40].

Bagul et al. reported the first NMP system [41]. The system uses improved pediatric cardiopulmonary circulation technology and adopts a pressure control mode. The perfusion fluid is mixed with red blood cells that clear white blood cells and crystal fluid, and anti-inflammatory drugs, antioxidants, and vasodilators are added. Subsequently, the research group reported the application of NMP in human kidneys [42]. The incidence of DGF in 18 cases of recipients who received expanded criteria donors' kidney and used this technology was 5.6%, while the rate is 36% in matched recipients with SCS [42].

At present, the research hotspots of NMP focus on optimizing solution, combining with hypothermic perfusion, and repairing long-term warm ischemic kidney. Regarding the individualized repair treatment of organs, such as drugs, stem cells, gene therapy, and other methods, because they are implemented in external organs and do not directly act on donors and recipients, they are expected to achieve higher safety and effectiveness.

4.3.3.2 Machine Perfusion of Liver

Ex vivo machine perfusion of donor livers is still in the verification stage of a large number of preclinical trials. There are also many controversies about the method, temperature, and time of perfusion. It is still a certain gap between the clinical application and now, but the existing experimental studies show that the ex vivo machine perfusion has a positive effect on the vitality maintenance and quality improvement of the isolated donor liver [43–45].

The current liver ex vivo perfusion system mainly consists of centrifugal pumps or roller pumps, heat exchangers, extracorporeal membrane oxygenators, liquid reservoirs, and organ reservoirs. In the existing animal experiments, the portal vein and hepatic artery dual perfusion system and the portal vein single perfusion system are used. Because the former can more simulate the liver blood perfusion in the body, it is widely used.

Normothermic machine perfusion of Liver: In vitro machine perfusion of the isolated liver at room temperature (37 °C) can re-establish a normal physiological environment while avoiding cold ischemia and hypoxia injury. The Berlin team described for the first time the application of NMP in an animal model of DCD liver transplantation [46]. The Oxford team successfully preserved the liver for 72 h with NMP [47]. In vitro NMP is the initial process of energy metabolism recovery and cell repair, and provides physiological conditions and required substrates for in vitro liver preservation. However, the composition of the NMP system is complex, difficult to operate and transport, and it requires more components of the solution.

Subnormothermic machine perfusion of Liver: Some studies have shown that 4–37 °C machine perfusion can significantly improve liver cell necrosis, apoptosis, energy conversion, portal vein resistance, and Kupffer cell activation compared with hypothermic perfusion. At the same time, the application of subnormothermic machine perfusion in DCD donor liver can ensure the function of transplantation and the integrity of sinusoidal epithelial cells after transplantation [48]. Studies have also shown that as the temperature increases, the better the bile production after transplantation.

Hypothermic machine perfusion of Liver: The temperature of the solution is controlled to 0–4 °C, and the hypothermic oxygenation perfusion provides a moderate oxygen supply and a reasonable low-temperature low-perfusion flow rate, which can permanently preserve the energy products generated by the electron transport chain. The production of ATP during hypothermic perfusion can restore the dynamic balance of cell energy metabolism and prevent the disintegration of mitochondria [49]. Improving the mitochondrial state is the key role of hypothermic perfusion. If the function of oxygen-treated organelles is improved, the cells can better deal with sudden oxidation after the transplant is reperfused. A study showed that the five-year graft survival rate of DCD liver transplantation after hypothermic oxygenation perfusion is similar to that of DBD and better than untreated DCD liver transplantation [50]. Hypothermic perfusion does not require additional equipment for heating, and can be achieved only by melting ice. In addition, oxygen consumption is significantly reduced under low-temperature conditions, and the perfusion solution does not require a specific oxygen carrier. Finally, bacteria grow slowly under low-temperature conditions and there are fewer graft-related infections.

Although the current research on in vitro liver machine perfusion is mainly focused on the animal experiment stage, due to the development and improvement of medical technology, a small number of clinical application reports have appeared. It is found that under HMP, the incidence of early non-function of the graft and biliary complications are reduced, and no primary non-function of the graft occurs [51] and liver inflammation and injury are significantly improved [52, 53]. The in vitro liver machine perfusion is expected to be put into the clinical application. When long-term machine perfusion becomes possible, the effect of machine perfusion is no longer just to improve the quality of the organ preservation process, and even the pre-transplantation preparation of the isolated liver can be used with the perfusion system. The most basic practice is the pre-use of drug intervention during the perfusion process to reduce postoperative reperfusion injury. Further consideration is the preoperative immunomodulation of the donor liver during in vitro perfusion, such as the application of CTLA4Ig transfection [54]. If the effect of machine perfusion to prolong liver viability is finally confirmed, those patients who are not suitable for solid organ transplantation can assist in improving liver function through extracorporeal liver perfusion system [55] or use the abandoned donor liver for perfusion, and then perform corresponding hepatocyte transplantation after improvement [56].

In short, in vitro liver machine perfusion is a new type of organ preservation method that is closer to physiology. Its successful application is bound to enable expanded criteria donors liver to be fully and rationally used, expand the source of donor liver, and further alleviate the dilemma of organ shortage.

4.3.3.3 Machine Perfusion of Heart/ Lung

Similar to the liver perfusion technology, the heart/lung perfusion technology has only animal experiments and sporadic clinical research reports confirming that in vitro machine perfusion can achieve higher graft survival and better graft function under extended storage conditions. The cost and management difficulties of infusion technology are considered disproportionate to the benefits of infusion. However, the shortage of organs makes us increasingly use expanded criteria donors, including DCD. Therefore, the application of machine perfusion in heart preservation has also received more and more attention. Unlike abroad, most of Chinese DCD are patients with severe brain injury or brain death who have cardiac arrest after removal of life support. Most of the donor's heart and lungs have no organic disease. Therefore, the application of machine perfusion technology is expected to significantly improve the quality of Chinese DCD donor heart. Unfortunately, there are no relevant animal experiments and clinical research reports in China.

The first clinical trials to evaluate the safety and effectiveness of the application of machine perfusion in cardiac preservation began in 2007 in the United States (PROCEED trial, Prospective Multicentre Safety and Effectiveness of the Organ Care System Device for Cardiac Use) and Europe (PROTECT-I, Prospective Multicentre European Trail to Evaluate the Safety and Performance of the Organ Care System for Heart Transplants). Both trials are prospective, multi-center studies using OCS heart perfusion system (TransMedics, Andover, MA, USA). The 30-day survival rate of 15 patients in the PROCEED trial was 93%. Five serious adverse events occurred, one died of cardiac insufficiency, and four recovered well after treatment [57]. The 30-day survival rate of 20 patients in the PROTECT-I trial was 100%, and none of the serious adverse events was related to the use of the perfusion device [58].

The clinical trial of lung machine perfusion started late, using the device from the same company of the cardiac perfusion device—OCS Lung. Preliminary test results show that after in vitro perfusion, the oxygenation index of the transplanted lung can be maintained at or even slightly higher than before donation Level. Subsequently, the research team started the INSPIRE trial. Although there was no short-term survival benefit reported, the safety and effectiveness of lung preservation by comparing machine perfusion and traditional SCS were verified [59]. Another EXPAND trial focused on extended criteria donors and DCD donor lungs, and it showed that 87% of donor lungs could be transplanted after perfusion with portable OSC Lung and 99% had survived at 30 days post-transplant [60].

Therefore, we have reason to expect that after continuous technological improvement, the application of mechanical perfusion technology to the preservation of heart and lungs will become a reality in the near future.

4.3.3.4 Machine Perfusion of Pancreases

Similar to the preservation of other organs, SCS is still the standard technology for pancreas preservation. SCS is sufficient for the pancreas with DBD, but for the more severely damaged DCD pancreas, machine perfusion may have a better repair effect.

The machine perfusion of the pancreas actually started in 1926. Researchers applied machine perfusion to evaluate the endocrine and exocrine function of the dog's pancreas [61]. However, because the blood vessels supplying the pancreas are more delicate and easy to damage than other organs, the application of machine perfusion in the preservation of the pancreas lags behind other organs. There are no reports of shaped external pancreatic perfusion. Machine perfusion was applied to the preservation of islets before isolation. Although HMP can cause pancreatic edema, it is beneficial to pancreatic quality [62]. Perfusion destroys the extracellular space of the pancreas, but can increase the number of islets and digest more evenly [63, 64], but this effect may cause serious complications in pancreatic transplantation. It is undeniable that the current pancreatic hypothermic mechanical perfusion technology is still far from mature, and the perfusion technology and method have not yet been concluded.

Compared with the HMP, the NMP of the pancreas is less mature. Idezuki et al. [65] used a blood-based isoperfusion solution to perfuse the dog's pancreas in a developed circuit, and added glucose to the perfusion solution to measure the quality of insulin produced by the pancreas to evaluate pancreatic function. They found that as the storage time increased, the amount of insulin production gradually decreased, and he could evaluate the preservation damage and vitality of the pancreas. Other researchers have reported more complicated perfusion systems [66, 67].

Although the mechanical perfusion technology of the pancreas is progressing slowly, the existing research results will provide an important basis for the design of more reasonable perfusion modes in the future.

References

1. Monbaliu D, Pirenne J, Talbot D. Liver transplantation using donation after cardiac death donors. J Hepatol. 2012;56(2):474–85.
2. Sui WG, Yan Q, Xie SP, Chen HZ, Li D, Hu CX, et al. Successful organ donation from brain dead donors in a Chinese organ transplantation center. Am J Transplant. 2011;11(10):2247–9.
3. He XS, Guo ZY, Ju WQ, Wang DP, Wu LW. Liver transplantation using donation after cardiac death donors: initial experience at a Chinese organ transplant center. Liver Transpl. 2013;19:S202.
4. Polyak MM, Arrington BO, Kapur S, Stubenbord WT, Kinkhabwala M. Donor treatment with phentolamine mesylate improves machine preservation dynamics and early renal allograft function. Transplantation. 2000;69(1):184–6.
5. Richter S, Yamauchi J, Minor T, Menger MD, Vollmar B. Heparin and phentolamine combined, rather than heparin alone, improves hepatic microvascular procurement in a non-heart-beating donor rat-model. Transpl Int. 2000;13(3):225–9.
6. Felker GM, Milano CA, Yager JE, Hernandez AF, Blue L, Higginbotham MB, et al. Outcomes with an alternate list strategy for heart transplantation. J Heart Lung Transplant. 2005;24(11):1781–6.
7. van der Kaaij NP, Kluin J, Lachmann RA, den Bakker MA, Lambrecht BN, Lachmann B, et al. Alveolar preservation with high inflation pressure and intermediate oxygen concentration reduces ischemia-reperfusion injury of the lung. J Heart Lung Transplant. 2012;31(5):531–7.
8. Pichlmayr R, Ringe B, Gubernatis G, Hauss J, Bunzendahl H. Transplantation of a donor liver to 2 recipients (splitting transplantation)—a new method in the further development of segmental liver transplantation. Langenbecks Arch Chir. 1988;373(2):127–30.
9. Busuttil RW, Goss JA. Split liver transplantation. Ann Surg. 1999;229(3):313–21.
10. Kilic M, Seu P, Stribling RJ, Ghalib R, Goss JA. In situ splitting of the cadaveric liver for two adult recipients. Transplantation. 2001;72(11):1853–8.
11. Urata K, Kawasaki S, Matsunami H, Hashikura Y, Ikegami T, Ishizone S, et al. Calculation of child and adult standard liver volume for liver transplantation. Hepatology. 1995;21(5):1317–21.
12. Strasberg SM, Lowell JA, Howard TK. Reducing the shortage of donor livers: what would it take to reliably split livers for transplantation into two adult recipients? Liver Transpl Surg. 1999;5(5):437–50.
13. Colledan M, Andorno E, Valente U, Gridelli B. A new splitting technique for liver grafts. Lancet. 1999;353(9166):1763.
14. Gundlach M, Broering D, Topp S, Sterneck M, Rogiers X. Split-cava technique: liver splitting for two adult recipients. Liver Transpl. 2000;6(6):703–6.
15. Rela M, Vougas V, Muiesan P, Vilca-Melendez H, Smyrniotis V, Gibbs P, et al. Split liver transplantation: King's College Hospital experience. Ann Surg. 1998;227(2):282–8.
16. Brüggenwirth IMA, Martins PN. RNA interference therapeutics in organ transplantation: the dawn of a new era. Am J Transplant. 2020;20(4):931–41.
17. Reich DJ, et al. ASTS recommended practice guidelines for controlled donation after cardiac death organ procurement and transplantation. Am J Transplant. 2009;9:2004–11.
18. Zhang S, Yuan J, Li W, Ye Q. Organ transplantation from donors (cadaveric or living) with a history of malignancy: review of the literature. Transplant Rev (Orlando). 2014;28:169–75.
19. Tang Y, et al. Donor indocyanine green clearance test predicts graft quality and early graft prognosis after liver transplantation. Dig Dis Sci. 2017;62:3212–20.
20. Hoffman A, Burger C, Persky L. Extracorporeal renal storage. Invest Urol. 1965;2:567–73.
21. Carrel A, Lindbergh CA. The culture of whole organs. Science. 1935;81(2112):621–3.
22. van der Vliet JA, Vroemen JP, Cohen B, Lansbergen Q, Kootstra G. Preservation of cadaveric kidneys. Cold storage or machine perfusion? Arch Surg. 1983;118(10):1166–8.
23. Muhlbacher F, Langer F, Mittermayer C. Preservation solutions for transplantation. Transplant Proc. 1999;31(5):2069–70.
24. Olschewski P, Hunold G, Eipel C, et al. Improved microcirculation by low-viscosity histidine-tryptophan-ketoglutarate graft flush and subsequent cold storage in University of Wisconsin solution: results of an orthotopic rat liver transplantation model. Transpl Int. 2008;21(12):1175–80.
25. Bachmann S, Bechstein WO, Keck H, et al. Pilot study: Carolina rinse solution improves graft function after orthotopic liver transplantation in humans. Transplant Proc. 1997;29(1–2):390–2.

26. Moers C, Smits JM, Maathuis MH, et al. Machine perfusion or cold storage in deceased-donor kidney transplantation. N Engl J Med. 2009;360(1):7–19.
27. Wight JP, Chilcott JB, Holmes MW, Brewer N. Pulsatile machine perfusion vs. cold storage of kidneys for transplantation: a rapid and systematic review. Clin Transpl. 2003;17(4):293–307.
28. Balupuri S, Buckley P, Snowden C, et al. The trouble with kidneys derived from the non heart-beating donor: a single center 10-year experience. Transplantation. 2000;69(5):842–6.
29. Moers C, Pirenne J, Paul A, Ploeg RJ. Machine preservation trial study G. Machine perfusion or cold storage in deceased-donor kidney transplantation. N Engl J Med. 2012;366(8):770–1.
30. Sandal S, Luo X, Massie AB, Paraskevas S, Cantarovich M, Segev DL. Machine perfusion and long-term kidney transplant recipient outcomes across allograft risk strata. Nephrol Dial Transplant. 2018;33(7):1251–9.
31. Jochmans I, Moers C, Smits JM, et al. Machine perfusion versus cold storage for the preservation of kidneys donated after cardiac death: a multicenter, randomized, controlled trial. Ann Surg. 2010;252(5):756–64.
32. Watson CJ, Wells AC, Roberts RJ, et al. Cold machine perfusion versus static cold storage of kidneys donated after cardiac death: a UK multicenter randomized controlled trial. Am J Transplant. 2010;10(9):1991–9.
33. Chen GD, Shiu-Chung Ko D, Wang CX, et al. Kidney transplantation from donors after cardiac death: an initial report of 71 cases from China. Am J Transplant. 2013;13(5):1323–6.
34. Summers DM, Johnson RJ, Hudson A, Collett D, Watson CJ, Bradley JA. Effect of donor age and cold storage time on outcome in recipients of kidneys donated after circulatory death in the UK: a cohort study. Lancet. 2013;381(9868):727–34.
35. Kayler LK, Magliocca J, Zendejas I, Srinivas TR, Schold JD. Impact of cold ischemia time on graft survival among ECD transplant recipients: a paired kidney analysis. Am J Transplant. 2011;11(12):2647–56.
36. Sung RS, Guidinger MK, Christensen LL, et al. Development and current status of ECD kidney transplantation. Clin Transpl. 2005:37–55.
37. Koetting M, Frotscher C, Minor T. Hypothermic reconditioning after cold storage improves post-ischemic graft function in isolated porcine kidneys. Transpl Int. 2010;23(5):538–42.
38. McAnulty JF. Hypothermic organ preservation by static storage methods: current status and a view to the future. Cryobiology. 2010;60(3 Suppl):S13–9.
39. Hosgood SA, Thompson E, Moore T, Wilson CH, Nicholson ML. Normothermic machine perfusion for the assessment and transplantation of declined human kidneys from donation after circulatory death donors. Br J Surg. 2018;105(4):388–94.
40. Hosgood SA, Saeb-Parsy K, Hamed MO, Nicholson ML. Successful transplantation of human kidneys deemed Untransplantable but resuscitated by ex vivo normothermic machine perfusion. Am J Transplant. 2016;16(11):3282–5.
41. Bagul A, Hosgood SA, Kaushik M, Kay MD, Waller HL, Nicholson ML. Experimental renal preservation by normothermic resuscitation perfusion with autologous blood. Br J Surg. 2008;95(1):111–8.
42. Nicholson ML, Hosgood SA. Renal transplantation after ex vivo normothermic perfusion: the first clinical study. Am J Transplant. 2013;13(5):1246–52.
43. de Rougemont O, Breitenstein S, Leskosek B, et al. One hour hypothermic oxygenated perfusion (HOPE) protects nonviable liver allografts donated after cardiac death. Ann Surg. 2009;250(5):674–83.
44. Gringeri E, Bonsignore P, Bassi D, et al. Subnormothermic machine perfusion for non-heart-beating donor liver grafts preservation in a Swine model: a new strategy to increase the donor pool? Transplant Proc. 2012;44(7):2026–8.
45. Xu H, Berendsen T, Kim K, et al. Excorporeal normothermic machine perfusion resuscitates pig DCD livers with extended warm ischemia. J Surg Res. 2012;173(2):e83–8.
46. Schon MR, Kollmar O, Wolf S, et al. Liver transplantation after organ preservation with normothermic extracorporeal perfusion. Ann Surg. 2001;233(1):114–23.
47. Butler AJ, Rees MA, Wight DG, et al. Successful extracorporeal porcine liver perfusion for 72 hr. Transplantation. 2002;73(8):1212–8.
48. Olschewski P, Gass P, Ariyakhagorn V, et al. The influence of storage temperature during machine perfusion on preservation quality of marginal donor livers. Cryobiology. 2010;60(3):337–43.
49. Changani KK, Fuller BJ, Bryant DJ, et al. Non-invasive assessment of ATP regeneration potential of the preserved donor liver. A 31P MRS study in pig liver. J Hepatol. 1997;26(2):336–42.
50. Schlegel A, Muller X, Kalisvaart M, et al. Outcomes of DCD liver transplantation using organs treated by hypothermic oxygenated perfusion before implantation. J Hepatol. 2019;70(1):50–7.
51. Guarrera JV, Henry SD, Samstein B, et al. Hypothermic machine preservation in human liver transplantation: the first clinical series. Am J Transplant. 2010;10(2):372–81.
52. Henry SD, Nachber E, Tulipan J, et al. Hypothermic machine preservation reduces molecular markers of ischemia/reperfusion injury in human liver transplantation. Am J Transplant. 2012;12(9):2477–86.
53. op den Dries S, Karimian N, Sutton ME, et al. Ex vivo normothermic machine perfusion and viability testing of discarded human donor livers. Am J Transplant. 2013;13(5):1327–35.
54. Lu S, Yu Y, Gao Y, Li GQ, Wang XH. Immunological inhibition of transplanted liver allografts by adeno-associated virus vector encoding CTLA4Ig in rats. Hepatobiliary Pancreat Dis Int. 2008;7(3):258–63.
55. Pascher A, Sauer IM, Hammer C, Gerlach JC, Neuhaus P. Extracorporeal liver perfusion as hepatic

assist in acute liver failure: a review of world experience. Xenotransplantation. 2002;9(5):309–24.
56. Gerlach JC. Bioreactors for extracorporeal liver support. Cell Transplant. 2006;15(Suppl 1):S91–103.
57. McCurry K, Jeevanandam V, Mihaljevic T, et al. 294: prospective multi-center safety and effectiveness evaluation of the organ care system device for cardiac use (PROCEED). J Heart Lung Transplant. 2008;27(2 Suppl):S166.
58. Tenderich G, El-Banayosy A, Rosengard B, et al. 10: prospective multi-center European trial to evaluate the safety and performance of the Organ Care System for heart transplants (PROTECT). J Heart Lung Transplant. 2007;26(2 Suppl):S64.
59. Warnecke G, Van Raemdonck D, Smith MA, et al. Normothermic ex-vivo preservation with the portable organ care system lung device for bilateral lung transplantation (INSPIRE): a randomised, open-label, non-inferiority, phase 3 study. Lancet Respir Med. 2018;6(5):357–67.
60. Loor G, Warnecke G, Villavicencio MA, et al. Portable normothermic ex-vivo lung perfusion, ventilation, and functional assessment with the Organ Care System on donor lung use for transplantation from extended-criteria donors (EXPAND): a single-arm, pivotal trial. Lancet Respir Med. 2019;7(11):975–84.
61. Babkin BP, Starling EH. A method for the study of the perfused pancreas. J Physiol. 1926;61(2):245–7.
62. Taylor MJ, Baicu S, Leman B, Greene E, Vazquez A, Brassil J. Twenty-four hour hypothermic machine perfusion preservation of porcine pancreas facilitates processing for islet isolation. Transplant Proc. 2008;40(2):480–2.
63. Taylor MJ, Baicu SC. Current state of hypothermic machine perfusion preservation of organs: the clinical perspective. Cryobiology. 2010;60(3 Suppl):S20–35.
64. Leeser DB, Bingaman AW, Poliakova L, et al. Pulsatile pump perfusion of pancreata before human islet cell isolation. Transplant Proc. 2004;36(4):1050–1.
65. Idezuki Y, Goetz FC, Kaufman SE, Lillehei RC. In vitro insulin productivity of preserved pancreas: a simple test to assess the viability of pancreatic allografts. Surgery. 1968;64(5):940–7.
66. Eckhauser F, Knol JA, Porter-Fink V, et al. Ex vivo normothermic hemoperfusion of the canine pancreas: applications and limitations of a modified experimental preparation. J Surg Res. 1981;31(1):22–37.
67. Kowalewski K, Kolodej A. Secretory function of isolated canine pancreas perfused with fluorocarbon emulsion. Surg Gynecol Obstet. 1978;146(3):375–8.

Liver Transplantation from Cardiac Death Donors

5

Ming Han

Abstract

DCD donor is a valuable organ source for liver transplantation, which is helpful to reduce the mortality of patients with end-stage liver disease and increase the availability of organ transplantation. The future development prospect of DCD liver transplantation is good [1]. With the continuous improvement of surgical skills and relevant clinical assistant techniques for DCD liver transplantation, its clinical effects have been continuously improved, but generally speaking, it is still not as good as donation after brain death (DBD) liver transplantation. The survival rate of patients after DCD liver transplantation at 1 and 3 years was lower than that of DBD liver transplantation, and the incidence of postoperative complications was higher than that of DBD liver transplantation. DCD graft is prone to postoperative complications such as ischemic bile duct stricture, primary graft nonfunction, hepatic artery, and portal vein thrombosis [2, 3].

M. Han (✉)
Organ Transplant Center, The First Affiliated Hospital of Sun Yat-sen University, Guangzhou, China

5.1 Indications and Timing of Liver Transplantation

5.1.1 Acute Liver Failure (ALF)

ALF has a sudden onset, severe illness, rapid progression, and high mortality. It is generally believed that ALF patients who have failed medical treatment or whose condition are still progressing after medical treatment should be included in the liver transplantation waiting list after exclusion of contraindications and given priority in donor liver allocation. These include primary explosive hepatic failure, primary graft nonfunction, graft arterial embolization, and acute decompensated Wilson's disease.

5.1.2 Chronic Cirrhosis

They include viral cirrhosis, alcoholic cirrhosis, primary biliary cirrhosis, primary sclerosing cholangitis, cryptogenic cirrhosis, secondary biliary cirrhosis, Budd–Chiari syndrome, etc. Cirrhosis is a benign disease with a good prognosis. In the decompensated stage, progressive jaundice, hepatic encephalopathy, intractable ascites, and coagulation mechanism disorders were the main manifestations, and the timing of surgery could be determined according to MELD

X. He (ed.), *Organ Donation and Transplantation after Cardiac Death in China*,
https://doi.org/10.1007/978-981-16-0815-5_5

score and Child–Pugh classification, so as to avoid the occurrence of serious complications affecting the surgical effect.

5.1.3 Malignant Liver Disease

Including primary hepatocellular carcinoma, bile duct cell carcinoma, children hepatoblastoma, and so on. In the face of tumor recurrence and low graft survival rate after liver transplantation for malignant tumor recipients, it is necessary to choose carefully. Reference to Milan standard, UCSF standard, and Hangzhou standard can effectively improve the survival rate of transplant recipients and determine the prognosis of recipients.

5.1.4 Congenital Metabolic Disease of the Liver

These include Wilson's disease, glycogen accumulation disease, hemochromatosis, -antitrypsin deficiency, hypertyrosinemia, polycystic liver disease, etc. If congenital metabolic disease progresses slowly and active medical treatment fails to improve the symptoms such as liver decompensation or abdominal distension, liver transplantation may be considered.

5.2 Preoperative Evaluation and Preparation of the Recipient

Comprehensive evaluation and preparation of patients are important for successful operation. Preoperative evaluation included indications and timing of surgery, tolerability and contraband of surgery, compatibility between donors and recipients, and psychosocial and ethical issues of patients and their families. Treatment during liver transplantation involves improving the function of the liver and other organs to sustain life and improve surgical tolerance, as well as the treatment of primary diseases to improve surgical efficacy.

5.2.1 Preoperative Evaluation

5.2.1.1 Surgical Indications and Timing Evaluation

The first step is to determine whether the patient must be treated with a liver transplant. At present, a variety of scoring criteria are used to determine the liver reserve function of patients, mainly including CTP grade, prognostic model of end-stage liver disease (MELD), model of pediatric end-stage liver disease (PELD), etc. The above model can be used to determine the natural course of liver disease and the expected survival time after transplantation. In addition, patients older than 70 years, who were obese, and those with a history of upper abdominal surgery, especially those with a history of portal shunt or portal devascularization, were significantly more at risk.

5.2.1.2 Evaluation of Surgical Tolerance and Contraindications

Cardiac Function

Intraoperative bleeding or clamping/opening of the inferior vena cava may result in reduced or rapidly increased preload, and hepatic reperfusion syndrome can also severely inhibit myocardial function, so adequate cardiac reserve is required. A history of smoking, high blood lipids, and risk factors associated with coronary heart disease, such as diabetes and hypertension, and various arrhythmias increase the risk of heart accidents. It is recommended to perfect the cardiac color Doppler ultrasonography for an accurate evaluation of cardiac function.

Respiratory System

In patients with chronic liver disease, hypoxemia due to abnormal ventilation, namely hepatopulmonary syndrome (HPS), has a poor prognosis after conservative treatment, and some HPS can be reversed by transplantation. Liver transplantation is not suitable for patients with severe progressive primary pulmonary disease and pulmonary dysfunction that cannot be cured, or with definite pulmonary infection.

Renal Function

Liver transplantation should be performed as soon as possible in patients with type I hepatorenal syndrome, and combined liver and kidney transplantation should be performed in patients with primary kidney disease. The timing of combined liver and kidney transplantation has not been determined yet. Some scholars have reported that combined liver and kidney transplantation is more effective than simple liver transplantation or staging liver and kidney transplantation for patients with serum creatinine >2 mg/dL.

Infectious Diseases

All tuberculin-positive patients (except those with BCG), with or without active TB, required anti-TB treatment postoperatively. Suppurative infection is contraindicated in liver transplantation and fungal infection should be treated thoroughly before operation. Human immunodeficiency virus infection is a relative contraindication for surgery.

Coagulation Function

In patients with cirrhosis, coagulation factor I and fibrinogen synthesis are reduced, and fibrinolysis is enhanced. At the same time, it is often associated with hypersplenism, thrombocytopenia, and dysfunction, resulting in abnormal coagulation function, which should be carefully evaluated and corrected before liver transplantation. In principle, preoperative prothrombin time activity (PTA) should be corrected to more than 30% or other measures should be taken.

Nutritional Status

About 80% of patients with end-stage liver disease have malnutrition and muscle wasting and were prone to have ventilator dependence and infectious complications after surgery. The perioperative risk was significantly higher than that of patients without malnutrition. Therefore, nutritional status should be evaluated before liver transplantation and appropriate supportive treatment should be given.

Evaluation of Primary Disease

Antiviral therapy is required for hepatitis B and C. Excessive hepatitis B virus (HBV) DNA load is an important cause of hepatitis B recurrence after surgery, which should be reduced to less than 10 copies/mL before surgery. At present, the treatment effect of hepatitis C is good, and taking medicine within half a year can turn negative. Autoimmune hepatitis suggests that postoperative anti-rejection drugs may need to be added. Patients with alcoholic cirrhosis must abstain from alcohol for at least 3–6 months before liver transplantation is considered. Fulminant liver failure is rarely self-healing, so liver transplantation should be performed as soon as possible. Retransplantation is suitable for some patients with primary graft nonfunction, acute hepatic artery embolization, severe rejection, or recurrent liver disease.

5.2.1.3 Surgical Feasibility and Imaging Assessment

Reevaluation of Primary Disease in Recipients

All candidates for liver transplantation need to be reevaluated for primary disease before transplantation. Especially for patients with liver cancer, comprehensive treatment may be required before and during the operation, so it is more necessary to carry out preoperative evaluation again to make sure whether the diagnosis of liver cancer is correct and whether there is tumor invasion of blood vessels and distant metastasis during the waiting period. The presence of extrahepatic metastasis and invasion of portal vein or inferior vena cava are contraindications for liver transplantation.

Imaging Assessment of Recipients

The vascular conditions of the recipient have an important impact on liver transplantation, and any lesion of the liver vessels will increase the difficulty of the operation. Therefore, imaging assessment is significant. For example, thrombosis of hepatic vein and inferior vena cava in patients with Budd–Chiari syndrome, portal vein thrombosis, cancer thromboembolism and spongy changes in patients with liver cirrhosis and liver cancer, metal stents may be left in portal vein and inferior vena cava after TIPS, which will affect the vascular reconstruction during liver transplantation and easily cause intraoperative massive hemorrhage and insufficient blood supply of transplanted liver.

Patients with liver disease often have liver atrophy and enlarged spleen, which may cause abdominal closure difficulty or abdominal compartment syndrome, and the spleen should be removed if necessary.

5.2.1.4 Recipient Compatibility Assessment

General Evaluation

Liver size is proportional to height, and the relationship between fat and thin is uncertain. The donor liver should be matched to the recipient, which may cause large liver syndrome (especially in children) and may also cause abdominal hypertension. Attention should also be paid to the donor liver vessel variation and whether it can match with the recipient. Liver texture should also be evaluated, and liver with malignant tumor should not be used as a donor. Livers with steatosis are prone to primary nonfunction after liver transplantation, so livers with steatosis exceeding 30% are not suitable for liver transplantation in principle.

Evaluation of Immune Compatibility

Liver is a relatively immune-exempted organ, which does not require strict HLA matching. The recipient's blood type can be supplied as long as it conforms to the principle of blood transfusion.

Virological Assessment

Serum HbsAg-positive donor liver is generally recommended for hepatitis B patients only. It is controversial whether the liver of patients with hepatitis C can be used as a donor for liver transplantation, such as the liver is of good quality and function, so that it can be used as a recipient for hepatitis C or advanced cancer.

5.2.1.5 Treatment of Liver Transplantation Recipients During Waiting Period

In the process of waiting for donor liver, maintaining liver function, treating various complications, and improving patients' surgical tolerance are important contents of waiting period treatment.

Treatment of Bleeding from Gastric Fundus and Esophageal Varices

Varicose vein hemorrhage is one of the most serious complications caused by portal hypertension in patients with end-stage liver disease. Endoscopically sclerosing agent injection or ligation therapy is feasible for patients with tolerability. Patients who are about to undergo liver transplantation can be temporarily treated with tri-lumen compression combined with drug therapy, such as pituitrin and somatostatin.

Correct Abdominal and Circulatory Disorders

Patients with end-stage liver disease are characterized by high low resistance and portal hypertension. Colloid solution can be used to dilate, prostagtin and other drugs can be used to improve the blood flow of the glomerular artery, abdominal puncture to release ascites in severe abdominal distension, or long-term catheter drainage. At the same time, it can improve the oxygen supply of local tissues, remove inflammatory mediators from blood and maintain the stability of the internal environment.

Protect Renal Function

Maintain effective circulation capacity is the most important. Appropriate use of diuretics, and avoid using nephrotoxic drugs. If preoperative renal function is impaired, continuous hemofiltration (CVVH) is feasible if necessary.

Prevention and Treatment of Hepatic Encephalopathy

Hepatic encephalopathy is a common complication of cirrhosis, which can be induced by bacterial peritonitis, gastrointestinal bleeding, massive diuresis and puncture ascites, electrolyte disturbance, etc. Treatment includes removal of triggers, laxative enema, reduction of protein content in food, intravenous acid medication, and adequate energy support. If hepatic encephalopathy is in stage III or IV, emergency liver transplantation should be performed.

Improve Coagulation Function

Vitamin K may be given to patients with mild clotting abnormalities. Fresh frozen plasma or prothrombin complexes and fibrinogen should be supplemented when PTA is less than 40%. Plasmapheresis in the treatment of coagulation disorders can significantly improve INR, increase fibrinogen levels, and reduce bilirubin. For patients with decreased platelets, if the count is less than 30 × 10^9/L, which should be supplemented. In the case of liver transplantation, the platelet count should be increased to more than 50 × 10^9/L before implantation.

5.2.1.6 Treatment of Patients with Liver Malignant Tumor Waiting for Liver Transplantation

Patients with liver cancer may be treated with tumor resection, TACE or local liver cancer therapy (such as radiofrequency or microwave therapy) to delay tumor progression and prolong the waiting time for liver transplantation.

Recently, with the increasing development of new targeted drugs, targeted therapy before liver transplantation has played a good role in delaying tumor growth and reducing the level of tumor markers. At the same time, targeted therapy after liver transplantation after tumor gene detection can effectively delay tumor recurrence and prolong patients' and grafts' survival time.

5.2.1.7 Antiviral Therapy Before Liver Transplantation

HBV-related liver diseases account for the majority of liver transplantation in China. If no preventive measures are taken, the HBV reinfection rate after liver transplantation can be as high as 80%. In recent years, the postoperative reinfection rate has been significantly reduced due to the prophylactic application of hepatitis B immunoglobulin (HBIG) and perioperative nucleotide analog. Entecavir and tenofovir, as novel nucleocapsid analogs, had strong inhibitory effects on HBV DNA replication.

With the development of anti-Hepatitis C drugs, currently, more than 90% of patients with hepatitis C virus (HCV) related end-stage liver diseases can turn from hepatitis C to negative after taking medicine for 3–6 months, and the recurrence rate of hepatitis C after liver transplantation has been significantly reduced.

5.2.1.8 Preparation Before Liver Transplantation

First of all, patients should be prepared psychologically and financially. The physician should evaluate the patient thoroughly, understand the surgical approach of the previous liver transplant, control all site infections including biliary tract infection, and eliminate fungal colonization as much as possible. Virus replication should be suppressed in patients with recurrent hepatitis. The dosage of immunosuppressant should be reduced from 2 weeks before surgery and could be completely discontinued from 5 to 7 days before surgery.

5.2.2 Donor Evaluation and Selection

5.2.2.1 Hot Ischemia Time

It is generally believed that after removal of the life support system, the time to confirm cardiac death is too long, such as 30 min for the liver and 60 min for the kidney, then these organs are no longer suitable for transplantation. It is currently believed that when systolic blood pressure <50 mmHg, there will be a hot ischemic injury to the organ. Once systolic blood pressure is <50 mmHg (or hemoglobin oxygen saturation <70%) for at least 2 min, a "functional hot ischemia time" is considered to have begun.

5.2.2.2 Donor Selection

Donor Screening

Strict donor characteristics include: age <50; Liver function is basically normal; Body mass <100 kg; ICU stay time <5 days; Hot ischemia time <20 min; Cold ischemia time <8 h, no steatosis or bullae steatosis liver volume ratio <15%; No high dose booster drug support; Hepatitis B or C virus serologically negative; No active infection.

Current single-center studies and large registry analyses have confirmed that older donors are at higher risk of recipient complications such as ischemic cholangiopathy, transplant failure, and death [4]. In the case of long-term donor ischemia, the donor body mass >100 kg, or body mass index (BMI) >30 kg/m, is also a high risk factor for increased transplant failure and death rate. The hemodynamic instability of the donor during extubation is also a risk factor for a poor prognosis [5]. The irreversible damage to the biliary tract caused by hypotension and/or hypoxia during extubation is still being investigated. Prolonged functional hot ischemia also increases the risk of ischemic cholangiopathy and graft failure in the recipient. Prolonged cold ischemia increases the recipient's risk of biliary complications, including ischemic cholangiopathy, graft failure, and death. The exact critical time of cold ischemia was 6–8 h.

DCD achieved the same transplant success rate as DBD donor liver using strict donor criteria, including BMI <29 kg/m, functional hot ischemia time <20 min (systolic blood pressure <50 mmHg), and time from donor cardiac arrest to start perfusion <10 min.

Marginal Donor Liver

In the case of the current shortage of donor organs, "marginal donor" can be used as a source of donor livers. Its features include: age 50 to 65 years old, BMI > 30 kg/m, hepatitis virus serological positive, high doses of blood pressure drug support, the split graft, serum sodium >155 mmol/L, serum creatinine >106 μmol/L, ICU stay time >5 days, warm ischemia time 20–30 min, cold ischemia time 8–15 h, steatosis degeneration of liver volume and big bubble ratio is 15–60%. Especially under the condition of long functional hot and cold ischemia time >12 h, the graft quality was poor [6–8].

Because DCD donors are in intensive care, their risk of potential infection is greater than that of living organ donation. Blood culture, cerebrospinal fluid culture, urine culture, sputum culture, and other cavity and humoral cultures that may be infected are recommended before donation.

Contraindication of DCD Donor Liver

In addition to absolute contraindications for general organ donation (i.e., invasive or hematologic malignancy, untreated systemic infection, prion infection, and human immunodeficiency virus infection), DCD donors also had absolute contraindications for: (1) end-stage liver disease (chronic liver disease, cirrhosis, and portal hypertension); (2) Acute liver failure (drugs, viruses, etc.); (3) severe steatosis (bullae steatosis liver volume proportion > 60%); (4) Acute liver injury that cannot be improved [7–10].

5.2.3 Liver Lavage, Preservation, and Repair

Effective perfusion of hepatic microvessels is crucial to the preservation of DCD donor liver. At present, there is no consensus on the perfusion selection of DCD donors, and it is generally believed that low-viscosity preservation solutions (such as HTK solution and Marshall solution) are more effective for liver preservation than high-viscosity solutions (such as UW solution). Systemic heparinization must be administered before donor liver is obtained to prevent the formation of microthrombus in the liver.

At the same time of liver preservation with conventional UW solution, mechanical perfusion preservation has attracted more and more attention recently. It tries to simulate liver perfusion under physiological conditions to reduce liver damage caused during preservation. Many experimental studies have proved that mechanical perfusion preservation has better preservation effect for marginal donor liver, especially for DCD donor liver. Due to the potential organ repair ability of normal temperature mechanical perfusion, it is currently favored by the transplantation community. Tolboom et al. proved through rat experiments that DCD donor liver can be effectively repaired after simple cryopreservation and then subjected to normal temperature mechanical perfusion preservation, thus improving the prognosis of the recipients [11]. The team of Professor XSH has successfully tried and implemented the normal temperature mechanical perfusion of the liver without ischemia transplantation and had achieved a good clinical efficacy [12]. However, there are still many difficulties to be solved in normal temperature mechanical perfusions, such as the choice of perfusion fluid, and higher requirements for the perfusion device.

Extracorporeal membrane oxygenation (ECMO) for cardiac death donor liver can effectively reduce heat ischemia injury, and its effectiveness has been reported in many institutions. In 1997, Johnson et al. in the United States first reported a case of DCD liver donor with 29 days of ECMO support. The recipient recovered and was discharged 3 weeks after the operation [13]. Subsequently, many studies reported the marginal donor liver application of ECMO, most of which obtained good results.

5.3 Liver Transplantation

Liver transplantation is one of the largest and most technically difficult operations in abdominal surgery. At present, with the improvement and perfection of surgical techniques such as anesthesiology and vascular anastomosis, liver transplantation has been carried out as a routine operation in many transplant centers in the world. Liver transplantation has become the only effective treatment to save the life of patients with acute liver failure, prolong the survival time of patients with end-stage liver disease, and improve their quality of life. Liver transplantation is divided into the following categories according to different surgical methods.

5.3.1 Classic Orthotopic Whole Liver Transplantation

Standard Orthotopic Liver Transplantation (OLT) was the first Orthotopic Liver Transplantation performed in the world by Professor Starzl, the "father of Liver Transplantation" in the United States in 1963.

5.3.1.1 Resection of Diseased Liver

Liver transplantation recipients often have severe cirrhosis and/or portal hypertension, hypersplenism, as well as systemic metabolic disorders and other basic diseases, so patients may be associated with abnormal liver function, coagulation mechanism disorders, electrolyte, and other unstable internal environment factors. In addition, some recipients may have other surgical histories before surgery (including cholecystectomy, splenectomy, portal-cavity shunt, etc.), and often have extensive intraperitoneal tissue adhesion. These are the main risk factors for uncontrolled bleeding during hepatectomy. Therefore, the risk of major bleeding should be fully assessed and prepared before surgery.

Specific steps: The patient shall be placed in the supine position, and the skin shall be disinfected from the neck to the upper 1/3 of the thigh. The right incision should extend to the midaxillary line and the left incision to the outer edge of rectus abdominis. A suspended abdominal cavity retractor is installed to fully expose the surgical field of vision. Careful investigation of abdominal organs, for severe portal hypertension, multiple surgical history, thrombocytopenia, abnormal coagulation function, should be appropriately supplemented with prothrombin complex, human fibrinogen and platelets, etc., to correct the coagulation function. Patients with malignant liver tumors should be carefully examined for extrahepatic metastasis and vascular cancer thrombus.

Free the liver from the superior and inferior vena cava, break the round ligaments, and sew the broken ends on both sides. The sickle ligament was cut off with the electric knife until it was close to the superior and inferior vena cava of the liver. The left coronal ligament and the left deltoid ligament were broken off. The venous branches at the junction of the left deltoid ligament and the tip of the left outer lobe should be properly ligated. The left outer lobe was turned to the right to expose the hepatogastric ligament, and the right deltoid ligament, the right coronal ligament, the ligaments of liver and colon and liver and kidney were further broken. Pull down and turn the liver left and right, expose the left and right diaphragmatic veins respectively. Fully expose the superior and inferior vena cava. The anterior fascia of the superior and inferior vena cava was carefully separated, the posterior wall was gradually obtuse, and the preset blocking band was used for reserve. The hepatoduodenal ligament was pulled to the left to expose the posterior subhepatic inferior vena cava, which was carefully separated on the upper plane of the renal vein and then the preblocking band was placed for use. At this point, the prepositioning of the superior, inferior hepatic vena cava and the first hepatic hilar occlusions has been completed.

Dissection of hepatoduodenal ligament by dissociating the first hepatic hilum and confirming the common bile duct. The exposed common bile duct is separated from the hepatic hilum to avoid damaging the distal blood supply. If there is no history of hilar surgery, the bile duct can be separated at the confluence of left and right hepatic ducts. The hepatic artery was identified in the left side of the common bile duct, and dissected retrograde until the common hepatic artery divided into the right hepatic artery and the distal gastroduodenal artery. To dissect the hepatic hilum to the left and right hepatic artery bifurcation, as close as possible to the hepatic hilum ligation of the hepatic artery. Finally, the portal vein should be separated, and the hepatic artery should be retracted to the left. The portal vein should be exposed and carefully separated. Portal vein should be kept to 3–5 cm, and ready to be cut off near the hepatic portal during resection of the diseased liver.

The diseased liver was resected and the portal vein and the subhepatic inferior vena cava were placed as close to the liver as possible and cut off with vascular blocking forceps. At least 1.5 cm free length was reserved for each vessel for vascular anastomosis. At this point, the recipient enters the liver-free stage. Stay away from the vascular forceps to cut off the superior and inferior vena cava. Treatment of hepatic bed after removal of diseased liver is the best time to thoroughly treat hepatic bed bleeding. The right deltoid ligament was sutured, the left deltoid ligament and the sickle ligament were sutured, and the inferior vena cava exfoliated surface was sutured. After the wound hemostasis, the superior and inferior vena cava of the liver were repaired for liver implantation. The septum between the left hepatic vein, the right hepatic vein, and the middle hepatic vein should be cut to form a large opening.

5.3.1.2 Anastomosis of Hepatic Superior and Inferior Vena Cava

After the donor liver was obtained and trimmed in vitro, the donor liver was placed in situ in the recipient liver bed, and the posterior wall of the superior and inferior vena cava was anastomosed first. First, both sides of the blood vessels were fixed with 4-0 Prolene line to fully expose the posterior wall of the blood vessels. During the anastomosis, attention should be paid to the following: the blood vessels between the donor and the recipient should not be reversed; otherwise, poor blood flow and high pressure of the inferior vena cava will be easily caused. During the anastomosis, the suture line should not be stretched too tight to avoid damaging the intima of the blood vessel.

5.3.1.3 Subhepatic Inferior Vena Cava Anastomosis

Finally, anastomosis of subhepatic inferior vena cava was performed. The anastomosis method and procedure were the same as that of the superior and inferior vena cava. Care should be taken to avoid injury to the right renal artery when the posterior wall is sutured. The length of inferior vena cava should not be too long, so as not to distort.

5.3.1.4 Portal Vein Anastomosis

In adults, 5-0 noninvasive suture is generally used for fixed traction, and inferior vena cava anastomosis is adopted. The posterior wall of the portal vein is sutured first, and then the anterior wall is anastomosed, and a continuous valvular suture is adopted. In children portal vein anastomosis, 7-0 noninvasive sutures can be used for intermittent suture. Note that the suture should not be pulled too tight to prevent anastomotic stenosis. Flush the portal vein with heparin saline before suturing the last two stitches in the anterior wall. The length of the donor and recipient portal vein should not be too long, so as not to distort the portal vein thrombosis.

5.3.1.5 Restore Blood Supply of Transplanted Liver

After the completion of the recipient portal vein anastomosis, the portal vein forceps can be opened to free the blood supply of the transplanted liver, and the liver-free period will be ended. At this time, the suprahepatic and inferior vena cava blocking forceps are not loosened temporarily. The preservation fluid with high potassium in the transplanted liver and blood containing a large amount of acid metabolites in the body are released through the inferior vena cava of the donor liver (250 mL), and then the inferior vena cava is blocked again with vascular blocking forceps.

5.3.1.6 Hepatic Artery Anastomosis

Hepatic artery reconstruction is the most critical step in the process of vascular reconstruction, which directly affects the function of the transplanted liver. Since there is a high possibility of variation in the hepatic artery, the surgeon must perform angioplasty according to the specific variation to obtain a larger arterial vessel for anastomosis as far as possible. Hepatic artery anastomosis was usually performed with 7-0 or 8-0 noninvasive vascular suture line and continuous or intermittent suture was performed.

After the completion of hepatic artery anastomosis, the recipient hepatic artery occlusion forceps were opened to restore all the blood supply of the transplanted liver. Under normal circumstances, the graft liver color gradually ruddy, tissue tension is normal, bile duct began to have golden bile outflow.

5.3.1.7 Reconstruction of Bile Duct

There are two ways to reconstruct the bile duct: end-to-end anastomosis of the common bile duct of donor and recipient and roux-en-Y anastomosis of bile duct with jejunum.

End-to-end anastomosis of the common bile duct is the most commonly used method of bile duct reconstruction in liver transplantation. After the resection of the donor liver and gallbladder, the common bile duct should be cut off at the proximal end of the gallbladder tube. The proper length of the common bile duct should be preserved, and the bile duct must be kept tenseless during the anastomosis. 6-0 or 7-0 absorbable suture (or PDS) was used for continuous suture (or continuous suture of the back wall and intermittent suture of the front wall), and the suture should be mucosa to mucosa. T tubes are usually not placed.

Bile duct with jejunum Roux-en-Y anastomosis is commonly used in the following situations: excessive tension during the anastomosis of the common bile duct, and the common bile duct of the recipient is too thin; Poor blood supply to distal common bile duct; Recipient choledochal lesions such as sclerosing cholangitis; The lateral veins around the common bile duct are abnormally rich. Before the anastomosis, T tube can be placed in the common bile duct, and it can be extracted from the jejunum 10 cm away from the choledochostomy, so as to facilitate the observation of bile characteristics and drainage volume after the operation. In the case of choledochojejunostomy, the jejunum is generally cut at 20–30 cm from the Treitz ligament, and an end-to-side anastomosis is performed by the common bile duct and the roux-en-Y intestinal loop at the distal end of the jejunostomy.

5.3.1.8 Place the Drainage Tube

Making sure that there was no active bleeding in the abdominal cavity. Three drainage tubes were placed under the right diaphragm near the right inferior vena cava, under the liver portal, and under the left liver. Close abdomen layer by layer. After operation, drainage volume and characteristics were closely observed and treated in time.

5.3.2 Piggyback Orthotopic Liver Transplantation

Piggyback Liver Transplantation is also known as in situ liver transplantation with prior inferior vena cava. It was first reported by Tzakis in 1989 that after continuous improvement of inferior vena cava anastomosis, the occurrence of hepatic venous reflux disorder was greatly reduced and orthotopic liver transplantation has become the mainstream operation in many large centers. The whole length of the recipient inferior vena cava and the hepatic vein was preserved, and the hepatic vein was anastomosed with the superior and inferior vena cava of the donor liver. The ligation or closure of the posterior inferior vena cava end of the donor liver and the reconstruction of other canals are the same as standard liver transplantation. Piggyback liver transplantation is limited by the technique of liver resection. When the recipient disease has caudate lobe hypertrophy (especially in some patients with Bader–Giari syndrome), the inferior vena cava is surrounded and it is extremely difficult to retain the inferior vena cava, and it is easy to cause massive bleeding due to reluctant retention. In addition, due to incomplete liver resection of the disease, it is not suitable for some liver malignant tumors, such as liver malignant tumors that have invaded the inferior vena cava, or close to the second and third hepatic hilum, cannot be separated from the inferior vena cava, and the tail has wrapped part of the inferior vena cava and cannot be separated.

5.3.3 Reduced Volume Liver Transplantation

Reduced-size Liver Transplantation (RLT) can be established by comparison of liver volume between donor and recipient when their body weight is significantly different. Such problems often arise when the donor liver of a normal size adult is provided to a child or to some smaller adult receptors. In this case, if total liver transplantation is still performed, the donor liver will be larger than the recipient needs. In space, it is unable to close the abdomen or abdominal difficulty; Functionally, the compression of the recipient into the hepatic vessel or inferior vena cava resulted in the obstruction of blood flow into the liver and the obstruction of vena cava reflux, leading to the insufficiency of donor liver perfusion, abnormal systemic circulation, and other problems, which will further result in the quality of the recipient's surgery decreased or even death.

Bismuth, a prominent French liver transplant scientist, first performed a volume-based liver transplant in a child with congenital biliary atresia in the 1980s. Later, global transplant centers are gradually carried out the operation, the commonly used with vessel pedicle of left liver (II–IV section) and left lobe (II–III section) and right half liver (V–VII section).

5.3.4 Split Liver Transplantation (SLT)

The way of one liver and one recipient cannot alleviate the global problem of donor Liver shortage. SLT is of great significance to alleviate the shortage of donor liver and shorten the waiting time of recipients under the condition of limited donor liver.

This method was first developed by Pichmayr of The University of Hanover in Germany in 1988 and has been gradually transplanted to various major universities around the world. As the name implies, a split liver transplant involves dividing one donor liver into two or more parts. There are two common ways to split the liver: one is to divide a donor liver from a normal-sized adult into the left outer lobe and the right three lobes; the left donor liver is transplanted to a child or newborn recipient, and the right donor liver is transplanted to a normal-sized adult recipient. Second, the donor liver of a normal size adult was divided into the left and right halves, the left was transplanted to a small size adult or child recipient, and the right was transplanted to a normal size adult recipient. As much as possible in order to avoid any receptor graft is too small, cause small liver transplantation syndrome (small for size syndrome, SFSS). You also need to determine to transplant to the recipient for the weight ratio of liver weight and the receptor (graft to recipient weight the wire, GRWR) is generally thought that the ratio of at least needs more than 1% is the acceptable safety limits.

In addition, it is necessary to ensure that each part of the donor liver has an independent and complete portal vein, hepatic artery, hepatic vein, and bile duct system. Preoperative for donor CT three-dimensional reconstruction and biliary imaging is very important, which will make sure the parts after the split graft of the division of vascular and bile duct, and we can find some rare vascular and bile duct variation, and to make a plan and adjust in time.

Cardiac death donors can only perform the external split. Attention should be paid to the distribution of hepatic artery, portal vein, hepatic vein, and bile duct during splitting.

5.4 Postoperative Management of Liver Transplantation

Posttransplant management includes intensive care after liver transplantation and routine management after return to the general ward. ICU treatment after liver transplantation is one of the key links in reducing postoperative mortality. Multidisciplinary and collaborative postoperative care can provide better clinical treatment and prognosis for transplant recipients. With the development of technology in the field of transplantation, postoperative treatment of liver transplantation has become more systematic and standardized.

5.4.1 ICU Treatment After Liver Transplantation

For patients with smooth recovery after transplantation, the length of stay in ICU was 24–48 h. The main objectives of intensive care treatment after liver transplantation are: (1) To maintain vital signs and stable internal environment; (2) To evaluate the patient's overall status and graft function, and to predict possible risk factors; (3) Monitoring and prevention of complications after liver transplantation.

5.4.1.1 Immediate Treatment After ICU Admission

After the patient is transferred to the intensive care unit, the following steps should be completed simultaneously or sequently, and the postoperative condition of the patient should be first evaluated as soon as possible: (1) Connect all monitoring leads to monitor vital signs; (2) Check the position and patency of endotracheal intubation and connect with mechanical ventilation; (3) Connect the liquid pathway, check and adjust the infusion speed of liquid and vasoactive drugs; and (4) Check the position of the marked drainage tube and fix it properly, and accurately record the amount of liquid and the characteristics of drainage fluid. Collect blood, urine, and other laboratory specimens; Bedside chest - abdominal X-ray and/or abdominal Doppler ultrasound should be performed when necessary.

5.4.1.2 Evaluation and Monitoring of Organ Function

The main purpose of the initial evaluation of patients after admission to ICU is to establish and maintain stable hemodynamics, oxygenation, and internal environment. A comprehensive assessment of the patient's general condition should then be conducted to assess organ function and to predict the risk of complications. (1) Monitoring of cardiovascular function; (2) Respiratory support and respiratory function monitoring; (3) Renal function and electrolyte balance monitoring; and (4) Monitoring of nervous system function.

5.4.1.3 Early Evaluation of Graft Function

The surgeons may evaluate the graft function from the description of the perfusion and biliary secretion in the graft liver. At the same time, detection of liver function and coagulation function, nerve and spirit change of patients, circulation stability, bile secretion quantity, renal function and so on which are all helpful to understand and judge the function of transplanted liver.

Typical graft PNF includes graft reperfusion edema, uneven color, poor quality of bile, disturbance of consciousness, low temperature, cycle is not stable, oliguria, low blood sugar, high potassium, lactic acidosis, stubborn, metabolic acidosis, blood coagulation function deterioration, etc., this is the most serious liver function is abnormal, need to retransplant.

Therefore, although the time from the diagnosis of PNF to the decision of retransplantation can vary from 24 h to 10 days, there is no dispute that the selection of retransplantation before the occurrence of multiple organ failure can improve the efficacy of retransplantation.

5.4.1.4 Prevention of Complications in ICU

Coagulation Function

The pathophysiological process of abnormal coagulation function in liver transplantation recipients is complicated, and intraoperative and postoperative hemorrhage is often occurred in some recipients due to a variety of factors such as lack of coagulation factor, abnormal platelet quantity and quality, increased endogenous anticoagulant substance, and hyperfibrinolysis. Other patients showed a tendency of hypercoagulability due to a large amount of procoagulant supplementation, improvement or splenectomy of hypersplenism, recovery of transplanted liver function, and lack of antithrombin III leading to heparin resistance, etc.

Prevention points:

1. In case of postoperative hemorrhage and suspected coagulation abnormality, dynamic coagulation test method is recommended to replace the traditional static coagulation test.
2. Even if the early postoperative coagulation function is still poor, if there is no obvious clinical bleeding tendency, the coagulation substance can be temporarily not supplemented.
3. High coagulation tendency, should promptly remove the etiology. Heparin anticoagulant therapy is helpful to prevent vascular complications and other thrombotic diseases of the transplanted liver.
4. Monitor infection and clinical medication. In addition to the influence of liver function and spleen function, infection and drug-induced bone marrow suppression are the most common causes of early coagulation abnormalities after transplantation.

Respiratory System

The delay of extubation after liver transplantation and pulmonary infection are the main reasons for prolonged ICU stay and the influence of perioperative survival rate.

Prevention Points

1. When mechanical ventilation is applied, auxiliary ventilation mode should be selected as far as possible to preserve the patient's spontaneous breathing.
2. Monitor and remove the influencing factors affecting offline extubation. Pleural effusion is not the main cause of extubation.
3. Intermittent noninvasive ventilation support is helpful to extubate patients with sleep apnea and chronic obstructive pulmonary disease (COPD) as soon as possible.
4. Patients with delayed wet-off extubation need strict respiratory care and monitor the microbiological changes of respiratory secretions.

Circulation System

Early systemic circulation resistance after liver transplantation is low, and vasoactive drugs are sometimes needed to maintain blood pressure. Thereafter, a sustained increase in central venous pressure (CVP) may occur. Electrolyte disturbances, vasoactive agents, myocardial ischemia, and cardiac dysfunction may all trigger arrhythmias.

Prevention Points

1. According to the fluid balance in the early postoperative period, appropriately limit the fluid intake and apply diuretics to control CVP <10 mmHg. CRRT is used when necessary.
2. Anti-arrhythmia therapy should first emphasize the elimination of incentives and should try to maintain its sinus rhythm. It is safe and effective for synchronous direct current cardiology with hemodynamic instability.

3. Postoperative hypertension is the result of multiple factors. High blood pressure is a controllable factor leading to cerebrovascular events in liver transplant recipients. On the basis of organ perfusion, it is recommended to gradually control the blood pressure level below 140/80 mmHg.

Renal Function

The risk factors for early postoperative acute renal failure (ARF) in liver transplant recipients were approximately the same as in non-transplant recipients.

Prevention Points

1. Maintain stable circulation and mean arterial pressure (MAP) >65 mmHg.
2. Follow the principle of combined immunosuppressive drugs. At the same time, avoid the combination of other nephrotoxic drugs.
3. Monitoring and control of systemic infections.
4. Large dose of diuretics is not recommended for patients with oliguria. CVVH or hemodialysis should be performed for severe electrolyte acid–base balance disorder and significant hyperazoemia. Gastrointestinal function common gastrointestinal symptoms include gastro-intestinal bleeding, gastric retention, abdominal distension, and diarrhea.

Gastroenteric Function

Common gastrointestinal symptoms include gastrointestinal bleeding, gastric retention, abdominal distension, and diarrhea.

Prevention Points

1. The principles of diagnosis and treatment of upper gastrointestinal bleeding are similar to those of non-transplant patients.
2. Monitor the blood concentration of immunosuppressant drugs.
3. The preoperative nutritional status was good, but parenteral nutrition was not needed in the early postoperative period. Early recovery of enteral nutrition.
4. Long-term use of broad-spectrum antibiotics should be avoided to cause intestinal flora disorder.

Neuropsychiatric System

Early neuropsychiatric complications of liver transplantation recipients may be clinically manifested as varying degrees of consciousness impairment, peripheral nerve dysfunction, mental disorders, epilepsy, etc.

Prevention Points

1. Maintain stable circulation and normal cerebral perfusion pressure. Avoid overdose of sedatives and prolonged hyperventilation.
2. Correct metabolic abnormalities such as hypoxia, hypoglycemia, electrolyte, and acid–base balance disorder.
3. Reducing the frequency of medical intervention in ICU and ensuring sufficient sleep are the basic measures to prevent and treat mental symptoms.
4. CsA and FK506 should be administered orally as far as possible, and blood drug concentration should be monitored, and blood magnesium and serum cholesterol levels should be maintained.
5. Any new neurologic signs and mental or psychiatric abnormalities are indicative of head CT or MRI examination.

5.4.2 Routine Management After Liver Transplantation

After liver transplantation, patients returned to the general ward from ICU and their condition was relatively stable, and their liver function indexes gradually improved. However, the status of transplanted liver should be closely monitored, various complications should be prevented, and the concentration of immunosuppressive agents should be adjusted so that the patient can be discharged from hospital successfully.

5.4.2.1 Monitoring of Transplanted Liver Function

Clinical Observation

Patients were transferred from the ICU to the general ward and the abdominal drainage tube or T tube was retained. The amount of discharge and the color character of bile should be recorded every day. When acute rejection occurs, there is a lightening, thinning, and reduction in the amount of bile.

Laboratory Inspection

1. Detection of liver function
2. Blood routine and coagulation indexes
3. Monitoring of blood drug concentration

Imaging Examination

1. Ultrasound

   Some complications may occur after liver transplantation, such as thrombosis or stenosis of hepatic artery, portal vein, hepatic vein and inferior vena cava, stenosis or biliary leakage of anastomotic stoma of biliary tract, etc. And various secondary changes caused by these lesions, such as hepatic parenchymal ischemia necrosis, peritoneal effusion, and biliary tumor, etc. Imaging examination plays an important role in the diagnosis of these complications.
2. CT examination

   In cases where the presence of vascular complications is suspected by ultrasound examination, enhanced CT examination may be performed.

Liver Biopsy

The gold standard for distinguishing acute rejection from preserved injury is liver biopsy. If there is no improvement or deterioration in biochemical indicators of liver function after liver transplantation, a biopsy should be performed.

5.4.2.2 Postoperative Drug Therapy

Selection of Immunosuppressive Regimen

The types of rejection after liver transplantation usually include hyperacute rejection, acute rejection, and chronic rejection. Liver is an immune-exempted organ, and the chance of hyperacute rejection is extremely low, but retransplantation is the only effective treatment once it occurs. Acute rejection is the most common type after liver transplantation and usually occurs 1–2 weeks after transplantation. The clinical manifestation lacks specificity, some patients may not have any symptoms, the common manifestation with the pain, jaundice, the fever, the abdominal distension uncomfortable, and so on. Liver biopsy is the most valuable method for the diagnosis of acute rejection. Histologically, inflammatory cells infiltrate the biliary epithelium, portal vein, and hepatic venous endothelium.

Routine perioperative immunosuppressive regimens are based on calcineurin inhibitor (CNI) combined with two or three immunosuppressive regimens of corticosteroids and mycophenol esters. Patients with advanced malignancy may be switched to Sirolimus 1 month or more after surgery.

Use of Anti-infective Drugs

Patients who recover well after liver transplantation can stop using prophylactic antibiotics 5–7 days after the operation. For those who still have infection, targeted treatment can be continued based on bacterial culture.

Fungal prophylaxis: Intestinal candida migration, surgical mucosal barrier destruction, and the use of broad-spectrum antibiotics after transplantation are important factors for invasive fungal infection.

Prevention and treatment of cytomegalovirus (CMV) infection focuses on prevention.

Others: patients with hepatitis B cirrhosis should receive anti-hepatitis B treatment after surgery. In China, entecavir or tenofovir combined with low-dose human hepatitis B immunoglobulin is the most commonly used prevention program.

5.5 Management of Postoperative Complications After Liver Transplantation

Postoperative complications of liver transplantation mainly include postoperative infection, bleeding, rejection, bile duct complications, and vascular complications, which will not only negatively affect the survival rate of patients but also affect the normal quality of life of patients. Most literatures have reported that the main factors affecting the long-term prognosis of DCD liver transplantation are postoperative primary graft nonfunction, hepatic artery thrombosis, early cholestasis, high incidence of ischemic bile duct stricture and rejection, especially high incidence of biliary complications, such as an ischemic biliary stricture [14–18].

5.5.1 Primary Liver Nonfunction (PNF) and Early Liver Insufficiency (EAD)

Among the concerns about complications after DCD liver transplantation, the first discovery was that the incidence of PNF and EAD in the transplanted liver increased significantly. Existing studies have shown that the incidence of PNF and EAD is similar to that of hepatic artery thrombosis.

5.5.1.1 Risk Factors of PNF and EAD

Studies have shown that ischemia-reperfusion injury, liver fat degeneration, advanced age of the donor, prolonged cold ischemia time, immune infection factors of the recipient, and decreased platelet level after liver transplantation are associated with poor recovery after liver transplantation [19–21].

5.5.1.2 Prevention and Treatment of PNF and EAD

1. Strictly control the cold and warm ischemia time of the donor to reduce the ischemia-reperfusion injury
2. Grasp the indications of the use of fatty liver donors, especially the donor liver with fatty >30%, and perform liver biopsy when necessary
3. Elderly donor liver has poor tolerance to cold and warm ischemic injury, and liver function can be evaluated in detail by imaging methods before acquisition
4. To select the appropriate recipient for marginal donor liver and attach importance to the individualized recipient immunosuppression program.

5.5.2 Infection After Liver Transplantation

The incidence of infection after liver transplantation is 30–70%, and the sites of infection are common in biliary tract, respiratory tract, urinary tract, various puncture sites and drainage sites, blood, abdominal cavity and so on. The pathogens were mainly bacteria, followed by fungal and viral infections.

5.5.2.1 Risk Factors for Infection

Risk factors for infection after liver transplantation mainly involve three aspects: donor, transplantation environment, and recipient.

Donor factors: major trauma, surgery, long stay in intensive care unit, ventilator use, and various invasive procedures increased the risk of donor infection before donation. Studies have shown that donor fatty liver, cold ischemia time, and total bilirubin are independent risk factors for infection after liver transplantation.

Factors of transplant tings: Pathogenic bacteria in the environment or carried by other patients can be transmitted to transplant recipients by medical staff, medical devices, public goods or air, causing serious infection.

Receptor factors: Receptor factors mainly include preoperative, intraoperative, and postoperative factors.

5.5.2.2 Specific Measures for Postoperative Infection Management Include

1. DCD donors should timely collect body fluid specimens and submit them for examination. Broad-spectrum antibiotics should be administered early in donors with existing or suspected infection. According to the results of the donor etiology examination, the recipient's anti-infection plan will be guided.
2. Attach importance to physical measures such as strengthening lung care and keeping abdominal drainage unobstructed.
3. To improve surgical techniques, shorten operation time and blood loss as much as possible, and shorten the duration of cold, ischemia-free donor period.

4. Closely monitor and strictly control blood sugar to avoid an increased risk of infection due to high blood sugar.
5. To improve the evaluation of various immune status and to reduce the use of immuno- suppressive drugs as long as the rejection reaction can be controlled.
6. Attention should be paid to the detection of procalcitonin (PCT), CRP, G, and GM test M.

5.5.3 Postoperative Abdominal Hemorrhage

Liver transplantation is complicated and traumatic, and postoperative abdominal bleeds are not rare, which is often one of the main causes of early death after liver transplantation. Postoperative celiac hemorrhage occurred within 3 weeks, most frequently within 24 h [22, 23].

5.5.3.1 The Causes of Abdominal Hemorrhage Mainly Include Two Aspects

Coagulation disorders: In the early postoperative period, the function of the new transplanted liver has not been completely recovered, leading to the synthesis of coagulation factors. At the same time, early postoperative thrombocytopenia and other factors affect the state of blood coagulation, which can lead to wound oozing or small blood vessel bleeding. Surgical factors: mainly after the operation of the ligation of small vessels incomplete, vascular anastomotic bleeding and electrocoagulation eschar off caused by bleeding.

5.5.3.2 The Treatment of Abdominal Hemorrhage After Liver Transplantation Should Focus on Prevention

Once the diagnosis of abdominal hemorrhage after liver transplantation is confirmed, regular nonsurgical treatment should be given immediately. If the bleeding is still uncontrollable or worsens, surgical exploration and hemostasis should be performed as soon as possible.

5.5.4 Bile Duct Complications After Liver Transplantation

The incidence of bile duct complications after liver transplantation is as high as 10–30%. More and more scholars have reported a consensus that biliary complications after DCD liver transplantation are the most common and fatal complications [24]. In addition to bile leakage, anastomotic stenosis, bile duct stones, ischemic bile duct stricture, and other ischemic bile duct diseases are still urgent complications requiring close attention at present.

5.5.4.1 Pathogenesis of Biliary Disease

Although the pathological mechanism of ischemic biliary stricture remains to be studied, the patency of hepatic artery, ischemia-reperfusion injury, cytomegalovirus infection, chronic rejection, ABO incompatibility, and other factors are considered to be important causes of biliary stricture. In addition, changes in bile composition caused by the increased time of warm ischemia are also thought to be another important mechanism for bile duct stricture. Therefore, the increased ratio of bile salts/phospholipids after reperfusion suggests the possibility of biliary system injury. Therefore, any operation to prolong the time of warm ischemia will cause injury to DCD transplant recipients.

5.5.4.2 Diagnosis of Biliary Complications

The clinical manifestations of biliary complications vary widely, ranging from absence of clinical symptoms or mild liver dysfunction to fatal cholangitis or septic shock. Doppler ultrasonography and magnetic resonance cholangiopancreatography (MRCP) can quickly and noninvasively diagnose and differentiate the bile duct complications.

5.5.4.3 Prevention and Treatment of Bile Duct Complications

It should be first focused on prevention, and standardize the acquisition of high-quality donor liver and minimize the duration of warm and cold ischemia time. During the operation, the blood supply of the bile duct should be protected to the maximum extent when the donor liver is removed, and the anastomosis of the hepatic artery should be emphasized. Bile duct anastomotic stricture is the most common reason, so nonsurgical treatment should be considered first. Most patients with early anastomotic stricture can obtain satisfactory curative effects by ERCP or PTCD drainage. For complex biliary tract diseases such as diffuse biliary stricture or graft biliary tree damage secondary to hepatic artery thrombosis, retransplantation should be performed [25–27].

5.5.5 Rejection After Liver Transplantation

5.5.5.1 Types of Rejection

Hyperacute rejection: Postoperative rejection of liver transplantation can be divided into hyperacute phase, acute phase, and chronic phase, among which acute phase is the most common. Hyperacute rejection occurs several hours to several days after liver transplantation, when the recipient has specific antibodies against the donor antigen, which is mainly manifested as bleeding and necrosis of the transplanted liver, resulting in immediate graft loss and extremely dangerous prognosis. Liver is a special organ for human immunity, and superacute rejection is very rare.

Acute rejection: As the most important and common rejection reaction in liver transplantation, it usually occurs after the recovery of liver function after transplantation. It is an immune response mediated by killer cells produced in the recipient body. Acute rejection usually occurs within 30 days postoperatively, and generally occurs within 5–15 days. The clinical manifestations were nonspecific, including fever, drowsiness, liver transplantation swelling and pain, leukocytosis, and other changes. Routine liver function tests may show abnormal elevation of serum transaminase and bilirubin. But only tube biopsy can provide clear evidence of rejection.

Chronic rejection: Recurrent episodes of acute rejection usually occur in the weeks, months, or even years after transplantation. It is an immune response mediated by both cells and body fluids. Patients usually have no obvious symptoms in the early stage, only AKP, γ-GGT continuously elevated, and gradually develop jaundice. The pathology presented progressive vascular structural damage. In the late stage of the disease, the bile duct in the transplanted liver disappears, also known as "bile duct disappearance syndrome." At this time, a second liver transplantation is generally required [28–30].

5.5.5.2 Treatment of Rejection After Liver Transplantation

Acute rejection: Principles of treatment. The diagnosis of acute rejection should be defined first, with pathological diagnosis as the gold standard. The effective blood concentration of immunosuppressive agents should be maintained. Methylprednisolone is the standard regimen for the treatment of acute rejection. Shock therapy, namely 500–1000 mg intravenous drip, decreases day by day after continuous 3 days.

Chronic rejection: Chronic rejection has a complex mechanism and is not sensitive to immunosuppressive therapy. Secondary transplantation is the best treatment.

5.5.6 Vascular Complications After Liver Transplantation

5.5.6.1 Arterial Complications

Arterial complications are the most common vascular complications after liver transplantation, including hepatic artery thrombosis, hepatic artery stenosis, and aneurysms.

Hepatic artery thrombosis: Hepatic artery thrombosis is the most serious vascular complication after liver transplantation, with an incidence of 3–5% and a fatality rate of 20–60%. DCD donors had a significantly higher incidence than DBD donors. The clinical features of early hepatic artery thrombosis include acute hepatic necrosis, delayed biliary fistula, and interstitial bacteremia. Advanced hepatic artery thrombosis is rarely reported in the literature and is characterized by fever, jaundice, bile duct and/or intrahepatic abscess, and biliary leakage (due to bile duct ischemia and necrosis). It is now recognized that its occurrence is associated with arterial thrombosis during hot ischemia, which leads to decreased blood flow in the liver, vascular endothelial injury, and further increases the chance of thrombosis. The risk of hepatic artery thrombosis can be reduced if heparin is administered immediately before discontinuation of donor support therapy [31–33].

Doppler ultrasonography is the preferred diagnostic method for hepatic artery thrombosis. Angiography is still the gold standard for the diagnosis of hepatic artery thrombosis. If hepatic artery thrombosis is found, active treatment should be given as soon as possible, interventional thrombolysis or emergency laparotomy, thrombectomy and reconstruction of hepatic artery should be performed.

Hepatic artery stenosis: The main related factors were the anastomosis conditions and techniques, liver extraction or transplantation injuries, postoperative rejection, etc. Angiography should be performed in patients with suspected hepatic artery stenosis. Once the diagnosis is made, correct treatment should be performed according to the degree of arterial stenosis and influence on the transplanted liver, and interventional therapy or reoperation of vascular reconstruction should be performed when necessary.

Aneurysms and pseudoaneurysms: Hepatic artery aneurysms and pseudoaneurysms are very rare complications after liver transplantation, but the fatality rate is high, about more than 50%. As soon as it is found clinically, it needs to be treated in advance. Open surgery and vascular interventional therapy can be used.

5.5.6.2 Venous Complications

Venous complications after liver transplantation are less common than arterial complications, and are more common in hepatic vein, portal vein system, and inferior vena cava, including Portal vein thrombosis (PVT), portal vein stenosis (PVS), hepatic vein, inferior vena cava stenosis or occlusion.

Portal vein complications: Mainly including portal vein thrombosis and portal vein stenosis. For the treatment of portal vein thrombosis, if extensive collateral circulation of portal vein has been established after liver transplantation, or portal vein stenosis is mild, without accompanying clinical symptoms, and liver function is not obvious abnormal, close observation can be made. Without special treatment, some patients can achieve long-term survival. Interventional therapy can be considered for portal vein complications in the late postoperative period, but retransplantation is required for patients with graft loss and other conditions.

Inferior vena cava complications: The incidence of inferior vena cava complications is extremely low, mainly including inferior vena cava thrombosis and inferior vena cava stenosis. Percutaneous angioplasty and stent placement are the preferred methods for the treatment of inferior vena cava stenosis.

References

1. Meurisse N, Vanden Bussche S, Jochmans I, et al. Outcomes of liver transplantations using donations after circulatory death: a single center experience. Transplant Proc. 2012;44(9):2868–73.
2. Le Dinh H, Roover A, Kaba A, et al. Donation after cardiocirculatory death liver transplantation. World J Gastroenterol. 2012;18(33):4491–506.
3. Bradley JA, Pettigrew GJ, Watson CJ. Time to death after withdrawal of treatment in donation after death (DCD) donors. Curr Opin Organ Transplant. 2013;18(2):133–9.
4. Denecke C, Yuan X, Ge X, et al. Synergistic effects of, warmischemia, and donor age on the immune response following donation after cardiac death kidney transplantation. Surgery. 2013;153(2):249–61.
5. Mathur AK, Heimbach J, Steffick DE, et al. Donation after cardiac death livertors of outcome. Am J Transplant. 2010;10(11):2512–9.
6. Jay C, Ladner D, Wang E, et al. A comprehensive risk assessment of mortality following donation after cardiac death liver transplant-an analysis of the National Registry. J Hepatol. 2011;55(4):808–13.
7. Dubbeld J, Hoekstra H, Farid W, et al. Similar liver transplantation survival with selected death donors and brain death donors. Br J Surg. 2010;97(5):744–53.
8. Fujita S, Mizuno S, Fujikawa T, et al. Liver transplantation from donation after cardiac death: a single center experience. Transplantation. 2007;84(1):46–9.
9. de Vera ME, Lopez-Solis R, Dvorchik I, et al. Liver transplantation using donation after cardiac death donors: long term follow up from a single center. Am J Transplant. 2009;9(4):773–81.

10. Foley DP, Fernandez LA, Leverson G, et al. Donation after cardiac death: the University of Wisconsin experience with liver transplantation. Ann Surg. 2005;242(5):724–31.
11. Tolboom H, Milwid JM, Izamis ML, et al. Sequential storage and normothermic pick of the rat liver. Transplant Proc. 2008;40(5):1306–9.
12. He X, Guo Z, Zhao Q, et al. The first case of free organ transplantation in humans: a proof of concept. Am J Transplant 2017.
13. Johnson LB, Plotkin JS, Howell CD, et al. Successful emergency transplantation of a liver allograft from a donor; maintain on extracorporeal membrane oxygenation. Transplantation. 1997;63(6):910–1.
14. Foley DP, Fernandez LA, Leverson G, et al. Biliary complications after liver transplantation from donation after cardiac death donors: an analysis of risk factors and long term outcomes from asingle center. Ann Surg. 2011;253(4):817–25.
15. Taner CB, Bulatao IG, Willingham DL, et al. The events in procurement as risk factors for ischemic cholangiopathy in liver transplantation using donation after cardiac death donors. Liver Transpl. 2012;18(1):100–11.
16. Skaro AI, Jay CL, Baker TB, et al. The impact of complicate medicine in liver transplantation using donors after Cardiacdeath: the complicate story. Surgery. 2009;146(4):543–53.
17. Mateo R, Cho Y, Singh G, et al. Risk factors for graft survival after liver donors: an analysis of OPTN/UNOS data. Am J Transplant. 2006;6(4):791–6.
18. Lee KW, Simpkins CE, Montgomery RA, et al. Economic organ survival after liver transplantation from donation after death organ. Transplantation. 2006;82(12):1683–8.
19. Chan EY, Olson LC, Kisthard JA, et al. One thing that sells blood to the donor is a blood donor death organ. Liver Transpl. 2008;14(5):604–10.
20. Hong JC, Yersiz H, Kositamongkol P, et al. Liver transplantation using outraged donation after cardiac death: a clinical predictiveindex for graft failure free survival. Arch Surg. 2011;146(9):1017–23.
21. Muiesan P, Girlanda R, Jassem W, et al. Single center experience with liver transplantation from controlled non heartbeating donors: a viable source of grafts. Ann Surg. 2005;242(5):732–8.
22. Ho KJ, Owens CD, Johnson SR, et al. Donor postextubation hypotension and age correlate with outcome after donation after cardiac death transplantation. Transplantation. 2008;85(11):1588–94.
23. Monbaliu D, Pirenne J, Talbot D. Liver transplantation using donation after death donors. J Hepatol. 2012;56(2):474–85.
24. Pirenne J, Van Gelder F, Coosemans W, et al. Type of donor aortic preservation solution and not cold time is a major determinant of biliary strictures after liver transplantation. Liver Transpl. 2001;7(6):540–5.
25. Dubbeld J, Hoekstra H, Farid W, et al. Similar liver transplantation survival with selected death donors and brain death donors. Br J Surg. 2010;97(5):744–53.
26. Foley DP, Fernandez LA, Leverson G, et al. Donation after cardiac death: the University of Wisconsin experience with liver transplantation. Ann Surg. 2005;242(5):724–31.
27. Grewal HP, Willingham DL, Nguyen J, et al. Liver transplantation using controlled donation after cardiac death organ: an analysis of a large single center experience. Liver Transpl. 2009;15(9):1028–35.
28. Pine JK, Aldouri A, Young AL, et al. Liver transplantation following donation after cardiac death: an analysis using matched pairs. Liver Transpl. 2009;15(9):1072–82.
29. De Vera ME, Lopez-Solis R, Dvorchik I, et al. Liver transplantation using donation after cardiac death donors: long-term follow-up from a single center. Am J Transplant. 2009;9(4):773–81.
30. Nguyen JH, Bonatti H, Dickson RC, et al. Long-term out comes of donation after death liver allografts from a single center. Clin Transpl. 2009;23(2):168–73.
31. Broom Head RH, Patel S, Fernando B, et al. Resource implications of the use of donation after circulatory determination of death in liver transplantation. Liver Transpl. 2012;18(7):771–8.
32. Mascia L, Mastromauro I, Viberti S, et al. Management to optimize organs procurement in brain dead donors. Minerva Anestesiol. 2009;75(3):125–33.
33. Rostrona AJ, Avlonitisa VS, Kirbya JA, et al. The hemodynamic commentary of the brain-dead organ donor and the potential role of vasopressin. Transplant Rev. 2007;21:34–42.

Kidney Transplantation from Cardiac Death Donors

6

Guodong Chen and Qihao Li

Abstract

Donation after cardiac death (DCD) kidney transplantation developed rapidly in recent years, because of the shortage of deceased donors. DCD donation process should be performed according to the guidelines of different countries. DCD kidneys are associated with higher risk of primary non-function (PNF) and delayed graft function (DGF) compared to donation after brain death (DBD) kidneys; however, long-term patient and graft survival, as well as graft function were all comparable between DCD and DCD kidneys. Donor age, body mass index (BMI), hypertension, diabetes, high donor creatinine, cause of death, and cold ischemia time may affect the outcome of a DCD kidney transplant. Hypothermic machine perfusion (HMP) and normothermic machine perfusion (NMP) may reduce the PNF and DGF rate after transplant. Carefully selection of the DCD donor kidneys, pre-transplantation (zero time) biopsy, carefully management of fluid and monitor of immunosuppressive drugs, such as using ATG and low dose calcineurin inhibitor (CNI) may reduce DGF and improve the long-term outcome of DCD kidney transplantation.

G. Chen (✉) · Q. Li
Organ Transplant Center, The First Affiliated Hospital of Sun Yat-sen University, Guangzhou, China

Kidney transplantation is the best treatment for patients with end-stage kidney diseases (ESRD). However, due to the shortage of donors, many patients died while waiting for suitable donors. In 2017, about 136,000 kidney transplants were performed worldwide, but according to WHO estimates, this activity is sufficiency only to meet 10% of transplant need. The average waiting time for a deceased donor kidney transplant in the UK is over 3 years. Owing to ill health, 12% of listed patients die or are removed from the waiting list within 3 years of listing [1]. In China, it is estimated that the ratio of donors and patients on the waiting list is about 1:30 [2]. Therefore, how to increase the deceased donors source for saving the lives of patients on the waiting list is a major problem worldwide.

Traditionally, the deceased donors were divided into donation after brain death (DBD) donors and donation after cardiac death (DCD) donors. The majority of kidney transplant recipients receive their kidney from brain dead (DBD) donors, but in recent years there has been a marked increase in the number of transplants using kidneys from donation after cardiac death (DCD) donors. In the UK, DCD donor numbers increased sixfold within ten years from 84 cases in 2004 to 527 cases in 2013 [1]. DCD donors has become a major way to expand the deceased donor pool over the last decade.

However, DCD kidney transplantation is associated with a higher risk of primary non-function

X. He (ed.), *Organ Donation and Transplantation after Cardiac Death in China*,
https://doi.org/10.1007/978-981-16-0815-5_6

(PNF) and delayed graft function (DGF), although the higher incidence of DGF after DCD kidney transplantation is not associated with the poorer graft survival as in DBD grafts [3, 4]. Meanwhile, the methods to improve the quality of DCD kidneys keep developing over the past decades, including hypothermic machine perfusion (HMP), premortem cannulation, normothermic machine perfusion (NMP) [5].

6.1 Current Situation and Trends of Kidney Transplantation from Cardiac Death Donors

In recent years, DCD kidney transplantation has developed rapidly worldwide. In Europe, especially the UK, the Netherlands, and Belgium have very successful DCD donor programs with 7.0–9.5 DCD donors per million population (pmp) in 2013. The USA, Australia, and Croatia also have well-developed DCD programs with 2.1–3.8 DCD donors per million population. DCD kidneys accounted for 11% of all kidney transplants in the USA and make up 30–50% of all deceased donors in some European countries. From 2006 to 2017, the proportion of DCD donors increased dramatically in both the UK and the USA (Fig. 6.1) [6]. However, there is still huge potential for expanding DCD donor pool. In Europe, there are approximately 350,000 cases of cardiopulmonary resuscitation a year. Only 40% of such cases are successfully resuscitated. However, for the remaining 60% that do not recover, these deaths become a potential for DCD donors. In a study in the USA between 2013 and 2016, it was estimated that there were 9828 potential DCD donors per year in the USA. If only 15% of the potential DCD donors could donate their kidneys, that would increase about 3000 cases of DCD kidney transplantation [7]. In China, DCD donor programs have begun in 2005 and developed rapidly in the last decade. In 2010, there were only 0.17 DCD donors per million population in DCD donor programs, while in 2019, the number increased to about 0.8 DCD donors per million population. Although there is still a huge gap in the DCD donor program between China and the Western countries, there is large potential for further increasing the DCD donation rate in China in the future.

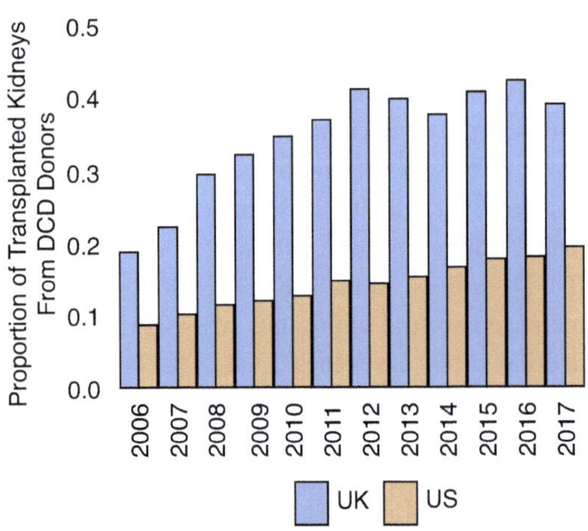

Fig. 6.1 Proportion of transplant kidneys from DCD donors, US vs UK (2006–2017)

6.2 Classification of Donation After Cardiac Death

DCD donors are divided into four categories according to Maastricht classification of DCD donors [8]. Category I is defined as dead on arrival. Patients are from out-of-hospital accidents who are not resuscitated. Category II is defined as unsuccessful resuscitation. Patient is brought to the emergency room while being resuscitated by the emergency medical services (EMS), and is declared dead after cardiopulmonary resuscitation (CPR) is unsuccessful. Category III is defined as awaiting cardiac or circulatory death. Patient occurs circulatory death after a planned withdrawal of life-sustaining therapies (WLST). Category IV is defined as cardiac arrest in a brain dead donor. Patients suffer an unexpected cardiac arrest after diagnosis of brain death and during donor management but prior to the organ retrieval. Category I and II are defined as uncontrolled DCD donors, while category III to IV are defined as controlled DCD donors. The majority of DCD donors in Belgium, The Netherlands, the UK, and the USA are category

III, whereas category II donors predominate in France and Spain. In China, there is a special category for DCD donors. China Category III. Organ donation after brain death is followed by circulatory death. Donor in this category has been diagnosed of brain death and organ procurement is conducted when cardiac arrest appears after a planned withdrawal of life-sustaining therapies because the relatives of the donor do not accept brain dead [9].

6.3 Donation Process of Cardiac Death Donors

Donation process of DCD donors includes withdrawal of life support from donors and harvesting the kidneys. Withdrawal of life-supporting treatment typically involves discontinuation of inotropes and ventilatory support. In China, a period of 5 minutes of observation is required after cardiac arrest before death can be confirmed and organ retrieval can be begun [9]. The time period deemed necessary from cessation of circulation to the start of organ procurement varies from 2 to 20 min internationally [10, 11].

Currently, the acceptable criteria for DCD donors in most of Chinese hospitals were as follows: (I) age <60; (II) warm ischemia time <25 min; (III) agonal time from withdrawal of mechanical, ventilated, or organ-perfusion support treatment to cardiac arrest <4 h and (IV) no history of systemic sepsis, diabetes mellitus, malignancy, or renal diseases [9].

Procurement of the kidneys from DCD donors in China is undertaken similar to that used in most other countries. Rapid laparotomy and arterial cannulation is performed, the abdominal organs are perfused with cold organ preservation solution such as UW or HTK solution, and ice slush is placed intraperitoneally to aid topical cooling of the organs. The warm ischemic time is controlled within 20 minutes. After in situ cooling, the kidneys are excised and delivered to the organ retrieval team, then are subjected to further cold perfusion on the back-table before cold storage. After procurement, the majority of DCD kidneys are subjected to simple static cold storage, and about 20% DCD kidneys in China undergo hypothermic machine perfusion, according to the preference of the retrieving and implanting surgeons [11].

There are three perfusion techniques including rapid laparotomy with direct aorta cannulation, in situ perfusions, and extracorporeal regional perfusion, which are commonly used to preserve kidneys before procurement. After the consent for donation is obtained and withdrawal of life support is performed, rapid laparotomy and direct aorta cannulation can be performed in Maastricht category III donors [12]. Before laparotomy is done and topical cooling of the organs is performed, in situ perfusion can be used in both controlled donors and uncontrolled donors, if consent for donation has been obtained [13]. Regional perfusion uses extracorporeal machine oxygenation circuit to selectively perfuse the abdominal organs after cannulation of the femoral vessels. This technique can be used to cool organs down both in uncontrolled DCD donors and DBD donors [14]. In recent years, it has been used to reperfuse the organs at body temperature (normothermic machine perfusion, NMP). This technique can further reduce the warm ischemia time of donor kidneys and reduce the PNF and DGF rate after DCD kidney transplantation [15].

6.4 Early Graft Function of DCD Kidney Transplantation

Delayed graft function (DGF) is the most striking difference in outcome between DCD and DBD donor kidneys, which is most commonly defined as the need for dialysis in the first 7 days post-transplant. Uncontrolled DCD kidneys have a much higher incidence of delayed graft function rate than controlled DCD kidneys and controlled DCD kidneys have a higher DGF rate compared to DBD kidneys. In a French study of uncontrolled DCD, delayed graft function occurred in 92% of recipients. The incidence of DGF after controlled DCD kidney transplantation in the UK is 49%. Hoogland reported that the incidence of PNF and DGF was substantially high in both type II (n = 128) and the type III (n = 208) groups

(22% vs. 21% and 61% vs. 56%, respectively) [16]. Analyzing an American database of 78,001 kidney donations, of which 2136 were from DCD donors, the results showed that although delayed graft function was more common in kidneys from DCD donors, particularly if the donation was uncontrolled, the 1-year graft survival was similar in all groups [17]. Primary non-function (PNF) rate after kidney transplant was low in controlled DCD kidneys. A study analyzing the data from the UK showed that the rate of PNF for both controlled DCD and DBD kidneys was similarly low, although the incidence was slightly higher for DCD than for DBD kidneys (4 vs. 3%, respectively, adjusted odds ratio of 1.49, $P = 0.04$) [18]. Our initial 71 DCD kidney transplants showed that the incidence of PNF and DGF were 2.8% and 28.2%, respectively. The PNF and DGF rates were significantly higher in DCD kidney transplants than DBD kidney transplants, which were lower than 1% and 10%, respectively [19].

In order to reduce the DGF rate of DCD kidney transplantation, usage of hypothermic machine perfusion (HMP) is increased for preserving the DCD kidneys in the recent years. A meta-analysis including both DBD and DCD kidneys suggested that HMP was associated with a relative risk of DGF of 0.804 (0.672–0.961) and that the reduction in DGF associated with HMP predicted a modest improvement in 10-year graft survival of 3% [20]. However, more randomized controlled trials of machine perfusion for DCD kidneys have produced conflicting results with respect to DGF. The results of two large, randomized controlled trials of static storage vs. machine perfusion of human DCD kidneys, in which one kidney from each donor was stored without perfusion, and the other was machine perfused, confirmed that pretransplant machine perfusion had no effect on 1-year patient, graft survival, and estimated post-transplant GFR. Decreased incidence and duration of DGF after machine perfusion was identified in 82 pairs of DCD kidneys [21], whereas the other study showed no beneficial effect on DGF [22]. A meta-analysis of multiple studies of hypothermic machine perfusion in DCD showed reduced DGF rates than kidneys placed in cold storage (Odds ratio = 0.64, $P = 0.03$) but no difference in 1-year graft survival [23]. Another meta-analysis comparing 175 machines perfused DCD kidney grafts with 176 cold storage grafts showed that machine perfused kidneys suffered less DGF (Odds ratio = 0.56, $P = 0.008$) but no differences in PNF and 1-year graft or patient survival [24]. Given the increased cost of machine perfusion, similar intermediate-term graft, and patient survival, the benefit of machine perfusion is unclear. Therefore, further studies are required before machine perfusion could be recommended over static cold storage as a better way to reduce DGF.

6.5 Graft and Patient Survival of DCD Kidney Transplantation

DCD kidneys show a comparable patient and graft survival to DBD kidneys and show a survival benefit to recipients over waiting for DBD kidneys [25]. A study from the UK including 739 DCD and 6759 DBD kidney transplant recipients, showed no difference in graft survival up to 5 years (hazard ratio = 1.01, $P = 0.97$) or in eGFR at 1 to 5 years after transplantation (at 12 months: −0.36 ml/min per 1.73 m^2, $P = 0.66$) [26]. A cohort from US Mycophenolic Renal Transplant Registry including 133 DCD kidney transplants and 415 DBD transplants. The incidence of DGF was 29.4% and 23.5% in the DCD group and the DBD group, respectively ($P = 0.1812$). The incidence of BPAR at 12 months was 9.0% and 9.9% respectively ($P = 0.7713$). The 1-year graft loss rate in the DCD group was higher than that in the DBD group (7.5% vs. 3.1%, $P = 0.0283$), and the 4-year graft loss rate and patient death rate were not significantly different between the DCD and DBD groups [27]. By comparing the long-term outcome of kidney transplantation from uncontrolled ($n = 128$) and controlled ($n = 208$) DCD donor kidneys procured, Hoogland et al. found that ten-year graft and recipient survival are similar in both groups (50% vs. 46%, $p = 0.74$ and 61% vs. 60%, $p = 0.76$, respectively). The outcome of kidney transplantation from uncontrolled and controlled donors after cardiac death is equivalent [16]. Another study from the Netherlands, including 2711 DCD kidney transplants and 3611 DBD kidney transplants, showed that despite higher incidences of early graft loss (+50%) and delayed graft function (+250%) in DCD grafts, 10-year graft and recipient survival were similar for the two graft types (10-year graft survival: 73.9%, 10-year patient survival: 64.5%). Long-term outcome equivalence was explained by a reduced impact of delayed graft function on DCD graft survival (RR: 0.69, 95% CI 0.55–0.87, $p < 0.001$). Mid and long-term graft function (eGFR), and the impact of delayed graft function on eGFR were similar for DBD and DCD grafts [28]. Our data from 71 DCD kidney transplants showed that the 1- and 3-year graft survival was 95.7% and 92.4%, respectively, which were comparable to DBD kidney transplants [19].

6.6 Graft Function of Recipients of DCD Kidney Transplantation

Recipients with DCD kidneys have similar graft survival compared to DBD donor, which has been reported by many studies. There is still some concern by some clinicians that graft function may be inferior in recipients of DCD kidneys, because ischemic injury incurred at the time of donation and transplantation may affect the long-term outcome. A study from UK compared graft function between 1768 DCD and 4127 DBD kidney transplant recipients. The results showed that graft function (eGFR) at 1 year was lower in DCD kidneys group compared to DBD kidneys group (eGFR 48 ml/min per 1.73 m^2 vs. 50 ml/min per 1.73 m^2, $P = 0.01$). There was no difference in graft function between DCD and DBD groups at 5 years after transplantation (49.6 ml/min per 1.73 m^2 vs. 48.1 ml/min per 1.73 m^2, $P = 0.97$) [18]. In a Chinese cohort study compared 325 DCD kidney transplants with 409 living donors (LD) kidney transplant. The graft function in the DCD group was better than that of the LD group at 3 years after transplant (eGFR: 71.14 ± 22.28 vs. 64.29 ± 16.76 mL/min/1.73 m^2; $P < 0.001$). There was no significant difference between the paired DCD and LD group (eGFR: 62.22 ± 18.50 vs. 66.99 ± 17.81 mL/min/1.73 m^2; $P = 0.068$) when matching donor age [28]. Therefore, there is no evidence that long-term graft function is inferior in kidney recipients from DCD donors than DBD donors or living donors.

6.7 Risk Factors Associated with Outcome of DCD Kidney Transplantation

There are several risk factors that may affect the outcome of DCD kidney transplantation. Donor age is the most important factor, which may affect graft survival no matter the recipients received kidneys from DCD or DBD donors. In a study of deceased kidney transplantation, the recipients who received kidneys from donors >60 years had more than twice the risk of graft failure compared to those transplanted with kidneys from donors <40 years in 3 years of transplantation (HR 2.35, 95% CI 1.85–3.0, $P < 0.0001$) [18]. In a study from Italy including young (<60 years) and old (≥60 years) DCD kidney transplants and old DBD kidney transplants, the results showed that compared to young DCD recipients, old DCD kidney transplant recipients had lower patient survival (66% vs. 85%; $P = 0.014$), death-censored graft survival (63% vs. 83%; $P = 0.001$), and eGFR (34 ml/min per 1.73 m^2 vs. 45.0 ml/min per 1.73 m^2; $P = 0.021$) after 5 years. In addition, old DCD recipients had higher incidence of DGF (70% vs. 47.2%; $P = 0.029$) and graft thrombosis (12.5% vs. 1.4%; $P = 0.021$) than young DCD recipients. There was similar 5-year patient survival (66% vs. 67%; $P = 0.394$) and death-censored graft survival (63% vs. 69%; $P = 0.518$) when compared to old DCD kidneys and old DBD kidneys. However, old DCD transplant had higher DGF (70% vs. 37.5%; $P = 0.007$) and lower estimated glomerular filtration rate

(34 mL/min per 1.73 m^2 vs. 41 mL/min per 1.73 m^2; $P = 0.029$) than old DBD group [29].

High donor body mass index (BMI) is another risk factor for DGF and graft failure. A study showed that DCD kidneys from donors with BMI > 45 kg/m^2 had a 1.84 times higher risk of graft loss [30]. Hypertension, diabetes, high donor creatinine and donor cause of death may also affect the outcome of DCD kidney transplant; the donors with these risk factors are defined as expanded criteria donors (ECD). The ECD donors usually have a poor outcome after kidney transplants than standard donors. In a UK Transplant Registry analysis study, ECD donors occurred in 31.5% of DBD and 34.9% of DCD transplants. There was no difference in graft survival between DCD and DBD transplants, although recipients from ECD donors had inferior graft survival compared to recipients from standard criteria donors. In addition, the risk-adjusted analysis showed that there was no significant interaction between standard criteria donors/ECD status and donor type when adjusting with HLA mismatch, recipient age, CIT, and recipient cause of the renal disease ($P = 0.45$). The primary non-function rate was higher in ECD DCD kidneys group compared to the standard criteria DCD kidneys group (4.1% and 2.7%, respectively, $P = 0.02$) [18].

Cold ischemia time (CIT) is another important risk factor that affects the outcome of a DCD kidney transplant. Kidneys from DCD donors are particularly vulnerable to long cold ischemia time. A study from the UK showed that relative risk for graft loss was 2.36 times (HR 1.39–4.02, $P = 0.004$) higher in DCD kidneys with a CIT of >24 h compared to kidneys with CIT of <12 h. The graft survival at 5 years after transplant was also lower in recipients with >24 h of CIT compared to recipients with <12 h of CIT (82.6% and 88.6%, respectively). There was no significant interaction between prolonged CIT and increasing donor age ($P = 0.96$). There were 22% of DCD donor kidneys used cold pulsatile machine perfusion; however machine perfusion did not show the impact on improving graft survival for deceased donor kidneys (adjusted HR 0.97, 95% CI 0.8–1.2, $P = 0.80$) [18]. Because cold ischemia time greatly impacts graft loss in DCD kidney transplant, CIT should be kept as short as possible (preferably <12 h).

6.8 Selection of DCD Kidneys

DCD kidneys have higher PNF and DGF rates after transplant. How to select or decline a DCD kidney is an important question in clinic. The decision to accept or decline a DCD donor kidney is usually made by transplant surgeons in the transplant centers based on the quality of the DCD donor kidney. The most common reason to decline a kidney by a transplant surgeon is the donor age, particularly the donor is too elderly. In recent years, many transplant centers have relaxed their criteria for using DCD kidneys from marginal donors because the experience of using DCD kidneys has accumulated step by step. Many DCD kidneys from old donors and donors with diabetes or cardiovascular disease have been used in the experienced centers. However, the discard rate of kidneys from DCD donors is still high, especially for kidneys from the elderly and ECD donors. Other factors may also cause surgeons to decline DCD kidneys, such as a protracted agonal period before asystole, unfavorable gross appearance following perfusion, and high resistant index during cold pulsatile perfusion. We evaluated the quality of 58 DCD and ECD donor kidneys using hypothermic machine perfusion. The results showed that the parameters of hypothermic machine perfusion might be useful non-invasive tools for evaluating the quality of DCD/ECD kidneys. One hour resistant index (RI) of machine perfusion >0.4 is correlated with DGF rate and 1 year graft function in DCD or ECD kidney transplantation [31]. Other reasons to decline kidneys from DCD donors include surgical damage to the organs during procurement, having risk of transmitting infection or malignancy of donor.

Pre-transplantation (Zero time) biopsy histology is an important predictor for the outcome of

DCD kidneys and can improve transplant outcome if those kidneys are not transplanted that are identified as probable failures after transplant. The most commonly used criteria for pre-transplantation is "Remuzzi Score." The Remuzzi Score has four components, including glomerular sclerosis, tubular atrophy, interstitial fibrosis, and atherosclerosis. After histological evaluation, the severity of chronic kidney injury in DCD donor kidneys can be quantified from scoring for each of these four components. Each component is scored 0–3, and provide a summed composite Remuzzi score of 0–12. It was recommended that kidneys from DBD donors with a score of >6 should be discarded, those kidneys with a score of 4–6 should be used as dual kidney transplantation, and those kidneys with a score of 0–3 should be used as single transplants [32]. A large retrospective multicenter analysis from Italian transplant centers has confirmed the value of pre-transplantation biopsy in transplantation of marginal kidneys according to Remuzzi score [33]. It has been shown in several large cohort of marginal deceased donor kidneys that pre-transplantation donor biopsy allowed safe allocation and transplantation of marginal kidneys. Some of those marginal kidneys might have been discarded on the basis of their high kidney donor profile index, which usually indicating a higher risk of post-transplant graft failure. However, acceptable transplant outcomes have been accomplished.

6.9 Pediatric DCD Kidney Transplantation

DCD kidney transplantation is often associated with an inflammatory reaction and oedema due to longer warm ischemia time; therefore, DCD kidneys may need a higher arterial blood pressure to get an adequate perfusion pressure. Many research have shown that pediatric DCD kidney transplantation is associated with a higher rate of DGF and reduced graft survival rate compared to pediatric DBD kidneys, and the hazard ratio is more than doubled. A retrospective cohort study from the Netherlands comparing 91 pediatric DCD kidney transplants with 405 pediatric DBD kidney transplants [34]. The results showed that the grafts from DCD donors were associated with higher rate of delayed graft function (48% vs. 8%, $P < 0.001$) and primary non-function (9% vs. 2%, $P < 0.01$) compared to DBD donors. There was no difference in estimated glomerular filtration rate between the two groups (57 ± 17 vs. 58 ± 21 ml/min at 1 year and 62 ± 14 vs. 57 ± 22 ml/min at 5 years, respectively). The risk of graft failure was higher in the DCD group than the DBD group (HR 2.440, 95% CI 1.280–4.650, $P = 0.007$) after adjusting for several confounding variables. Patient survival was similar between two groups (HR 1.559, 95% CI 0.848–2.867, $P = 0.153$). Therefore, it should weigh the slightly higher risk of graft failure by accepting a DCD kidney against the risks of staying on the waiting list for a long period when the surgeons decide whether or not to allocate a DCD kidney to a child.

6.10 Postoperative Management of DCD Kidney Transplantation

6.10.1 Peri-Operative Fluid Management

Fluid depletion in peri-operative period of DCD kidney transplantation may decrease initial graft function and increase the DGF rate after transplant. It has been shown that pre-operative and operative fluid loading may reduce the DGF rate after transplant. In a study including recipients of DCD kidneys, the results showed that for those recipients from DCD kidneys, low central venous pressure and low blood pressure during operation might increase the risk of PNF [35]. Therefore, it is important to monitor venous pressure immediately after the surgical procedure, keep the recipients well hydrated, and avoid immediate post-transplant dialysis. These methods may reduce the DGF and PNF rate after a DCD kidney transplant.

6.10.2 Post-Transplant Monitoring

After DCD kidney transplantation, patients with DGF should undergo regular ultrasonography, renal angiography, or both to rule out other causes other than acute tubular necrosis, usually due to temporary renal insufficiency. In addition, it is difficult to diagnose rejection in patients with DGF. Therefore, biopsies should be performed when necessary. In our center, Acute rejection was clinically diagnosed if serum creatinine increased 10% or more per day, and at the same time, ultrasound examination for the allograft showed the resistant index greater than 0.8. Most patients with the clinical diagnosis of acute rejection were further proven by standard percutaneous kidney allograft biopsy [19].

6.10.3 Immunosuppressive Therapy Protocol

DCD kidneys are more susceptible to calcineurin inhibitor (CNI) nephrotoxicity compared to DBD kidneys. Immediately use of CNI after transplant may exacerbate ischemic injury of DCD kidneys, increase DGF rate, delay recovery from DGF and impair long-term graft function. Therefore, it is better to avoid or postpone the use of CNI drugs or use low dose CNI immediate after transplant. In some patients with severe CNI nephrotoxicity, mTOR inhibitors may be used to replace CNI. Polyclonal antibodies may be used in order to postpone the immediate use of CNI after DCD kidney transplants. Some studies showed that anti-thymocyte globulins (ATG) can protect donor kidneys from ischemia-reperfusion injury during operation [36]. In our center, patients were given rabbit anti-thymocyte globulin and methylprednisolone as induction therapy during the operation and the first two days after kidney transplantation. In our experience, thymoglobulin seemed to be more effective than ATG-F on reducing DGF in patients with increased risk factors for DGF. For the patients with increased risk factors for DGF, the DGF rate was 22.5% in the thymoglobulin group vs. 56.3% in the ATG-F group ($P = 0.015$) [37]. For the recipients who received DCD kidneys from old donors, the maintenance CNI dose should be kept in relatively low level, because these kidneys are more susceptible for CNI nephrotoxicity.

References

1. Callaghan CJ, Harper SJF, Saeb-Parsy K, et al. The discard of deceased donor kidneys in the UK. Clin Transpl. 2014;28:345–53.
2. Huang J. The "Chinese Mode" of organ donation and transplantation. Hepatobil Surg Nutr. 2017;6(4):212–4.
3. Weber M, Dindo D, Demartines N, et al. Kidney transplantation from donors without a heartbeat. N Engl J Med. 2002;347:248–55.
4. Brook NR, Waller JR, Nicholson ML. Non heart-beating kidney donation: current practice and future developments. Kidney Int. 2003;63:1516–29.
5. Tavares-da-Silva E, Figueiredo A. Renal procurement: techniques for optimizing the quality of the graft in the cadaveric setting. Curr Urol Rep. 2020;21(2):12.
6. Ibrahim M, Vece G, Mehew J, et al. An international comparison of deceased donor kidney utilization: what can the United States and the United Kingdom learn from each other? Am J Transplant. 2020;20:1309–22.
7. Boyarsky BJ, Jackson KR, Kernodle AB, et al. Estimating the potential pool of uncontrolled DCD donors in the United States. Am J Transplant. 2020 May 5; https://doi.org/10.1111/ajt.15981.
8. Thuong M, Ruiz A, Evrard P, et al. New classification of donation after circulatory death donors definitions and terminology. Transpl Int. 2016;29(7):749–59.
9. Huang J, Wang H, Fan ST, et al. The national program for deceased organ donation in China. Transplantation. 2013;96(1):5–9.
10. Domínguez-Gil B, Haase-Kromwijk B, Van Leiden H, et al. Current situation of donation after circulatory death in European countries. Transpl Int. 2011;24:676–86.
11. Reich DJ, Mulligan DC, Abt PL, et al. ASTS recommended practice guidelines for controlled donation after cardiac death organ procurement and transplantation. Am J Transplant. 2009;9:2004–11.
12. Snoeijs MG, Dekkers AJ, Buurman WA, et al. In situ preservation of kidneys from donors after cardiac death: results and complications. Ann Surg. 2007;246:844–52.
13. Garcia-Rinaldi R, Lefrak EA, Defore WW, et al. In situ preservation of cadaver kidneys for transplantation: laboratory observations and clinical application. Ann Surg. 1975;182:576–84.
14. Koyama I, Shinozuka N, Miyazawa M, Watanabe T. Total body cooling using cardiopulmonary bypass for procurement from non-heart-beating donors. Transpl Proc. 2002;34:2602–3.

15. Net M, Valero R, Almenara R, et al. The effect of normothermic recirculation is mediated by ischemic preconditioning in NHBD liver transplantation. Am J Transplant. 2005;5:2385–92.
16. Hoogland ERP, Snoeijs MGJ, Winkens B, et al. Kidney transplantation from donors after cardiac death: uncontrolled versus controlled donation. Am J Transplant. 2011;11:1427–34.
17. Gagandeep S, Matsuoka L, Mateo R, et al. Expanding the donor kidney pool: utility of renal allografts procured in a setting of uncontrolled cardiac death. Am J Transplant. 2006;6:1682–8.
18. Summers DM, Johnson RJ, Hudson A, et al. Effect of donor age and cold storage time on outcome in recipients of kidneys donated after circulatory death in the UK: a cohort study. Lancet. 2013;381:727–34.
19. Chen GD, Ko S-CD, Wang C, Qiu J, Han M, He X, Chen L. Kidney transplantation from donors after circulatory death: an initial report of 71 cases from China. Am J Transplant. 2013;13(5):1323–6.
20. Wight JP, Chilcott JB, Holmes MW, et al. Pulsatile machine perfusion vs. cold storage of kidneys for transplantation: a rapid and systematic review. Clin Transpl. 2003;17:293–307.
21. Jochmans I, Moers C, Smits JM, et al. Machine perfusion versus cold storage for the preservation of kidneys donated after cardiac death: a multicenter, randomized, controlled trial. Ann Surg. 2010;252:756–64.
22. Watson CJ, Wells AC, Roberts RJ, et al. Cold machine perfusion versus static cold storage of kidneys donated after cardiac death: a UK multicenter randomized controlled trial. Am J Transplant. 2010;10:1991–9.
23. Bathini V, McGregor T, McAlister VC, et al. Renal perfusion pump vs. cold storage for donation after cardiac death kidneys: a systematic review. J Urol. 2012;189:2214–20.
24. Deng R, Gu G, Wang D, et al. Machine perfusion versus cold storage of kidneys derived from donation after cardiac death: a meta-analysis. PLoS One. 2013;8:e56368.
25. Snoeijs MG, Schaubel DE, Hene R, et al. Kidneys from donors after cardiac death provide survival benefit. J Am Soc Nephrol. 2010;21:1015–21.
26. Summers DM, Johnson RJ, Allen J, et al. Analysis of factors that affect outcome after transplantation of kidneys donated after cardiac death in the UK: a cohort study. Lancet. 2010;376:1303–11.
27. Zhu D, McCague K, Lin W, et al. Outcome of kidney transplantation from donor after cardiac death: reanalysis of the US mycophenolic renal transplant registry. Transplant Proc. 2018;50(5):1258–63.
28. Zhang X, Lyu J, Yu X, et al. Comparison of graft outcome between donation after circulatory death and living-donor kidney transplantation. Transplant Proc. 2020;52(1):111–8.
29. Favi E, Puliatti C, Iesari S, et al. Impact of donor age on clinical outcomes of primary single kidney transplantation from Maastricht category-III donors after circulatory death. Transplant Direct. 2018;4(10):e396.
30. Ortiz J, Gregg A, Wen X, et al. Impact of donor obesity and donation after cardiac death on outcomes after kidney transplantation. Clin Transpl. 2012;26:E284–92.
31. Chen G, Wang C, Zhao Y, et al. Evaluation of quality of kidneys from donation after circulatory death/ expanded criteria donors by parameters of machine perfusion. Nephrology (Carlton). 2018;23(2):103–6.
32. Remuzzi G, Grinyò J, Ruggenenti P, et al. Early experience with dual kidney transplantation in adults using expanded donor criteria. Double Kidney Transplant Group (DKG). J Am Soc Nephrol. 1999;10:2591–8.
33. Gandolfini I, Buzio C, Zanelli P, et al. The kidney donor profile index (KDPI) of marginal donors allocated by standardized pretransplant donor biopsy assessment: distribution and association with graft outcomes. Am J Transplant. 2014;14:2515–25.
34. de Vries EE, Hoogland PE, et al. Transplantation of kidneys from paediatric DCD donors: a comparison with DBD donors. Nephrol Dial Transplant. 2013;28(1):220–6.
35. Snoeijs MG, Wiermans B, Christiaans MH, et al. Recipient hemodynamics during non-heart-beating donor kidney transplantation are major predictors of primary nonfunction. Am J Transplant. 2007;7:1158–66.
36. Jose Perez-Saez M, Montero N, Redondo-Pachon D, et al. Strategies for an expanded use of kidneys from elderly donors. Transplantation. 2017;101:727–45.
37. Chen GD, Lai XQ, Ko DS, et al. Comparison of efficacy and safety between rabbit anti-thymocyte globulin and anti-T lymphocyte globulin in kidney transplantation from donation after cardiac death: a retrospective cohort study. Nephrology (Carlton). 2015;20(8):539–43.

7 Lung Transplantation from Cardiac Death Donors

Jingyu Chen, Chunxiao Hu, and Guohui Jiao

Abstract

Lung transplantation in China has developed rapidly with advances in organ preservation and surgical techniques as well as perioperative management. Wuxi lung transplantation center has been among the top lung transplantation centers with lung transplantation volume of over 100 cases per year since 2015. Donated lungs from cardiac death (DCD) donors and brain death donors have been accepted following specific criteria. Lung transplantation recipients receiving DCD donated grafts have comparable outcomes to DBD grafts. DCD donors could provide more transplantable lungs, thus alleviating the shortage of the donated lungs. Further research on DCD lungs, such as long-term benefit of the recipients, effect of ex vivo lung perfusion in lung repair is extremely needed. By virtue of the Green Channel of organ transportation, best matching recipients and donors will be extensively considered nationwide, more listed candidates could be transplanted and survived.

J. Chen (✉) · C. Hu · G. Jiao
Wuxi Lung Transplant Center, Wuxi People's Hospital, Nanjing Medical University, Wuxi, China
e-mail: chenjy@wuxiph.com

Globally, more than 4600 lung transplantations were reported to be performed annually [1]. Lung transplantation (LTx) has developed rapidly, which has been attributed to advances in organ preservation and surgical techniques, immunosuppressive regimens, and criteria refinement [2, 3]. LTx is developing in China and it is still challenging to maintain a sustainable LTx program to diminish the geographic disparity and balance the supply and demand covering a wide range of organ donation, allocation, and service area.

7.1 Overall Introduction of Lung Transplantation in China

The legal basis to support the development of volunteered organ donation is the Regulations on Human Organ Transplantation announced in the year 2007. The policy of donation-after-cardiac-death (DCD) was initiated in 2010. Thereafter, in the year 2013, Interim Provisions on Human Organ Procurement and Allocation were implemented by the National Health and Family Planning Commission. The high level of supervision on the process of organ donation and transplantation, especially on prohibiting transplant tourism and regulating living donor organ transplantation was strengthened. Ever since the full establishment of the China Lung Transplantation Registry (CLuTR) and National Lung Transplantation Data Center, with the support of

X. He (ed.), *Organ Donation and Transplantation after Cardiac Death in China*,
https://doi.org/10.1007/978-981-16-0815-5_7

the government, lung donation and transplantation activities have been managed and supervised according to the regulations. The year 2015 brought positive changes marked by government announcements stating that voluntary donation from the citizens is the sole legal source of human organs [4].

With propaganda from the official organization on the volunteered organ donation and transplantation, the Chinese public has increased awareness and acceptance of the issue and showed strong willingness to be volunteered donors. Meanwhile, with the improvement of post-LTx survival and medical insurance coverage, more candidates have been referred to qualified centers for assessment and listing. CLuTR contains data from 1542 lung transplants performed through December 31, 2019 (Fig. 7.1).

Wuxi center (WX) has been among the top lung transplantation centers with LTx volume of over 100 cases in an average of consecutive years. Following were China-Japan Friendship Hospital (CJ), First Affiliate Hospital of Guangzhou Medical University (GZ), and Shanghai Pulmonary Hospital (SHP). However, the volume distribution was far more than balanced in China, reflected by over 80% transplanted cases contributed by the four largest centers (WX, CJ, GZ, and SHP). According to the statistics up to December 31, 2019, CLuTR included recipients who had a median age of 59 years old (IQR: 49–65).

The largest category of diagnosis before transplantation was idiopathic interstitial pneumonitis (IIP), followed by chronic obstructive lung disease (COPD). Occupational lung diseases (OLD) included pneumonoconiosis and lymphangioleiomyomatosis (LAM). Single LTx cases were preferred to be considered in patients with pneumoconiosis, ILD (including IIP and ILD-not IIP). However, more bilateral LTx has been performed in pulmonary hypertension, LAM, and bronchiectasis patients. Currently, over 40% of candidates were transplanted at the age beyond 60 years old. Previously, before 2020, the estimated percentage of ECMO bridging was 4.9% and mechanical ventilation rate was 5.5%. However, in the year 2020, considering the special condition of COVID-19, more critically severe patients got listed with support by ECMO and MV, their short-term outcome was not compromised being considered in critical and urgent conditions.

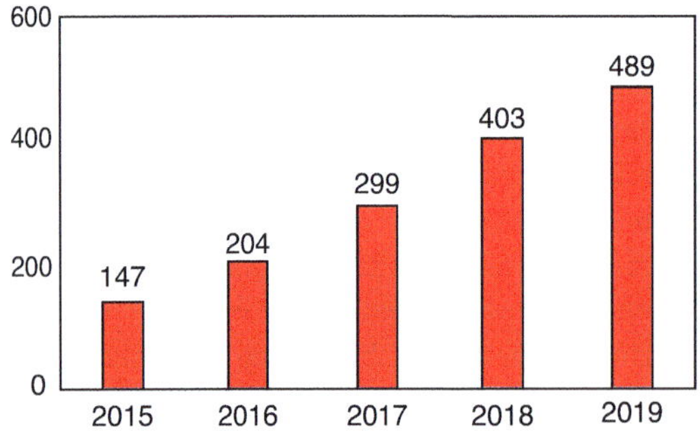

Fig. 7.1 Number of reported LTx cases from January first, 2015 to December 31st, 2019

According to the statistics from 2015 to 2018, the median donor age was 36 years old, 83.5% of the donors were from the 18- to 49-years-old age group and 88.7% were male donors. DBD donors have been increased to be used for LTx. In the CLuTR cohort, the median allograft cold ischemic time for SLT was 360.0 (247.5–430.0) min and BLT 480.0 (360.0–570.0) min [5]. As the surgeons performed more numbers of transplants, there was a clear trend in diminishing cold ischemic time in recent years.

7.2 Donor Selection Criteria

For donors admitted in intensive care units, prolonged mechanical intubation, extracorporeal circulation life support, and hospital-acquired pneumonia were common with an ever-increasing rate of prolonged support time. Currently, not only donated lungs compatible with "ideal criteria" but also "marginal" donated grafts have been accepted in donor selection and matching process. Criteria when considering acceptance of donated lungs from cardiac death donors and brain death donors demonstrated as follows.

The ideal criteria for donated lungs:

a. ABO blood type compatible between donors and recipients.

b. Age < 60 years old.
c. Smoking history <400 cigarettes per year.
d. Duration of mechanical ventilation <1 week.
e. Partial pressure of oxygen (PaO_2)/Fraction of inspiration O_2 (FiO_2) > 300 mmHg (Condition, positive end-expiratory pressure (PEEP) 5 cmH_2O);
f. Clear manifestation on chest imaging.
g. No significant effusions seen in bronchoscopy.
h. No drug-resistant microbiology results from sputum culture.

Criteria of "acceptable" marginal lungs:

a. ABO blood type compatible between donors and recipients.
b. Age < 70 years old.
c. Smoking history <400 cigarettes per year.
d. No specific exclusion criteria on duration of mechanical ventilation.
e. PaO_2/FiO_2 > 250 mmHg (PEEP, 5 cmH_2O);
f. Mild or moderate effusion on chest imaging.
g. When considering volume reduction or lung lobe transplantation, matching between donors and recipients should be discussed with experts.
h. No specific exclusion criteria of trauma on the chest.
i. Grafts acceptable after proper management of aspiration or sepsis.
j. Grafts acceptable after effusions in trachea cleared.
k. No pan-resistant microbiology results from sputum culture.
l. No serious primary diseases on donated lungs, such as active tuberculosis, lung cancer, donors with a history of asthma could be acceptable.
m. Grafts reach the standard of donor acceptable criteria after ex vivo lung perfusion recovery.
n. Cold ischemic time no more than 12 h.

As is shown from the reports and our practice, recipients transplanted with marginal donated grafts showed comparable short- and long-term results to those who were transplanted with "ideal grafts." New arising ex vivo lung perfusion techniques have shown promise in recovering marginal lungs, with respect to existed grafts infection and deteriorated oxygenation function [6].

7.3 Management of Deceased Cardiac Death Donors

After the consent procedures are fully conducted, the withdrawal of life-sustaining therapy, confirmation of death, and procurement of organs are done in the operation room. All the procurement surgeons get prepared and after the final farewell of family and donor, the patient is extubated with all inotropic medications ceased but palliative sedation for symptom control continued. After deceased status was confirmed, the patient is re-intubated and ventilated, bronchoscopy is performed to examine and rule out the aspiration of gastric content. Sternotomy is performed with pulmonary cannulation. Upon pleural cavities are open, lungs are inspected and examined. Tidal volume is expected to be maintained at 6–8 mL/kg. PEEP is set on 5 cm H_2O. Bilateral bronchoscopy examination with lavage is performed in the region of lung contusion or suspected aspiration. Sputum culture is acquired before antibiotics are adopted. Cardiac output, central venous pressure, and extravascular lung water are monitored and evaluated for body fluid balance. Diuretics are injected to maintain a negative balance when necessary. Corticoid is administered according to body weight.

For the lung procurement and recovery procedure, Raffinose-low-potassium dextran solution is prepared and perfused after heparin is injected into pulmonary artery. Ante-grade perfusion is performed with a pressure of 30–40 cm H_2O, at the fluid volume of 40–60 mL/kg. After the grafts were resected, retrograde perfusion is performed from branches of pulmonary veins. Massage maneuver on the grafts is performed with inflation of lungs like the mechanism of normal breath action. The perfusion is not stopped until the efflux is seen to be clear. Hand check manipulation is then performed to ensure that no significant mass is palpated within the lung tissue. The resected lungs will be recovered and maintained in RLPD with lower-than-physical temperature. During the cold perfusion, the lungs are topically cooled with saline. Back-table anatomical resection, split and repair of resected lungs will be performed thereafter. Recipient management post-LT is not different for patients with DCD lungs or DBD lungs. Immunosuppressant regimens and drug concentration monitoring are performed, while antibiotics are continued especially in those recipients with donated lungs from marginal donors.

We have analyzed data from a group of 22 DCD donors. With an average PaO_2/FiO_2 value of 385.1 mmHg. Among those potential donors, 20 lungs were determined to be recovered in the initial evaluation. All the lungs were compatible with the "ideal" criteria of donated lung grafts. When performing the lung procurement, one grafted was failed to be procured due to extensive adhesion to the chest wall. The remained 19 DCD donated grafts were successfully recovered and transplanted. Average warm ischemic time of the donated lungs was 12.3 ± 7.1 min. The lungs were used in four single LTx with average cold ischemic time 258.7 ± 70.9 min, while the cold ischemic time for bilateral LTx was 299.6 ± 130.8 min and 439.8 ± 129.1 min. In the total of 21 recipients, 5 in-hospital death occurred and 2 of the death cases were due to pan-resistant drug infection, other death causes included 1 primary graft dysfunction, 1 acute rejection, and 1 pulmonary thrombosis. The average in-hospital stay was 42 days. One-year survival rate was approximately 76%.

7.4 Survival Status of Lung Transplant Recipients in China

Comparing to the follow-up data reported from global large lung transplant centers, Chinese recipients had a higher incidence of infection and acute injection early in postoperative periods. Common posttransplant morbidities, included infection, acute rejection, renal dysfunction, primary graft dysfunction (PGD), diabetes mellitus, broncho-pleural fistula, and bronchial anastomotic lesions. The total <30 days, 3 months, 6 months, 1-year, 2-year, and 3-year Kaplan–Meier survival rates in CLuTR were 81.45%, 74.97%, 72.24%, 70.11%, 64.85%, and 61.16% [5].

In terms of patient survival after lung transplant by disease category, patients who had LAM and pneumoconiosis had superior survival compared to other main diagnoses, such as pulmonary fibrosis. However, we found a higher percentage of >60 age patients in China. Age of 66+ patients had a shorter survival period and lower estimated rate in the follow-up. Age and pre-transplant indications were recognized otherwise, the crucial factors when considering the matching factors between recipients and donors. It was not the donation types, i.e., DCD or DBD, which decided the survival of the recipients. However, the pretransplantation graft status, reflected by oxygenation function and bacterial colonization, was the determinant of post-LTx survival. In the cohort, pulmonary infection occurred in a large portion of death cases within 30 days post-LTx. We have advanced tools, such as next-generation sequencing, thus to understand if there was donor–recipient transfer of microbiology ecology.

7.5 DCD and DBD Lungs in Transplantation

DCD donors could provide more transplantable lungs, thus alleviating the shortage of the donated lungs. However, there is still space to do more research on how to make the best use of the potential donors [7]. A previous study with the extracted data from the Scientific Registry of Transplant Recipients during the period of 2006–2014, only 2.1% of the DCD lungs were used, while 21.4% of the DBD lungs were transplanted in the same period [8].

As is commonly believed, LTx recipients receiving DCD donated grafts have comparable outcomes to DBD grafts. One-year survival rate could reach to more than 80% and 3-year survival at around 60%. Selection criteria of DCD donors are similar to that of DBD donors. In DCD donation, warm ischemic time (WIT) is defined as the time between cardiac arrest and cold perfusion. Pre-recover heparin and, agonal time and warm ischemic time are crucial for the quality of the donated grafts. As for the warm ischemic time, the starting point is when $SaO_2 < 85\%$ and SBP <50 mmHg. Prolonged warm ischemic time leads to low PaO_2/FiO_2 post transplantation. In our practice, within 60 min of maximum acceptable warm ischemic time, there was no significant impact on the graft function post transplantation. The length of cold ischemic time has an impact on graft function and contributes to the primary graft dysfunction (PGD) and anastomotic stenosis post transplantation, which is suggested to be optimized within 8 h.

During the period of cardiac death to lung procurement, blood gas analysis will help one understand the lung function. Proper management of mechanical ventilation will enhance the usage rate of the grafts. Tidal volume and PEEP are the most important factors in airway management during the donated lung maintenance. Stabilized hemodynamics could reduce the pulmonary edema, while the renal function was properly monitored. Heart failure could also compromise the status of hemodynamics. Diuretic is necessary for fluid balance maintenance in the procedure.

Neurogenic pulmonary edema, aspiration of gastric contents, pulmonary infections, contusion, and ventilation-associated lung injury constitute the main reason for low retrieval rate in DCD donors [9]. Steroids use further reduces the systemic inflammation reaction which causes injury to the lungs. Thrombosis formation is related to the PGD risk and reduced long-term survival. Heparin treatment is still controversial and lacks convincing evidence. Ethical concern of pre-cardiac death use of heparin and risk of intracranial hemorrhage remained to be further discussed.

Ex vivo lung perfusion (EVLP) could be used in lung repair, thus increasing the donated graft use. EVLP has a positive effect on intrapulmonary thrombosis and bronchial effusion clearance, as well as reducing pulmonary edema. DCD donations and other marginal donations could benefit from EVLP repair and we have published our initial results of animal studies [10, 11]. Experimental studies demonstrated acceptable grafts with up to 90 min warm ischemic time. EVLP has been used to assess uncontrolled DCD donor lungs before implantation.

Additional antibiotics treatment during EVLP adds more benefit to graft lungs with PaO_2 less than 300 mmHg, heavy lungs during palpation, massive blood transfusion (>10 units), poor lung compliance, suspicion of aspiration, and high C-reactive protein (CRP) related to a pulmonary infection. Non-portable EVLP and portable EVLP systems have been used to recondition the DCD lungs [12, 13]. Portable EVLP might provide the solution to enhance the donor lung quality, facilitating the logistical procedure and potentially reduce the cost of peri-procurement maintenance. After confirmed good lung function after EVLP, DCD lung transplantation can be done safely and recipients survived with acceptable midterm outcomes and quality of life. Decreased post-transplantation hospital stays and PGD occurrence rate were not the only benefits from the shortened cold ischemic time alone [14–16]. We are still waiting for the longitudinal results of the study on novel strategies of EVLP on donated lungs [17].

Global-wide practice has shown that for DCD and DBD recipients, post transplantation outcomes, including graft survival and rejection rate, were generally comparable. ISHLT DCD Registry demonstrated comparable 1- and 5-year survival between DCD and DBD lung recipients. There were some reports from large centers, which revealed that DCD donors might have a higher incidence of airway complications [18]. Larger cohort with prolonged follow-up, more important, the matching baseline factors, diminishing impact of confounding factors from both donors and recipients, will facilitate the more insightful recommendation on the use of DCD donations.

7.6 Lung Transplantation in China, Past and Future

The community-based citizens' donation has become the only legitimate source of transplantable organs in China ever since the year of 2015. China Organ Transplant Response System (COTRS) is the mandatory official organ allocation system, which performs automated patient-oriented organ match based on aboveboard scientific organ allocation policies. Legal implementation in the new era of volunteered organ donation has contributed enormously to increase deceased donor rates. The standard of "donation after brain plus cardiac death (DBCD)" has been established with legislation nurturing the development of organ transplantation affairs in China. However, the volume of accepted donated lungs was still below the average global level.

To guarantee the high quality of recovering the donated grafts, close cooperation between transplant surgeons and proficient organ procure organizations (OPOs) was outreached. Since May 6, 2016, the Codes of Organ Transportation has been enacted to guarantee a solid pathway for transportation of the "gift of life," coordinated by the National Health and Family Planning Commission, the Ministry of Public Security, the Ministry of Transport, Civil Aviation Administration of China, China Railway Corporation and the Red Cross Society of China. The recovered organs transported swiftly with significant shortened ischemic time, thus more feasible lungs could be transplantable even in the most complicated scenarios—patients with a long time use of mechanical ventilation or excorporaeal circulatory support, difficulties of clearing sputum or secretions with infections, multi-comorbidities, can be challengeable for both medical teams and patients [19, 20]. According to our observation, short- to long-term survival for indications are comparable to reported data from other countries, such as in IPF [21]. Since the establishment of "China Lung Transplantation Alliance" in September 2018, enhanced collaboration has been performed between transplantation and procurement surgeons, physicians, critical care intensivists, and coordinated staff [22]. Involved transplant teams in Alliance work in cooperation simultaneously on multi-organ procurement projects with concordant workflow and transported allocated organs, further reducing the ischemic time.

Organ donation and allocation are not limited to the local service area especially in lung transplantation per current practice in China. By virtue of the Green Channel of organ transportation, best matching recipients and donors will be extensively considered nationwide, after fully considering the allocation principle of proximity. Thus, more listed candidates could be transplanted and survived. In all, China with its largest population in Eastern Asia is continuously improving the lung transplantation registry and program, incorporating transplantation of ever-increasing lung grafts from both DBD and DCD donors.

References

1. Chambers DC, Cherikh WS, Goldfarb SB, et al. International Society for Heart and Lung Transplantation. The International Thoracic Organ Transplant Registry of the International Society for Heart and Lung Transplantation: thirty-fifth adult lung and heart-lung transplant report—2018; Focus theme: Multiorgan Transplantation. J Heart Lung Transplant. 2018;37(10):1169–83.
2. Gottlieb J, Smits J, Schramm R, et al. Lung transplantation in Germany since the introduction of the lung allocation score: a retrospective analysis. Dtsch Arztebl Int. 2017;114(11):179–85.
3. Klesney-Tait J, Eberlein M, Geist L, et al. Starting a lung transplant program: a roadmap for long-term excellence. Chest. 2015;147(5):1435–43.
4. Huang JF. The "Chinese Mode" of organ donation and transplantation. Hepatobil Surg Nutr. 2017;6(4):212–4.
5. Hu CX, Chen WH, He JX, et al. Lung transplantation in China between 2015 and 2018. Chin Med J. 2019;132(23):2783–9.
6. Tian D, Wang Y, Shiiya H, et al. Outcomes of marginal donors for lung transplantation after ex vivo lung perfusion: a systematic review and meta-analysis [published online ahead of print, 2019 Aug 25]. J Thorac Cardiovasc Surg. 2019;S0022-5223(19)31641-1.
7. Luc JGY, Jackson K, Weinkauf JG. Feasibility of lung transplantation from donation after circulatory death donors following portable ex vivo lung perfusion: a pilot study. Transplant Proc. 2017;49(8):1885–92.

8. Mooney JJ, Hedlin H, Mohabir PK, et al. Lung quality and utilization in controlled donation after circulatory determination of death within the United States. Am J Transplant. 2016;16:1207e15.
9. Inci I, Hillinger S, Schneiter D, et al. Lung transplantation with controlled donation after circulatory death donors. Ann Thorac Cardiovasc Surg. 2018;24(6):296–302.
10. Liu F, Lu Y, Wei D, et al. Effect of ex vivo lung perfusion on storage of isolated lungs. Ann Palliat Med. 2020;9(2):359–67.
11. Wei D, Gao F, Yang Z, et al. Ex vivo lung perfusion with perfusate purification for human donor lungs following prolonged cold storage. Ann Transl Med. 2020;8(3):38.
12. Cypel M, Yeung JC, Liu M, et al. Normothermic ex vivo lung perfusion in clinical lung transplantation. N Engl J Med. 2011;364:1431e40.
13. Warnecke G, Moradiellos J, Tudorache I, et al. Normothermic perfusion of donor lungs for preservation and assessment with the Organ Care System Lung before bilateral transplantation: a pilot study of 12 patients. Lancet. 2012;380:1851e8.
14. Tikkanen JM, Cypel M, Machuca TN, et al. Functional outcomes and quality of life after normothermic ex vivo lung perfusion lung transplantation. J Heart Lung Transplant. 2015;34:547e56.
15. Andreasson A, Karamanou DM, Perry JD, et al. The effect of ex vivo lung perfusion on microbial load in human donor lungs. J Heart Lung Transplant. 2014;33:910e6.
16. Sommer WKC, Tudorache I, Salman J, et al. Warm perfusion of the donor lung for preservation might have positive immunomodulatory effects after transplantation. Transplantation. 2012;94:943.
17. Jiao GH. Evolving trend of EVLP: advancements and emerging pathways. SN Compr Clin Med. 2019;1:287–303.
18. De Oliveira NC, Osaki S, Maloney JD, et al. Lung transplantation with donation after cardiac death donors: long-term follow-up in a single center. J Thorac Cardiovasc Surg. 2010;139(5):1306–15.
19. Huang L, Chen W, Guo L, et al. Scopulariopsis/microascus isolation in lung transplant recipients: a report of three cases and a review of the literature. Mycoses. 2019;62(10):883–92.
20. Gao F, Chen J, Wei D. Lung transplantation for bronchiolitis obliterans syndrome after allogenic hematopoietic stem cell transplantation. Front Med. 2018;12(2):224–8.
21. Dotan Y, Vaidy A, Shapiro WB, et al. Effect of acute exacerbation of idiopathic pulmonary fibrosis on lung transplantation outcome. Chest. 2018;154(4):818–26.
22. Wu B, Hu C, Chen W, et al. China lung transplantation developing: past, present and future. Ann Transl Med. 2020;8(3):41.

8 Pancreas and Islet Transplantation from Cardiac Death Donors

Zheng Chen and Peng Zhang

Abstract

Pancreas transplantation has become accepted as an effective treatment for diabetes mellitus (DM) to restores glycogenic control and also prevents or reverses the progression of secondary complications of DM. Due to the complexity of pancreatic exocrine management and the difficulty in the timely diagnosis of pancreas graft rejection, pancreas transplantation once lagged far behind kidney, heart, liver, and other organ transplants in terms of total number of transplants and transplantation outcome. With the clinical application of a new type of powerful immunosuppressant, organ preservation technology improvement and surgical technique mature, the results of pancreas transplantation have improved over time, and pancreas graft and patient survival rate of simultaneous pancreas and kidney transplantation (SPK) continuously improve, becoming an effective treatment of type 1 diabetes mellitus (T1DM) and part of type 2 diabetes mellitus (T2DM) with uremia. Pancreas transplantation involves multiple disciplines, including the immunological and non-immunological selection of the donor and recipient, incision, perfusion and preservation of the donor pancreas, donor pancreas implant, diagnosis, prevention, and treatment of rejection, use, monitoring and adjustment of immunosuppressant regimen, and long-term follow-up and management.

Z. Chen (✉) · P. Zhang
Organ Transplant Center, The Second Affiliated Hospital of Guangzhou Medical University, Guangzhou, China

8.1 Pancreas Transplantation

Pancreas transplantation is the most effective treatment for patients with diabetes mellitus (DM) to restores glycogenic control and also prevents or reverses the progression of secondary complications of DM [1]. Over the last 30 years, >31,000 pancreas transplants had been performed in the USA and >15,000 pancreas transplants in other countries [2]. Pancreas transplantation involves multiple disciplines, including the immunological and non-immunological selection of the donor and recipient, incision, perfusion and preservation of the donor pancreas, donor pancreas implantation, diagnosis, prevention, and treatment of rejection, use, monitoring and adjustment of immunosuppressant regimen, and long-term follow-up and management. Pancreas transplantation includes pancreas transplantation alone (PTA), pancreas after kidney transplantation (PAK), simultaneous pancreas and kidney transplantation (SPK), combined liver and pancreas transplantation (CLP), and liver and pancreas cluster transplantation (LPCT). In the USA,

X. He (ed.), *Organ Donation and Transplantation after Cardiac Death in China*,
https://doi.org/10.1007/978-981-16-0815-5_8

the 5-year patient survival rates are currently 93% for SPK, 91% for PAK, and 78% for PTA recipients, and the 5-year pancreas graft survival rates are currently 73% for SPK, 65% for PAK, and 53% for PTA [3]. PAK patients have previously undergone a kidney transplant with either a living or deceased donor and receive pancreas transplantation after renal function recovered. The transplanted pancreas and kidneys were from different donors. The pancreas is transplanted either in combination with a kidney, commonly called SPK. In SPK, both organs, the pancreas and the kidney, are procured from the same deceased donor. Pancreas graft and patient survival rates in SPK patients were superior to those patients undergoing PAK or PTA. Therefore, the majority of pancreas transplants have been performed SPK. Notably, SPK recipients' patient survival rates at 10 years were 66%, higher than the rates in PTA recipients with DM with end-stage renal disease (ESRD), which was 47%. In recent years, the proportion of type 2 diabetes mellitus (T2DM) patients receiving pancreas transplantation has been increasing year by year. In the USA in 2016, T2DM patients who received pancreas transplants accounted for only 4.7%. Long-term follow-up has shown that there was no statistically significant difference in 10-year patient and pancreas graft survival rate between SPK recipients with type 1 diabetes mellitus(T1DM) and T2DM [4]. In the last 4 years, 151 ipsilateral SPK transplants were performed by the Organ Transplant Center, the Second Affiliated Hospital of Guangzhou Medical University (Guangzhou, China).

8.1.1 Indications and Contraindications [5–7]

8.1.1.1 Indications

Indications for PTA: (a) T1DM patients with frequent episodes of severe hypoglycemia or hyperglycemia, insulin resistance and severe retinopathy. (b) Unstable diabetes mellitus with unexpected insulin treatment. (c) Insulin-dependent T2DM patients. (d) Total pancreatectomy for chronic pancreatitis or pancreatic cancer, with blood glucose control difficult to control or diabetic complications.

Indications for SPK: (a) T1DM patients with end-stage renal failure (uremia), and renal failure after kidney transplantation alone. (b) Insulin-dependent T2DM patients with end-stage renal failure (uremia). (c) Post-transplant diabetes mellitus, with insulin dependence and renal allograft failure.

Indications for CLP or LPCT: (a) End-stage liver disease with T1DM. (b) End-stage liver disease with uncontrollable, insulin-dependent T2DM with complications. (c) Lesions of liver and pancreas with no other effective treatment. (d) Malignant lesions involving liver, pancreas, duodenum, and other organs without systemic distant metastasis.

8.1.1.2 Contraindications

Uncontrolled systemic infections (including tuberculosis, active hepatitis, etc.); combined with serious organic lesions of heart, lung, brain, and other important organs, or poor general situation, intolerant to the transplant operation; recent(< 6 months) myocardial infarction history; the malignant tumor is not treated or cured for less than 1 year; an uncured ulcer; in AIDS active period; severe gastrointestinal dysfunction and immunosuppressant should not be used; accompanied by severe mental and psychological illness; a high degree of non-compliance that cannot be controlled by multidisciplinary intervention; a variety of progressive metabolic diseases(e.g. hyperoxaluria). The following conditions should be considered as contraindications for pancreatic bladder drainage: uncured urinary tract infection; lower urinary tract stenosis; neuropathic bladder voiding dysfunction, bladder contracture, or bladder dilatation caused by diabetes. The residual urine volume of the bladder was measured at >100 mL.

8.1.2 Surgical Technique

Over the years, different surgical techniques have been described for the management of exocrine pancreatic secretions. Two major approaches of pancreas transplantation are drainage of the duodenal segment to the bladder (bladder drainage) or to the small bowel (enteric drainage). In 1983, Sollinger first proposed that the donor pancreatic duct or the duodenal segment connected to the pancreas was anastomosed to the bladder, with the advantage of fewer intraabdominal suppurative infections and other surgical complications associated with pancreatic jejunal drainage, and enabling diagnosis of acute rejection by measuring urinary amylase. For this reason, bladder drainage became mainstream. However, its long-term complications, such as hemorrhagic cystitis, chronic urinary tract infection and metabolic acidosis, have become new problems. About 25% of the recipients of bladder drainage were forced to switch to enteric drainage due to urinary complications within 10 years after surgery [8]. Therefore, in the 1990s, the approach of enteric drainage was taken seriously again. The operative success rate of enteric drainage is close to that of bladder drainage, which can reach more than 90%. In general, there was no significant difference in the patient and pancreas graft survival regardless of the drainage. Despite this, most of the world's centers now regard enteric drainage as the first choice because it is more physiological.

Pancreas transplantation can be divided into systemic venous drainage and portal venous drainage according to different approaches of portal venous drainage. Theoretically, portal venous drainage is more in line with physiological characteristics and allows insulin to be metabolized through the liver first, which may avoid hyperinsulinemia and thus reduce complications such as glucose and fat metabolic disorders, progressive atherosclerosis as well as insulin resistance. However, portal venous drainage has not been shown to be superior to systemic venous drainage in terms of graft function and long-term survival. In contrast, the recipient has lower surgical risk because systemic venous drainage is technically easier. In 2011, the International Pancreas Transplantation Registry reported that 82% of SPK and 90% of PTA were performed with systemic venous drainage.

In 2003, The Emory Transplant Center reported a new technique that was utilizing a single arterial conduit to vascularize both organs, with donor pancreas and kidney placed in the same iliac fossa [9, 10]. The main points are as follows: while obtaining the donor organ, one side of the internal, external, and common iliac arteries, namely the so-called Y graft iliac artery, were taken. The kidney was first transplanted during the operation, and the end of the internal iliac artery of the Y graft iliac artery of the donor artery was anastomosed, while the end of the common iliac artery of the Y graft iliac artery was anastomosed with the external iliac artery of the recipient, and the blood flow of the kidney was opened. Then transplantation of the pancreas, the abdominal aortic sleeve piece containing the celiac trunk and superior mesenteric artery common flap was anastomosed end-to-end with the external iliac artery of the Y graft iliac artery, the portal vein of the donor pancreas was anastomosed end-to-side with the recipient's portal vein or inferior vena cava, and the duodenum was anastomosed laterally with the recipient's ileum to complete the pancreas transplantation. Later, the technique has been gradually developed and popularized in many centers, for example in the Organ Transplant Center of the Second Affiliated Hospital of Guangzhou Medical University in China, 151 cases of ipsilateral simultaneous pancreas and kidney transplantation were successfully performed in the past 4 years. The ipsilateral transplantation has certain advantages: (a) The other side of the iliac vessel can be reserved for the recipient; (b) The difficulty of anastomosis of transplanted pancreas artery was reduced after artery bypass; (c) Shortened the operation time and cold ischemia time of transplanted pancreas; (d) Lower the arterial pressure of the pancreas, which is more physiological; (e) The pressure of vena cava reflux is lower than that of the iliac vein, which reduces venous complications.

8.1.3 Postoperative Management

Due to diabetes patients' susceptibility and systemic vascular lesions, surgical trauma, pancreatic exocrine processing difficulties and postoperative stronger immune inhibitors and other factors, pancreas transplantation, especially SPK, has a higher incidence of surgical complications. Early postoperative strict monitoring, effective treatment and immunosuppressive therapy are crucial to help to improve the prognosis and reduce complications and mortality.

Postoperative patients should be monitored for vital signs, central venous pressure and fluid inflow and outflow. Amylase is the main index to monitor the exocrine function of the pancreas graft, which can be diagnosed comprehensively according to the levels of amylase in blood, urine, and peripancreatic drainage. Blood glucose level is an important indicator to monitor the endocrine function of the pancreas graft. When rejection is suspected, increase the number of blood glucose tests as appropriate. At 3–4 weeks after the transplantation, oral glucose tolerance test, serum insulin and C-peptide release test and hBA1c are examined when pancreas graft function was well restored, and the endocrine function of pancreas graft should be comprehensively evaluated. Color Doppler ultrasound and abdominal CT of pancreas graft should be regularly reviewed. Prophylactic use of broad-spectrum antibiotics for 1 week followed by ganciclovir for CMV infection in pancreas transplantation recipients. Use somatostatin to prevent pancreatitis. For the pancreas is a hypo-perfusion organ, anticoagulant therapy is often needed to prevent the thrombosis of the transplanted pancreas.

8.1.4 Immunosuppressant

On account of the particularity of diabetic lesions, high rate of graft rejection and graft loss, and side effects caused by postoperative immunosuppressive regimens, immunosuppressants in pancreas transplantation and SPK are more complicated than PTA. The basic principles of drug use are as follows: it can effectively prevent rejection, and at the same time minimize the toxic side effects of the drugs; drug combination is generally adopted; since the pancreas is a highly immunogenic organ, induction therapy is often needed in the early stage of SPK, and the dosage of immunosuppressive regimens is relatively large; avoid overuse of immunosuppressant to reduce infections and tumors caused by reduced immune function.

Common immunosuppressant: (a) Adrenal glucocorticoids, including methylprednisolone (MP), prednisolone (Pred); (b) Biological agents for induction therapy, including ATG, ALG, alemtuzumab, and basiliximab; (c) Other commonly used drugs include cyclosporin A(CsA), tacrolimus (Tac), mycophenolate Mofetil (MMF), mizoribine, azathioprine (Aza), sirolimus (SRL), etc. [10].

Maintenance medication regimens: (a) Tac + MMF+ steroids; (b) Tac + SRL+ steroids; (c) CsA + MMF+ steroids; (d) Tac + SRL. At present, the use of steroids in the maintenance of immunosuppressants is gradually decreasing, especially in patients with T2DM; steroids can be reduced until they are removed.

8.1.5 Complications

8.1.5.1 Rejection

Rejection is one of the main reasons leading to long-term pancreas allograft loss. Clinically, it is usually divided into hyperacute, accelerated, acute, and chronic rejection. The incidence of rejection in CLP or LPCT was significantly lower than that of SPK due to the immune protection of the transplanted liver [11].

Hyperacute Rejection [7]

Hyperacute rejection is more common within 24 h after the pancreas allograft to restore blood flow. It usually occurs intraoperatively, when the transplanted pancreas, after restoring blood supply, turns into flower mottling, with the color gradually becoming purplish-brown and losing luster, and the pancreas surface effuses more. At present, there is no effective treatment. If hyperacute pancreas allograft rejection is suspected, extensive microthrombus formation of the pancreas allograft is likely to occur, and the pancreas allograft should be removed as soon as possible.

Acute Rejection [12–14]

Acute rejection is most common, usually occurred in 1-week to 3-month post-transplantation. No subjective symptoms are found in PTA. The main clinical manifestations in SPK recipients were renal graft rejection, including decreased urine volume, weight gain, fever, and elevated blood pressure. Laboratory examinations show elevated blood glucose, amylase, or creatinine. Observation of changes in urine amylase and urine pH is helpful to diagnosis acute rejection in pancreas transplantation recipients with bladder drainage. DSA can be detected in peripheral blood when antibody-mediated rejection (AMR) occurs. But at present, graft biopsy is still the gold standard for the diagnosis of acute rejection.

Treatment in acute rejection: (a) High-dose methylprednisolone shock therapy; (b) Anti-lymphocyte antibodies should be used in response to the hormone-resistant or severe acute rejection; (c) Adjustment of the immunosuppressive regiments; (d) Suspected or clearly diagnosed as AMR, relevant measures may be taken as appropriate, including plasmapheresis or immunosorbent removal of antibodies, high-dose IVIG neutralizing and inhibiting antibodies in vivo; CD20 monoclonal antibody (rituximab) clearing B lymphocytes, proteasome inhibitors (bortezomib) inducing plasma cell apoptosis and reducing antibody production, the complement inhibitor eculizumab on the complement protein C5 and inhibiting antibody-dependent cell-mediated cytotoxicity. Appropriate anticoagulant drugs should be used to help the restoration of graft function.

Chronic Rejection [15–16]

Chronic rejection refers to chronic progressive pancreatic allograft dysfunction, which usually occurs at 3-month post-transplant. With clinical lack of specific symptoms, recipients can have fever, abdominal pain, and graft tenderness, with the change of biochemical indicators such as serum amylase and blood glucose increase, the pancreas allograft function gradually loses, and the disease is difficult to reverse. Rituximab may be used for mild antibody-induced chronic rejection. When the pancreas allograft function loss, insulin may be required. When the renal graft function is lost, dialysis is resumed, and re-transplantation was awaited.

8.1.5.2 Intraperitoneal Bleeding [15, 17]

Intraperitoneal bleeding usually occurs within 3 weeks post-transplant, and sudden dilatation pain in the transplanted pancreas extends to the lower abdomen and bladder, etc. When having more oozing of blood or active bleeding, obvious symptoms appear, which clinically manifests as cold sweat, fidgety, pulse fast, blood pressure drop, urine little or no urine, as well as drainage tube blood drainage material suddenly increased. Ultrasound can assist diagnosis. Generally, if intraperitoneal bleeding occurs, fluid replacement and blood transfusion should be carried out quickly, vital signs should be closely observed, and anticoagulant should be adjusted or stopped properly. On the condition that arterial or venous rupture or bleeds profusely or conservative transfusion treatment is ineffective, emergency surgical exploration should be conducted.

8.1.5.3 Thrombosis in Pancreas Allograft [15, 18]

The thrombosis of the pancreas allograft can be caused by many reasons, including hypercoagulability in DM recipients, easy blockage of blood flow in the pancreas with low perfusion, intraoperative pancreatic edema, and pancreas graft rejection. Arterial thrombosis usually has no local symptoms but is clinically manifested by a sudden increase in blood glucose and a decrease in serum and urinary amylase. Early venous thrombosis, as a result of pancreas graft congestion, swelling, in addition to blood glucose and serum amylase increase, can be accompanied by local pain and tenderness of transplanted pancreas. Color Doppler Ultrasonography, angiography, or CT, magnetic resonance angiography and other examinations can help to make a definite diagnosis. Surgical exploration should be carried out as soon as possible in case of suspected major vascular embolization of transplanted pancreas, supplemented by anticoagulation and thrombolytic therapy. The pancreas allograft should be surgically removed as soon as possible once arterial and/or venous thrombosis has completely blocked the vessel.

8.1.5.4 Pancreatitis in Pancreas Allograft [15, 19]

Pancreatitis in the pancreas allograft is often characterized by edema but can also progress to hemorrhage, necrotizing pancreatitis and graft function loss. The clinical manifestations are fever, persistent abdominal pain, abdominal distension, tenderness, and rebound pain at the graft, as well as significantly increased serum and urinary amylase, and sudden and rapid decrease of serum amylase from a high level or normal, indicating extensive bleeding and necrosis of the transplanted pancreas. Conventional treatments for pancreatitis include fasting, gastrointestinal decompression, parenteral nutrition, inhibition of pancreatic exocrine, and maintenance of water, electrolyte, and acid-base balance. If conservative treatment fails or bleeding necrotizing pancreatitis is suspected, surgery should be performed as soon as possible to remove the transplanted pancreas and its surrounding necrotic tissue, and partial or total pancreas allograft should be removed if necessary.

8.1.5.5 Pancreatic Leakage and Pancreatic Fistula [15, 17, 20]

Based on the site, time and the causes of pancreatic leakage, and the size of the leakage port, the clinical manifestations of pancreatic leakage are different. The common clinical manifestations include fever, local swelling pain and tenderness, and increased leucocyte and blood amylase. Detection of amylase in drainage is helpful in diagnosis, and ultrasound or CT examination shows perioperative effusion in the pancreas allograft. After the occurrence of pancreatic leakage, the surrounding pancreatic effusion should be timely to drainage. Control local infection, inhibit pancreatic fluid secretion, and indwelling catheter should be taken in recipients with bladder drainage. If peripancreatic drainage unobstructed, most pancreatic leakage can be closed by itself after a few weeks. It is feasible to repair the fistula if it does not heal for a long time.

8.2 Islet Transplantation

Clinical islet transplantation is performed by injection with less surgical trauma and good safety. After Edmonton protocol was successfully applied in clinical islet transplantation in 2000, clinical islet transplantation has been carried out in more and more international centers. Considerable progress has been made in islet isolation and purification, transplantation technology and post-transplantation management, which further improves the efficacy of islet transplantation [21]. At present in some experienced islet transplantation center, the proportion of exogenous insulin treatment ar 5 years after the islet transplantation can reach 50–70%, and the medium and long-term efficacy of islet transplantation has gradually close to the pancreas transplantation, which indicates that islet transplantation has transited from the experimental treatment into a routine treatment of refractory diabetes [22–26].

8.2.1 Indications and Contraindications

Indications for islet transplantation alone: (a) T1DM with poor therapeutic effect; (b) T2DM accompanied by islet failure; (c) undergoing total pancreatectomy in case of benign lesions such as chronic pancreatitis and benign pancreatic tumor [27, 28].

Indications for islet transplantation after other organ transplantation: (a) T1DM after liver, kidney, heart, and lung transplantation; (b) insulin-dependent T2DM after liver, kidney, heart, and lung transplantation; (c) insulin-dependent new-onset DM after liver, kidney, heart, and lung transplantation [29, 30].

Contraindications for islet transplantation are the same as for pancreas transplantation.

8.2.2 Quality Assessment of Donor Pancreas and Islets

8.2.2.1 Selected Criteria of Donor Pancreas

Meets the general criteria of organ transplant donors; the donor should be between 20 and 60 years old; no history of diabetes; no history of pancreatic trauma; BMI >20 kg/m^2; glycated hemoglobin (HbA1c) level <6% [31].

Clinical studies have confirmed that the higher the BMI of organ donors is, the better the success rate of islet preparation, and even some islet transplantation centers basically choose donors with BMI >27 kg/m^2. A comprehensive evaluation should be conducted in combination with blood glucose, fasting C-peptide and HbA1c level in the evaluation of donors.

8.2.2.2 Assessment of Donor Islet

Donor Islet quality assessment should be conducted before islet transplantation; the number of islets should be >5000IEQ/kg at the first islet transplantation and >4000IEQ/kg at the second transplantation; islet purity should be >30%; Islet activity should be >70%; microscopic examination of bacteria and fungi in islet culture medium should be negative, and endotoxin content in islet culture medium should be <5 U/kg [32].

8.2.3 Donor Pancreatic Procurement and Islet Preparation

Pancreas anatomy in islet transplantation is the same as in pancreas transplantation; however, the preservation of blood vessels from the pancreas is not required. The donor pancreas must be procured with great care to ensure the integrity of the pancreatic glands, but the processing time should be minimized to retain as much oxygenated blood as possible before the aorta closes. After the perfusion of University of Wisconsin Solution (UW), the whole pancreas and part of the duodenum shall be contained, placed in a sterile UW solution at 4 °C, and transported to the islet preparation center as soon as possible for islet preparation [33].

The whole process of clinical islet cell preparation should be completed in the Good Manufacturing Practices (GMP) laboratory. When the donor pancreas arrives at GMP laboratory, the pancreas is first checked for integrity, adequate perfusion, edema, fibrosis, etc. After confirming that the donor pancreas is suitable for islet cell isolation, the adipose tissue and lymph nodes around the pancreas should be removed as far as possible. However, the outer membrane of the pancreas should be completely preserved in this process so as to achieve good results when the digestive fluid is perfused. Islet preparation process includes pancreas perfusion with collagenase → pancreas digestion at about 37 °C → purification of islets by continuous density gradient centrifugation → islet culture in CMRL1066 culture medium at 37 °C (the longest culture time should not be >72 h) [31].

8.2.4 Procedures for Islet Transplantation

At present, clinical islet transplantation is routinely performed by percutaneous transhepatic portal vein puncture. The specific procedures are as follows: the patient is supine, and after local anesthesia, the puncture site is the right midaxillary line, the anterior axillary line 9–10 intercostal space or below xiphoid. The 22-g Chiba needle is selected to puncture to the liver under the guidance of ultrasound. After the contrast agent is injected and the Chiba needle is confirmed to enter the portal vein branch, the fine guidewire is injected into the portal vein trunk through the Chiba needle, and then the Chiba needle was replaced with a 4–6 French sheath. The portal vein pressure is measured. If the portal vein pressure is <20 mmHg, slow infusion of islet suspension containing heparin sodium could begin. The portal vein pressure should be measured every 5–10 min to prevent acute portal hypertension caused by too fast infusion speed. If the portal vein pressure is >20 mmHg, islet infusion should be suspended and wait until the portal vein pressure drops to <20 mmHg before slow infusion. When the catheter is removed, the puncture route of liver parenchyma should be embolized with a gelatin sponge, spring coil or even hemostatic gel to prevent liver puncture hole bleeding after islet transplantation [34, 35].

8.2.5 Postoperative Treatment and Immunosuppressive Regimens

After islet transplantation, patients should stay in bed for 8 h and receive short-term anticoagulant therapy, that is, pump heparin within 48 h, maintaining APTT in 50–60 s, and then giving low-molecular heparin sodium anticoagulant therapy within 1 week. Etanercept is administered before and after islet transplantation to treat blood-mediated inflammatory responses, and antibacterial, antifungal, and antiviral therapies are also needed to administer. It is generally believed that islet graft vascularization needs to be completed within 2–4 weeks to play a normal physiological function. Therefore, patients receiving islet transplantation therapy should continue to use insulin to control blood glucose after surgery, so as to help the islet graft avoid affecting its physiological function due to hyperglycemia. Islet transplantation requires ultrasound examination to confirm that there is no hematoma or portal venous thrombosis in the liver. Liver function, immune status (T cell subsets, PRA), and islet function (blood glucose, HbA1c, C-peptide) should be closely monitored [36].

Islet transplantation immunosuppressive therapy is currently based in Edmonton scheme, which does not use hormone drugs but use the rabbit anti-thymocyte immunoglobulin (ATG) or Basiliximab as induction therapy, low-dose tacrolimus (blood concentrations of 4–6 ng/mL) joint sirolimus (blood drug concentration 8–12 ng/mL) or MMF as immunosuppressive maintenance therapy.

8.2.6 Complications

The safety of islet transplantation is one of the important factors for the sustainable development of islet transplantation. At present, the vast majority of islet transplantation is percutaneous transhepatic portal vein puncture. Usually, the operation can be completed only under local anesthesia at the skin puncture point, with fewer traumas and a low incidence of complications. However, clinical studies have shown that the following complications may occur after islet transplantation.

(a) Bleeding: Clotting indexes should be closely monitored during anticoagulation therapy, heparin sodium should be stopped when clinical manifestations of bleeding occur, protamine therapy should be given according to coagulation indexes, and emergency surgical exploration should be performed when occurs large amount of blood loss or unsuccessful conservative transfusion treatment [37].
(b) Thrombosis: If the anticoagulant strength is insufficient or IBMIR is severe in patients during or after islet transplantation, a large number of local thrombosis may be formed in islet graft. In severe cases, a large number of thromboses may be formed in the portal vein system, and severe liver lesions may occur. Adequate anticoagulation should be administered during and after islet transplantation, and the level of IBMIR should be inhibited by the combination of antitumor necrosis factor and other drugs.
(c) Abnormal Liver Function: Alanine aminotransferase and aspartate aminotransferase show slow growth with an incidence of up to 50%, usually returning to normal completely after 1 month. Nearly 20% of islet transplantation recipients may occur liver microsteatosis [35].
(d) Infection: The recipient is infected when the islet graft is infected with a small amount of microbial contamination, so the patient was routinely given infection-prevention therapy after transplantation.
(e) Sensitization: After islet transplantation, there may be sensitization to donor HLA. Recipient's PRA should be routinely monitored before and after islet transplanta-

tion. If PRA is weakly positive before transplantation, donors with positive sites should be avoided, and islet transplantation can only be accepted if the CDC is negative. If PRA is neutral, islet transplantation should be suspended.

(f) Hypoglycemia: The occurrence of IBMIR after portal islet transplantation can lead to the destruction of a large number of islets in a very short time, and patients may have severe hypoglycemia reaction due to the release of insulin in large quantities. Symptomatic treatment should be given by intravenous glucose infusion.

(g) Gallbladder Perforation: At present, percutaneous transhepatic portal vein puncture is mainly performed under the guidance of an X-ray. Since the puncture needle cannot be precisely positioned during puncture, there will be the risk of accidental injury to the gallbladder, leading to gallbladder perforation. Therefore, X-ray and ultrasonic guidance should be combined to improve the accuracy of puncture.

8.2.7 Islet Auto Transplantation

So far, islet auto transplantation has been widely carried out in Europe and America, mainly for the treatment of patients with chronic pancreatitis who need total pancreatectomy [38, 39]. Indications for islet auto transplantation include recurrent acute pancreatitis, chronic pancreatitis complicated with abdominal pain, and failing to receive standard medical, endoscopic, or conventional surgical treatment. Contraindications include C-peptide negative diabetes, T1DM; portal venous thrombosis, portal hypertension, and severe liver disease; high risk of cardiopulmonary diseases; and known as pancreatic cancer. The branch of the mesenteric vein is usually selected for islet auto transplantation, and the unpurified islets are slowly transferred back after intubation. There is no need to take immunosuppressive drugs after islet auto transplantation, but short-term anticoagulant therapy is required, and insulin should be used as appropriate.

References

1. White SA, Shaw JA, Sutherland DER. Pancreas transplantation. Lancet. 2009;373:1808–17.
2. Dholakia S, Oskrochi Y, Easton G, Papalois V. Advances in pancreas transplantation. J R Soc Med. 2016;109(4):141–6.
3. Gruessner AC, Gruessner RWG. Pancreas transplantation for patients with type 1 and type 2 diabetes mellitus in the United States: a registry report. Gastroenterol Clin North Am. 2018;47(2):417–41.
4. Dholakia S, Mittal S, Quiroga I, Gilbert J, Sharpies EJ, Ploeg RJ, Friend PJ. Pancreas transplantation: past, present, future. Am J Med. 2016;129(7):667–73.
5. Al-Qaoud TM, Odorico JS, Redfield RR 3rd. Pancreas transplantation in type 2 diabetes: expanding the criteria. Curr Opin Organ Transplant. 2018;23(4):454–60.
6. Mittal S, Gough SC. Pancreas transplantation: a treatment option for people with diabetes. Diabet Med. 2014;31(5):512–21.
7. Shi C, Bingyi S. Clinical technical operation specifications-organ transplantation. Beijing: People's Medical Publishing House; 2010. p. 139–65.
8. Gruessner AC, Gruessner RWG. Pancreas transplantation of US and non-US cases from 2005 to 2014 as reported to the United Network for Organ Sharing (UNOS) and the International Pancreas Transplant Registry (IPTR). Rev Diabet Stud. 2016;13(1):35–58.
9. Fridell JA, Shah A, Milgrom ML, Goggins WC, Leapman SB, Pescovitz MD. Ipsilateral placement of simultaneous pancreas and kidney allografts. Transplantation. 2004;78(7):1074–6.
10. Heilman RL, Mazur MJ, Ks R. Immunosuppression in simultaneous pancreas-kidney transplantation: progress to date. Drugs. 2010;70(7):793–804.
11. Dean PG, Kukla A, Stegall MD, Kudva YC. Pancreas transplantation. BMJ. 2017;357:j1321.
12. Niederhaus SV, Leverson GE, Lorentzen DF, Robillard DJ, Sollinger HW, Pirsch JD, Torrealba JR, Odorico JS. Acute cellular and antibody-mediated rejection of the pancreas allograft: incidence, risk factors and outcomes. Am J Transplant. 2013;13(11):2945–55.
13. de Kort H, Roufosse C, Bajema IM, Drachenberg CB. Pancreas transplantation, antibodies and rejection: where do we stand? Curr Opin Organ Transplant. 2013;18(3):337–44.
14. Pelletier RP, Rajab AA, Diez A, DiPaola NR, Bumgardner GL, Elkhammas EA, Henry ML. Early immunosuppression treatment correlates with later de novo donor-specific antibody development after kidney and pancreas transplantation. Clin Transpl. 2015;29(12):1119–27.
15. Organ Transplantation Society of Chinese Medical Association. Chinese guidelines for the diagnosis and treatment of pancreas transplantation (2016 edition). Chin J Organ Transplant. 2016;37(10):627–34.
16. de Kort H, Mallat MJK, van Kooten C, de Heer E, Brand-Schaaf SH, van der Wal AM, Roufosse C, Roelen DL, Bruijn JA, Claas FH, de Fijter JW,

Bajema IM. Diagnosis of early pancreas graft failure via antibody-mediated rejection: single-center experience with 256 pancreas transplantations. Am J Transplant. 2014;14(4):936–42.
17. Troppmann C. Complications after pancreas transplantation. Curr Opin Organ Transplant. 2010;15(1):112–8.
18. Farney AC, Rogers J, Stratta RJ. Pancreas graft thrombosis: causes, prevention, diagnosis, and intervention. Curr Opin Organ Transplant. 2012;17(1):87–92.
19. Nadalin S, Girotti P, Konigsrainer A. Risk factors for and management of graft pancreatitis. Curr Opin Organ Transplant. 2013;18(1):89–96.
20. Nath DS, Gruessner A, Kandaswamy R, Gruessner RW, Sutherland DE, Humar A. Late anastomotic leaks in pancreas transplant recipients – clinical characteristics and predisposing factors. Clin Transpl. 2005;19(2):220–4.
21. Shapiro AM, Lakey JR, Ryan EA, Korbutt GS, Toth E, Warnock GL, Kneteman NM, Rajotte RV. Islet transplantation in seven patients with type 1 diabetes mellitus using a glucocorticoid-free immunosuppressive regimen. N Engl J Med. 2000;343(4):230–8.
22. Hering BJ, Kandaswamy R, Ansite JD, Eckman PM, Nakano M, Sawada T, Matsumoto I, Ihm SH, Zhang HJ, Parkey J, Hunter DW, Sutherland DE. Single-donor, marginal-dose islet transplantation in patients with type 1 diabetes. JAMA. 2005;293(7):830–5.
23. Bellin MD, Barton FB, Heitman A, Harmon JV, Kandaswamy R, Balamurugan AN, Sutherland DER, Alejandro R, Hering BJ. Potent induction immunotherapy promotes long-term insulin independence after islet transplantation in type 1 diabetes. Am J Transplant. 2012;12(6):1576–83.
24. Berney T, Ferrari-Lacraz S, Bühler L, Oberholzer J, Marangon N, Philippe J, Villard J, Morel P. Long-term insulin-independence after allogeneic islet transplantation for type 1 diabetes: over the 10-year mark. Am J Transplant. 2009;9(2):419–23.
25. Gibly RF, Graham JG, Luo X, Lowe WL Jr, Hering BJ, Shea LD. Advancing islet transplantation: from engraftment to the immune response. Diabetologia. 2011;54(10):2494–505.
26. Qi M, Kinzer K, Danielson KK, Martellotto J, Barbaro B, Wang Y, Bui JT, Gaba RC, Knuttinen G, Garcia-Roca R, Tzvetanov I, Heitman A, Davis M, McGarrigle JJ, Benedetti E, Oberholzer J. Five-year follow-up of patients with type 1 diabetes transplanted with allogeneic islets: the UIC experience. Acta Diabetol. 2014;51(5):833–43.
27. Hering BJ, Clarke WR, Bridges ND, Eggerman TL, Alejandro R, Bellin MD, Chaloner K, Czarniecki CW, Goldstein JS, Hunsicker LG, Kaufman DB, Korsgren O, Larsen CP, Luo X, Markmann JF, Naji A, Oberholzer J, Posselt AM, Rickels MR, Ricordi C, Robien MA, Senior PA, James Shapiro AM, Stock PG, Turgeon NA, Clinical Islet Transplantation Consortium. Phase 3 trial of transplantation of human islets in type 1 diabetes complicated by severe hypoglycemia. Diabetes Care. 2016;39(7):1230–40.
28. Ryan EA, Bigam D, James Shapiro AM. Current indications for pancreas or islet transplant. Diabetes Obes Metab. 2006;8(1):1–7.
29. Galindo RJ, Wallia A. Hyperglycemia and diabetes mellitus following organ transplantation. Curr Diab Rep. 2016;16(2):14.
30. Jenssen T, Hartmann A. Emerging treatments for post-transplantation diabetes mellitus. Nat Rev Nephrol. 2015;11(8):465–77.
31. Hanley SC, Paraskevas S, Rosenberg L. Donor and isolation variables predicting human islet isolation success. Transplantation. 2008;85(7):950–5.
32. James Shapiro AM, Pokrywczynska M, Ricordi C. Clinical pancreatic islet transplantation. Nat Rev Endocrinol. 2017;13(5):268–77.
33. Kin T, James Shapiro AM. Surgical aspects of human islet isolation. Islets. 2010;2(5):265–73.
34. Schuetz C, Markmann JF. Islet cell transplant: update on current clinical trials. Curr Transplant Rep. 2016;3(3):254–63.
35. Owen RJT, Ryan EA, O'Kelly K, Lakey JRT, McCarthy MC, Paty BW, Bigam DL, Kneteman NM, Korbutt GS, Rajotte RV, Shapiro AMJ. Percutaneous transhepatic pancreatic islet cell transplantation in type 1 diabetes mellitus: radiologic aspects. Radiology. 2003;229(1):165–70.
36. Changsheng M. Pancreas and combined pancreas-kidney. In: Suisheng X, editor. Chinese medicine of transplantation. Nanjing: Jiangsu Science and Technology Publishing House; 2011. p. 442–60.
37. Venturini M, Angeli E, Maffi P, Fiorina P, Bertuzzi F, Salvioni M, De Cobelli F, Socci C, Aldrighetti L, Losio C, Di Carlo V, Secchi A, Del Maschio A. Technique, complications, and therapeutic efficacy of percutaneous transplantation of human pancreatic islet cells in type 1 diabetes: the role of US. Radiology. 2005;234(2):617–24.
38. Beamish CA, Gaber AO, Afshar SF, Fraga DW, Hamilton DJ, Sabek OM. Variability in endocrine cell identity in patients with chronic pancreatitis undergoing islet autotransplantation. Am J Transplant. 2019;19(5):1568–76.
39. Desai CS, Vonderau JS, Ma X, Hanson M, Xu X, Khan A. The first report of total pancreatectomy and islet cell autotransplantation for pancreatic cystosis in patient with cystic fibrosis. Pancreas. 2019;48(6):e54–5.

9 Multiple Organ Transplantation from Cardiac Death Donors

Qiang Zhao and Weixin Luo

Abstract

Multiple organ transplant is the treatment for multiple abdominal organ failure. The term multiple organ transplantation or multiple visceral transplantations is defined as the en-bloc transplantation of three or more than three abdominal viscera that are related to each other in anatomy and function, such as hepatic pancreaticoduodenal transplantation, which has the advantages of comprehensive replacement of organ function and maintaining the normal anatomical and physiological structure between transplanted viscera. The multivisceral transplantation was pioneered by Thomas Starzl. In 1983, Starzl performed the first two multi-organ transplants in humans with en-bloc inclusion of the pancreas, liver, stomach, intestine, colon, and duodenum. Both cases were performed under cyclosporine-based immunosuppression in two children with gut and liver failure caused by short bowel syndrome. Later, with interleukin (IL)-2 receptor antibodies gradually being introduced into the clinical practice, the immunosuppressive protocols have undergone a major shift and have contributed to the further development of transplantation medicine. At the same time, a new understanding of the mechanisms of graft tolerance and allograft acceptance has guided the effective application of these agents in recipient or donor preconditioning and induction therapy. In addition, the accumulation of experience, the introduction of new diagnostic and biological tools, and the use of effective antimicrobials have contributed to the development of postoperative care.

Q. Zhao (✉) · W. Luo
The First Affiliated Hospital of Sun Yat-sen University, Guangzhou, China

9.1 Nomenclature

The multivisceral transplantation (MVTx) can be full or modified. A full MVTx means en-bloc transplantation of the pancreas, small bowel, stomach, duodenum, and liver (Fig. 9.1), while a modified MVTx does not include liver transplantation (Fig. 9.2) [1–3].

9.2 Indications and Contraindications

9.2.1 Indications

MVTx is indicated for those who have undergone complex abdominal diseases, including extensive mesenteric desmoid tumors, massive polyposis,

X. He (ed.), *Organ Donation and Transplantation after Cardiac Death in China*,
https://doi.org/10.1007/978-981-16-0815-5_9

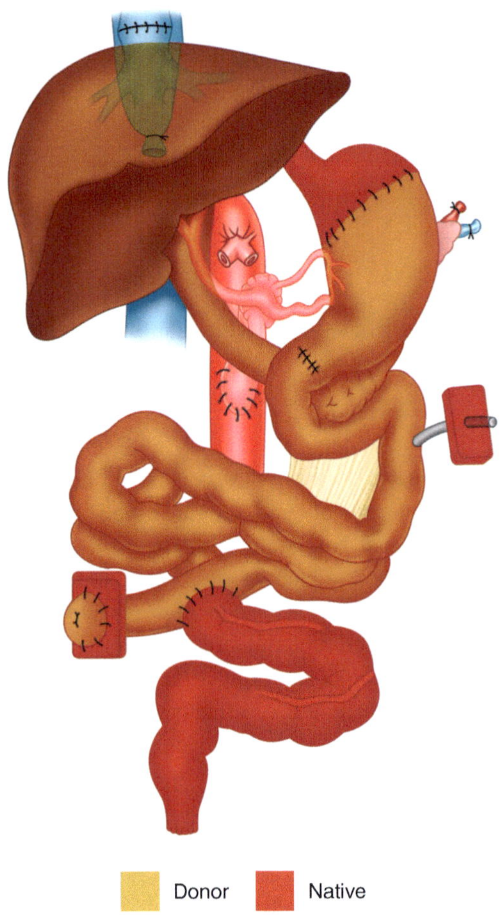

Fig. 9.1 Illustration depicts full MVTx. (From Rees, M.A., Amesur, N.B., Cruz, R.J., Borhani, A.A., Abu-Elmagd, K.M., Costa, G., and Dasyam, A.K. (2018). Imaging of Intestinal and Multivisceral Transplantation. Radiographics 38, 413–432)

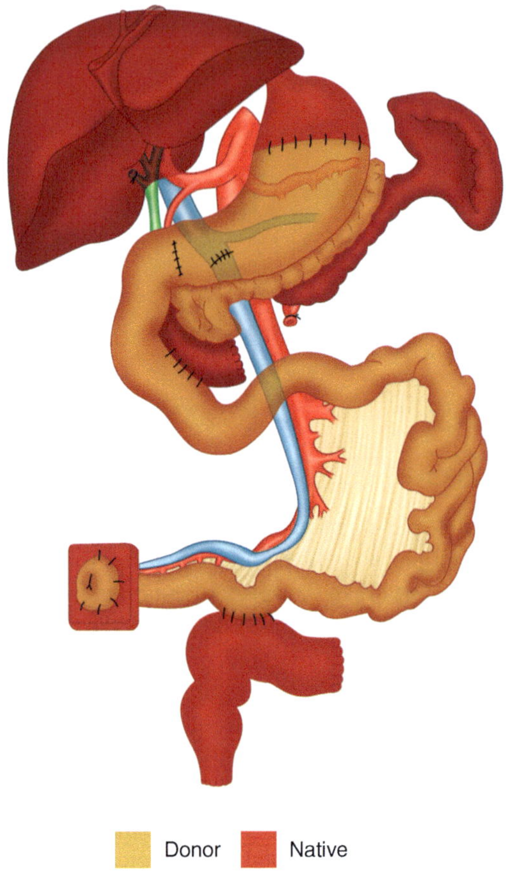

Fig. 9.2 Illustration depicts modified MVTx. (From Rees, M.A., Amesur, N.B., Cruz, R.J., Borhani, A.A., Abu-Elmagd, K.M., Costa, G., and Dasyam, A.K. (2018). Imaging of Intestinal and Multivisceral Transplantation. Radiographics 38, 413–432)

diffuse portomesenteric thrombosis (for which MVTx is the only treatment option), other locally aggressive neoplasms, vascular catastrophe, trauma, and generalized intestinal dysmotility due to neuropathy or myopathy [4, 5]. Based on the experience of the international Intestinal Transplant Registry and extensive single-center, the primary indication for MVTx is a short gut syndrome [1, 6]. The most common underlying causes in pediatric practice includes necrotizing enterocolitis gastroschisis, pseudo-obstruction, and volvulus. The most common causes in adults are Crohn's disease, dysmotility disorders, mesenteric, desmoid tumors, trauma, and vascular disease. Generally speaking, the procedure is not justified nowadays if patients remain stable on total parenteral nutrition (TPN) without any severe TPN-related complications and have a good life expectancy without transplantation. However, once the patients develop life-threatening complications, predominantly run out of sites for venous access, recurrent line sepsis or TPN-related liver disease, the role of the MVTx is clear [7].

9.2.2 Contraindications

Incurable tumor, persistent life-threatening intra-abdominal or systemic infections, severe cardiopulmonary insufficiency, and severe immune deficiency syndromes (SIS) in which successful stem cell transplantation is not possible before transplant are absolute contraindications to visceral transplantation [8, 9]. Poor psychosocial support has been identified as a relative contraindication because of the associated poor long-term survival. Conversely, the presence of controlled neuropsychiatric disorders should not preclude transplantation, since successful recovery from surgery has recently been reported in both children and adults [10]. Chemical dependency, locally advanced desmoid tumors, abdominal infection, and psychosomatic disorders are supposed to be managed and treated before being considered as a contraindication for transplantation. History of gut tumor, older age, and loss of central venous access should not be solely considered as a contraindication for transplant.

9.3 Preoperative Assessment

Patients who are going to receive MVTx usually require a thorough evaluation process, including assessing the type of required allograft, candidacy for transplant, extent of gut failure, and presence of contraindications for transplant. MVTx is a representative interdisciplinary specialty. In particular, initial advice is needed from surgeons, anesthetists, gastroenterologists, radiologists, hepatologists, pharmacists, specialist nurses in gastroenterology and transplantation, tissue typists, physiotherapists, dieticians, occupational therapists, psychologists, and psychiatrists. The evaluation covers clinical, endoscopic, biochemical, histologic studies, radiologic and so on. Equally important is the development of a thorough socioeconomic and psychiatric assessment with the establishment of management tactics, which aims to rescue candidacy for transplantation and address the potential pathologic conditions. As noted earlier, particular attention should be paid to relative and absolute contraindications of the transplantation.

Special laboratory, endoscopic and imaging examinations are required for the cause of gut failure. The adaptive and congenital immune status are supposed to be assessed in those with inborn or congenital diseases, with the aim of having an assessment on the potential risk of developing graft-versus-host disease after transplant. As for the patients having hereditary tumorous disorders, endoscopy is required to assess the extent of coexistent malignancy and dysplastic syndrome [11]. Before the transplant, adequate imaging is of great value. Furthermore, once selected for planning implantation, patients are necessary to receive thorough imaging of the surgical field related to the extent of remnant bowel, the arterial, venous and portal intra-abdominal vasculature. This is achieved by a variety of imaging methods, including computed tomography (+/− angiography), magnetic resonance imaging (especially MR enterograms and venograms), digital subtraction angiography, barium examination, and fistula angiography. An intensive assessment of organ function may also be dictated, for example evaluating the glomerular filtration rate is necessary for chronic renal impairment patients if they are to receive MVTx [7].

9.4 Donor Operation and Recipient Surgery

9.4.1 Donor Operation

The major factor of successful transplantation is the quality of the visceral allograft [12]. Briefly, as part of the standard multiorgan harvest procedure, the process of retrieval of the multivisceral allografts from deceased donors is of great importance [13]. The anatomy of the gut organs is the basement of the harvest technique. For both deceased and living donor allografts, it serves as a key factor to obtain high-quality arterial and venous-free vascular grafts for the back table and in situ vascular reconstructions.

9.4.2 Recipient Surgery

In the early 1990s, Starzl et al. established the most commonly used technique for MVTx, in other words, the retrieval and implantation of multiple grafts [14]. The main types of MVTx are shown in Figs. 9.1 and 9.2.

Figure 9.1 shows full MVTx, in which enteric anastomoses depicted include proximal end-to-end anastomosis between the native stomach and donor stomach and distal side-to-end anastomosis between the donor ileum and native colon sigmoideum. The chimney ileostomy and percutaneous jejunostomy tube are performed. Vascular anastomoses depicted include the arterial inflow of the Carrel patch to the native infrarenal aorta abdominalis and venous outflow of the segment of donor inferior vena cave (IVC), with a confluence of hepatic veins, anastomosed in a piggyback pattern to the native IVC. It should be noted that the donor superior mesenteric vein (SMV) and donor portal vein (not shown) are not interrupted in this type of transplant and do not need anastomosis. In some specific cases, in which preservation of the native colon is achievable, a primary ileocolic anastomosis can be performed and a temporary loop ileostomy can be made to defunction the anastomosis and allow frequent ileoscopy and biopsy of the transplanted bowel.

Figure 9.2 shows modified MVTx, in which enteric anastomoses depicted include side-to-side native-to-donor duodenoduodenostomy to accommodate pancreaticobiliary secretions; proximal end-to-end anastomosis between the native stomach and donor stomach; and distal side-to-side anastomosis between the donor ileum and oversewn native rectum. Vascular anastomoses of this operation consist of arterial inflow of the Carrel patch to the native infrarenal aorta abdominalis (not shown) and venous outflow of the donor SMV, which was directly anastomosed to the native portal vein.

During the procedure, preparing the recipient abdominal cavity for graft implantation and eventual abdominal wall closure is one of the most challenging components. In some cases, patients may have undergone multiple laparotomies before transplantation, where the abdominal cavity is often complex, for example, contraction, dense adhesions, fistulae, collections, and numerous stomata. Therefore, variable resection of the existing intraabdominal internal organs is necessary, aiming to make enough space for the graft and prepare recipient vessels for anastomosis [7]. In patients with short gut syndrome, the loss of the abdominal cavity is one of the most challenging problems. It has been reported that mortality and morbidity are commonly associated with exposed organs. To solve this problem, several innovative surgical strategies have been conducted in clinical practice, like the use of small-for-size allografts, component separation techniques, implantation of tissue expanders before transplant, visceral allograft reduction, myocutaneous flaps, synthetic mesh, acellular dermal allograft, and simultaneous vascularized abdominal wall or nonvascularized rectus fascia transplant [15–19].

9.5 Postoperative Care

Postoperative care serves as a vital part of the process of MVTx. After transplantation, how to manage immunosuppression, monitor the allograft function, and diagnose with prompt treatment of recipient microbial infection are the three key issues.

The use of novel immunosuppressive and immune-modulatory strategies has been one of the seminal contributions that increased the therapeutic efficacy of visceral transplantation. To date, immunology treatment has acquired great achievement in postoperative care like the introduction of induction therapy and receptor preconditioning to the tacrolimus-based immunosuppression regimen. In daily clinical practice, rabbit antithymocyte globulin (rATG), anti-IL-2 receptor humanized antibodies, alemtuzumab, and cyclophosphamide are the most used pharmacologic and biologic agents. Also, mammalian targets of rapamycin (mTOR) inhibitor, mycophenolate mofetil, and azathioprine have been used as adjunctive treatment. Some other immunomodulatory strategies have been used to improve the outcome of MVTx, like bone marrow augmentation, donor pretreatment, and allograft irradiation [20–23]. Besides, how to monitor the functions of allograft and the alloimmune response of recipient remain the central part issue of postoperative care. Progress has been made on monitoring of graft rejection like protocol ileoscopies with multiple random intestinal biopsies and serial measurement of circulating donor-specific antibodies (DSA) [21–23]. On the base of previously defined histopathologic criteria, the diagnosis of chronic rejection, humoral, and acute cellular is established [24, 25]. Patients with elevated transaminases and supported by histopathologic examination of the liver biopsy should be diagnosed as probable liver rejection. Receptors with significant elevation of serum lipase and amylase, without obvious causes of nonimmunologic pancreatitis are commonly accompanied by the rejection of the pancreatic allograft [11].

With the establishment of macrochimerism and microchimerism in the recipients, the graft-versus-host disease may occur, which should be confirmed by histopathologic and immunocytochemical examination including in situ hybridization, polymerase chain reaction (PCR) techniques, the immunohistologic staining of donor-specific HLA antigens, and the short tandem repeat technique [23, 26]. To achieve full nutritional autonomy, enteric feeding mostly begins during the early postoperative period while a reduction in intravenous nutrition is adopted [11].

In recent years, the outcome after MVTx has substantially advanced because ofthe introduction of new antimicrobial drugs, more and more clinical experience, and advanced molecular diagnostic techniques, which reduced the risks of posttransplant lymphoproliferative disorders (PTLD), cytomegalovirus, and fungal infections [6].

9.6 Post-Transplantation Complications

9.6.1 Early Post-Transplantation Complications

In the first few days after transplantation, graft thrombosis is a major risk, especially for patients with previous bowel infarctions, because many patients have a potential for thrombosis. Therefore, prevention and treatment of thrombosis should be started before surgery, including intravenous heparin, low molecular weight heparin, or an epoprostenol infusion [7]. Intestinal anastomotic leakage is more common after transplantation and is usually atypical in clinical manifestations and timing. In this case, inserting a jejunostomy tube at the distal end of the anastomosis during transplantation can provide a useful way for early enteral feeding. Accumulation in the abdominal cavity is common, usually a sterile hematoma or chyle collection, but it can also be inflammatory fluid, anastomotic leakage, intestinal perforation, or a lymphocele, requiring radiological or surgical intervention [7]. The fluid management after MVTx is one of the most challenging parts of postoperative care. The monitoring and replacement of water and electrolytes must be cautious because the huge body fluid losses from the transplanted bowel and the transfer from long-term TPN to enteral nutrition can be very variable and complicated. In particular, the risk of dehydration and acute renal failure still exists for many months after transplantation.

9.6.2 Immunosuppression and Rejection

The transplanted intestine is more likely to be rejected than any other solid organ, and the recipient needs a high level of early maintenance of immune suppression. In multiple organ transplantation, if a liver graft is included, the intestine can provide a certain degree of immune protection, although this effect is variable. Most centers adopt an induction therapy-based regimen that combines tacrolimus monotherapy with anti-lymphocyte monoclonal antibodies, like basiliximab, anti-thymocyte globulin, or alemtuzumab [27]. Post-transplant rejection is most common in the first 3 months after transplantation and requires frequent endoscopy and biopsy (1–2 times/week) for close monitoring. Increased stomal output, increased C-reactive protein, and changes in serum markers of intestinal absorption function (such as albumin) can be used as indicators of rejection, but endoscopy is still the gold standard. Rejection detected by endoscopy ranges from mild erythema to complete mucosal loss. Typical histological findings include apoptotic bodies, loss of crypt cells, and inflammatory infiltration of the lamina propria [7].

9.6.3 Infection

Sepsis is still the main cause of death after intestinal and multiple organ transplantation. In the early stages of transplantation, the burden of immunosuppression significantly increases the risk of postoperative infections and opportunistic infections, especially viral infections, such as cytomegalovirus (CMV) and fungal infections, such as Aspergillus. Preventive measures include broad-spectrum antibiotics and antifungal drugs during the perioperative period, as well as long-term prevention of Pneumocystis carinii (usually cotrimoxazole) and CMV disease (usually ganciclovir). However, refractory CMV infection is still the main cause of morbidity, especially among CMV-negative recipients who receive grafts from CMV-positive donors. This may be due to the overall increase in resistance to antiviral drugs, changes in serum drug levels caused by oral malabsorption of valganciclovir and significant fluctuations in renal function, and the potential role of the transplanted intestine as a site for virus replication [7].

9.7 Outcomes Following Transplantation

According to reports, the survival rates of patients and grafts at 1 year after intestinal and MVTx are 80% and 75%, respectively [28]. Indeed, the 1-year survival rate of isolated small bowel grafts reported by high-volume centers exceeds 90% [29]. The long-term results of MVTx are still relatively poorer. The 2011 International Transplant Registration Report showed that the patients and graft 5-year survival rates were 60% and 50% and continued to improve. Factors found to be related to the improvement of patient survival include the use of induction therapy, the use of sirolimus as maintenance immunosuppression, tacrolimus monotherapy as the main immunosuppression, admission to the hospital for transplantation, transplantation at the hospital with at least 10 cases experience and the age of the recipient [30].

References

1. Grant D, Abu-Elmagd K, Mazariegos G, et al. Intestinal transplant registry report: global activity and trends. Am J Transplant. 2015;15(1):210–9.
2. Abu-Elmagd KM. The small bowel contained allografts:existing and proposed nomenclature. Am J Transplant. 2011;11(1):184–5.
3. Cruz RJ Jr, Costa G, Bond G, Soltys K, Stein WC, Wu G, Martin L, Koritsky D, McMichael J, Sindhi R, et al. Modified "liver-sparing" multivisceral transplant with preserved native spleen, pancreas, and duodenum: technique and long-term outcome. J Gastrointest Surg. 2010;14:1709–21.
4. Nickkholgh A, Contin P, Abu-Elmagd K, et al. Intestinal transplantation: review of operative techniques. Clin Transplant. 2013;27(suppl 25):56–65.
5. Borhani AA, Dasyam AK, Papachristou G, et al. Radiologic features of pancreatic and biliary complications following composite visceral transplantation. Abdom Imaging. 2015;40(6):1961–70.
6. Abu-Elmagd KM, Costa G, Bond G, et al. Five hundred intestinal and multivisceral transplantations at a single center: major advances with new challenges. Ann Surg. 2009;250:567–81.
7. Harper SJF, Jamieson NV. Intestinal and multivisceral transplantation. Surgery (Oxford). 2017;35:391–6.
8. Abu-Elmagd K, Bond G, Reyes J, et al. Intestinal transplantation: a coming of age. Adv Surg. 2002;36:65–101.
9. Abu-Elmagd K, Khanna A, Fujiki M, et al. Surgery for gut failure: autoreconstruction and allotransplantation. In: Fazio V, Church JM, Delaney CP, et al., editors. Current therapy in colon and rectal surgery, vol. 42. Philadelphia: Elsevier; 2017. p. 372–84.
10. Abu-Elmagd KM, Kosmach-Park B, Costa G, et al. Long-term survival, nutritional autonomy, and quality of life after intestinal and multivisceral transplantation. Ann Surg. 2012;256(3):494–508.
11. Costa G, Parekh N, Osman M, Armanyous S, Fujiki M, Abu-Elmagd K. Composite and multivisceral transplantation: nomenclature, surgical techniques, current practice, and long-term outcome. Surg Clin North Am. 2019;99:129–51.
12. Nickkholgh A, Contin P, Abu-Elmagd K, et al. Intestinal transplantation: review of operative techniques. Clin Transpl. 2013;27:56–65.

13. Abu-Elmagd K, Bond G, Reyes J, et al. Intestinal transplantation: a coming of age. Adv Surg. 2002;36:65–101.
14. Starzl TE, Todo S, Tzakis A, et al. The many faces of multivisceral transplantation. Surg Gynecol Obstet. 1991;172:335–44.
15. Carlsen BT, Farmer DG, Busuttil RW, et al. Incidence and management of abdominal wall defects after intestinal and multivisceral transplantation. Plast Reconstr Surg. 2007;119:1247–55.
16. Mangus RS, Kubal CA, Tector AJ, et al. Closure of the abdominal wall with acellular dermal allograft in intestinal transplantation. Am J Transplant. 2012;12:S55–9.
17. Watson MJ, Kundu N, Coppa C, et al. Role of tissue expanders in patients with loss of abdominal domain awaiting intestinal transplantation. Transpl Int. 2013;26:1184–90.
18. Gondolesi G, Selvaggi G, Tzakis A, et al. Use of the abdominal rectus fascia as a nonvascularized allograft for abdominal wall closure after liver, intestinal, and multivisceral transplantation. Transplantation. 2009;87:1884–8.
19. Levi DM, Tzakis AG, Kato T, et al. Transplantation of the abdominal wall. Lancet. 2003;361:2173–6.
20. Abu-Elmagd KM, Costa G, Bond GJ, et al. Evolution of the immunosuppressive strategies for the intestinal and multivisceral recipients with special reference to allograft immunity and achievement of partial tolerance. Transpl Int. 2009;22:96–109.
21. Abu-Elmagd K, Reyes J, Bond G, et al. Clinical intestinal transplantation: a decade of experience at a single center. Ann Surg. 2001;234:404–16.
22. Grant D, Abu-Elmagd K, Masariegos G, et al. Intestinal transplant registry report: global activity and trends. Am J Transplant. 2015;15:210–9.
23. Abu-Elmagd KM, Wu G, Costa G, et al. Preformed and de novo donor specific antibodies in visceral transplantation: long-term outcome with special reference to the liver. Am J Transplant. 2012;12:3047–360.
24. Lee RG, Nakamura K, Tsamandas AC, et al. Pathology of human intestinal transplantation. Gastroenterology. 1996;110:2009–12.
25. Thiede C, Bornhauser M, Oelschlagel U, et al. Sequential monitoring of chimerism and detection of minimal residual disease after allogeneic blood stem cell transplantation (BSCT) using multiplex PCR amplification of short tandem repeat markers. Leukemia. 2001;15:293–302.
26. Abu-Elmagd KM, Costa G, Bond G, et al. Five hundred intestinal and multivisceral transplantations at a single center: major advances with new challenges. Ann Surg. 2009;250:567–81.
27. Mao Q, Li YS, Li JS. The current status of multivisceral transplantation. Hepatobiliary Pancreat Dis Int. 2009;8:345–50.
28. Hanto DW, Fishbein TM, Pinson CW, et al. Liver and intestine transplantation: summary analysis, 1994-2003. Am J Transpl. 2005;5:916–33.
29. Fishbein TM, Kaufman SS, Florman SS, et al. Isolated intestinal transplantation: proof of clinical efficacy. Transplantation. 2003;76:636–40.
30. Fishbein TM. Intestinal transplantation. N Engl J Med. 2009;361:998–1008.

Immunosuppressive Strategies in Transplantation Using Cardiac Death Donors

10

Xiaomin Shi

Abstract

Organs from donors after cardiac death can greatly relieve the critical organ shortage in transplantation. Such organs suffer a longer time of warm ischemia, which compromises organ quality and leads to more severe inflammation. Graft rejection is an unresolved issue that involves all kinds of immune responses. Whether or not the utilization of organs from donors after cardiac death affects graft rejection is incompletely defined. Mechanisms of rejection and the development of immunosuppressive protocols are discussed. Furthermore, current findings on the study of strategies against graft rejection involving organs from donors after cardiac death are summarized.

10.1 Introduction

Graft rejection is an unavoidable issue in transplantation since antigens from the host or donor activate immune responses, which can subsequently lead to dysfunction of the allograft [1]. Based on the origin of antigens, rejection can be divided into host versus graft rejection (HVGR) and graft-versus-host rejection (GVHD). GVHD mostly occurs in bone marrow transplantation while HVGR is the major obstacle in solid organ transplantation. According to the onset time, graft rejection can also be divided into hyperacute rejection (few minutes to few hours after transplantation), acute rejection (in weeks after transplantation), and chronic rejection (months and years after transplantation) [2, 3]. Thanks to the discovery and development of immunosuppressive drugs, the outcome of transplantation has been greatly improved. However, there are side effects of immunosuppressive drugs, such as susceptibility to infection and recurrence of cancer [4]. Therefore, how to generate an ideal immunosuppressive strategy for each patient is still under study [5, 6]. Organs from donors after cardiac death suffer from a longer time of warm ischemia. Whether usage of such organs affects rejection and choice of immunosuppressive strategies remains to be defined.

10.2 Mechanisms of Rejection in Transplantation

Diverse transplantation antigens have been described, including major histocompatibility complex (MHC) molecules, minor histocompatibility antigens, ABO blood group antigens, and monocyte/endothelial cell antigens. Among them, MHC molecules expressed on the surface

X. Shi (✉)
Organ Transplant Center, The First Affiliated Hospital of Sun Yat-sen University, Guangzhou, China
e-mail: shixm5@mail.sysu.edu.cn

X. He (ed.), *Organ Donation and Transplantation after Cardiac Death in China*,
https://doi.org/10.1007/978-981-16-0815-5_10

of the donor cells are the principal target of immune response [7]. In nature, graft rejection is a series of immune responses involving all kinds of immune cells and non-immune cells. Immune responses are a very complex system, which is supposed to be well-tuned as effector cells fight against foreign invaders while regulatory cells protect the body from overactive effector cells [8]. In the setting of transplantation, both inhibition of effector cells and induction of regulatory cells can inhibit rejection [9, 10].

10.2.1 Adaptive Immune Cells

10.2.1.1 T Cells

It is well accepted that T cells play an essential role in rejection. In mouse transplant models, when T cells are depleted, there is neither acute rejection nor chronic rejection [11]. Recipient T cells can be activated by donor antigens directly (by binding to MHC on the surface of donor antigen-presenting cells) and indirectly (by binding to MHC on the surface of recipient antigen-presenting cells). The former is majorly involved in acute rejection while the latter has a dominant role in chronic rejection [2]. CD4-positive T cells recognize MHC-II molecules and CD8-positive T cells recognize MHC-I molecules, while class III MHC genes encode several components of the complement system. The full activation of T cells requires both antigen recognition by TCR and costimulatory signaling. The engagement of costimulatory ligands and receptors promotes the proliferation, function, and survival of T cells, even affects T cell polarization [12]. Therefore, co-stimulation blockade is an important way to induce tolerance in transplantation. CD28 is the most effective and well-characterized costimulatory molecule in T cells. CD28 signaling is activated via binding to its ligand CD80/CD86, which amplifies TCR activation, promotes IL-2 production, inhibits apoptosis induction, prevents anergy, and supports germinal center formation [13]. CTLA-4 also binds to CD80/CD86. It is known that CTLA-4 Ig can induce transplant tolerance via inhibiting CD28 ligation. Another important costimulatory signal on T cells is CD40/CD40L (CD154) [14]. Likewise, anti-CD154 antibody is used to inhibit acute rejection and is widely used in animal chronic rejection models. Apart from effector T cells which promote rejection, there are regulatory T cells that suppress the activation and function of effector T cells and hence induce tolerance [15].

Collectively, to inhibit graft rejection and induce transplant tolerance via T cell modulation, three perspectives are considered: T cell depletion, blocking T cell activation and function, and increasing regulatory T cells [16].

T Cell Depletion

Currently, monoclonal/polyclonal antibodies are available in the clinic to deplete T cells, which include anti-CD3 monoclonal antibody, anti-lymphocyte globulin, both of which are effective in eliminating circulating T cells. Another monoclonal antibody called alemtuzumab (Campath), which is anti-CD52 specific (targeting T cells and B cells), can lead to depletion of both peripheral and central lymphoid (lymph nodes and spleen) lymphocytes as it has been shown that with a short course of alemtuzumab therapy, the peripheral depletion may maintain for up to a year. Clinically, depletion of peripheral leucocytes in the recipient decreases the rate of acute rejection and prolongs the survival of allograft [17].

Blocking T Cell Activation and Function

IL-2 is important for the proliferation and function of T cells. Therefore, blocking IL-2 signaling pathway is a useful way to prevent rejection. Different agents are available for this reason in the clinic, such as anti-CD25 monoclonal antibodies (basiliximab, daclizumab) and calcineurin inhibitors (ciclosporin, tacrolimus) [18]. Another way to inhibit T cells is a costimulatory blockade, such as CTLA4-Ig and anti-CD154 antibody.

Increasing Regulatory T Cells

In humans, the marker for regulatory T cells is $CD4^{+}CD25^{high}CD127^{low}FOXP3^{+}$. Regulatory T cells inhibit the activation and cytokine secretion of effector immune cells (such as T cells and B cells), hence are considered with great potential to induce transplant tolerance [16, 19, 20]. Until April 28, 2019, there are 19 registered clinical trials involving regulatory T cell therapy in transplantation on ClinicalTrials.gov. According to the protocols on the expansion of T regulatory cells, these trails can be divided into two groups: in vivo expansion and ex vivo expansion. However, the long-term safety and outcome of these trials are still under investigation [16, 21].

10.2.1.2 B Cells

Allograft rejection can be classified into three types: T cell-mediated rejection (TCMR), antibody-mediated rejection (AMR, previously named as humoral rejection), and mixed rejection (coexistence of both TCMR and AMR). On the one hand, to regulate TCMR, B cells play a role as antigen-presenting cells, which provide both costimulatory and cytokine signals to activate and stimulate T cells [22–24]. As a matter of fact, B cells consist of the largest population of antigen-presenting cells in the immune system. Under certain circumstances, B cells can enhance the generation of memory T cells [25]. In addition, B cells are able to form tertiary lymphoid organs, which are rich in T cells and B cells so that the interactions between T cells and B cells are strengthened. On the other hand, antibodies produced by B cells are the leading cause of AMR. Donor-specific antibodies can cause hyperacute rejection, which may even be considered as a contraindication to transplantation. Antibodies lead to graft injury and rejection through several different mechanisms, such as antibody-dependent cell cytotoxicity mechanism in which antibody-coated cells are eliminated by killer cells like natural killer cells, complement fixation, vascular injury, expression of adhesion molecules to recruit leukocytes, platelet activation and thrombotic occlusions. However, there are regulatory B cells as well, which have regulatory functions with the production of cytokines IL-10, IL-35, and TGFβ. Regulatory B cells also promote the generation of regulatory T cells via affecting the process of T cell differentiation.

In order to inhibit graft rejection by modulating B cells, interventions are designed from the following perspectives: eliminating/blocking alloantibodies, B cell depletion, suppressing B cell activation and function, plasma cell depletion, and increasing regulatory B cells [26, 27].

10.2.2 Innate Immune Cells

Apart from adaptive immune cells (T cells and B cells), innate immune cells are critically involved in graft rejection and transplant tolerance. Until now, immunosuppressive protocols are majorly aimed at inhibiting adaptive immune cells. However, as the study on adaptive immunity goes further and further, increasing evidences indicate that innate immune cells are affecting graft injury and rejection in previously unknown ways [28, 29].

10.2.2.1 Macrophages/Monocytes

Macrophages are of tremendous plasticity as there is a great overlap of the expressed surface markers between different subsets. Moreover, macrophages are very dynamic since the cytokine milieu can modulate the activity and polarity of macrophages. Currently, macrophages can be generally divided into two types: M1 macrophages (pro-inflammatory, previously referred to as classically activated macrophages) and M2 macrophages (anti-inflammatory, previously referred to as alternatively activated macrophages) [30, 31]. Once activated by LPS and IFN-γ, M1 macrophages produce pro-inflammatory cytokines, including IL-1, IL-6, and TNFα, which favors the differentiation of Th17 cells while inhibits the induction of T regulatory cells. M2 macrophages are activated by IL-4 and IL-13 and produce anti-inflammatory cytokines, such as IL-10 and TGFβ. M2 macrophages have a healing capacity and play an important role in processes like vascular stability, wound healing, and tissue regeneration [32, 33].

In transplant, macrophages and monocytes are rapidly recruited to the allograft and involved in both acute rejection and chronic rejection [34].

Macrophages are the largest population among allograft infiltrating leucocytes (38–80%) in human biopsies. In acute rejection, macrophages can function as antigen-presenting cells as well as pro-inflammatory cytokine-producing cells and adopt the M1 phenotype. However, studies have also shown that 1 year after transplantation, 92% of renal allograft infiltrating macrophages exhibited a $CD68^+CD206^+$ M2-like phenotype. In murine heart transplant model, inhibiting M2 macrophage differentiation suppressed chronic rejection and ameliorated graft vascular disease. Strategies for macrophage-centered immunosuppressive therapies include macrophage deletion, inhibiting macrophage recruitment and activation, modulating the polarization of macrophage subsets, and increasing regulatory macrophages [31].

10.2.2.2 Dendritic Cells (DCs)

As antigen-presenting cells, DCs are messengers that link innate and adaptive immune responses. DCs are categorized into conventional dendritic cells and plasmacytoid dendritic cells. Conventional DCs are further divided into myeloid DCs ($CD11c^+CD11b^+CD205^-$) and lymphoid DCs ($CD11c^+CD205^+CD11b^-$), both of which are potent stimulators for T cell proliferation and differentiation [35]. In addition to antigen presentation, DCs also regulate T cells via co-stimulation and cytokine production, which can modulate the activation and polarization of T cells. In transplant, DCs plays a role in both graft rejection and transplant tolerance. Protocols to induce regulatory DCs (which lead to graft tolerance) have been developed both in vitro and in vivo. In the in vitro protocols, both genetic (transgenic expression of coinhibitory molecules and regulatory immune cytokines) and pharmacological (mTOR inhibitors) interventions are utilized, which have demonstrated efficacy in prolonging graft survival in combination with co-stimulation blockade [36–39].

10.2.2.3 Natural Killer (NK) Cells

NK cells are frequently found in rejecting grafts. It has been demonstrated that NK cells modulate both graft rejection and transplant tolerance in various transplant models [28, 35]. NK cells have a unique self and non-self recognition system. Both stimulatory and inhibitory receptors are expressed on the surface of NK cells and the signals from both types of receptors are required to make NK cells tolerant of autologous cells. An essential feature in the system is that the ligands of inhibitory receptors are self MHC class I molecules and MHC class I molecules are expressed on all nucleated cells. Thanks to this setting, NK cells do not attack self cells. In transplant, NK cells can recognize donor cells vis such "missing self" or "missing ligand" recognition system since donor cells lack self MHC class I molecules to engage with inhibitory receptors. Once activated by allogeneic cells, NK cells acquire abilities to perform cytolytic function and produce pro-inflammatory cytokines. Another unexpected role of NK cells is the induction of tolerance in transplantation. The mechanism is that NK cells recognize and kill allogeneic donor antigen-presenting cells, which are required for the priming of alloreactive T cells in a direct way. Likewise, the elimination of other donor cells can also inhibit the activation of T cells in an indirect way [40–43].

10.3 The History of the Development of Immunosuppressive Drugs

As mentioned above, the development of immunosuppressive drugs plays a pivotal role in the progression of organ transplantation. Undoubtedly, each groundbreaking discovery on immunosuppressive drugs in history significantly advanced the development and application of transplantation. Up to date, there are three kinds of representative immunosuppressive drugs as they have changed immunosuppressive strategies in the clinic [44].

10.3.1 Azathioprine

Azathioprine was developed in 1961. Together with glucocorticoid, Azathioprine led to the long-term survival of allograft, which pioneered the application of immunosuppressive drugs in transplantation and laid the foundation of immunosuppressive strategies till now. Azathioprine functions metabolically to inhibit the synthesis of DNA, which limits cell proliferation and leads to apoptosis. Azathioprine suppresses cellular immunity as well as humoral immunity. Upon the development of Azathioprine, the immunosuppressive strategy at that time was to adjust the usage of glucocorticoid on the basis of the application of Azathioprine. However, the effect of Azathioprine is not specific, which may result in metabolic disorder, such as high blood glucose, high blood lipid, and high blood pressure. Later in the 1980s, it was found that mycophenolic acid (MPA) specifically inhibits DNA synthesis in T cells and B cells. In the early 1990s, the precursor of MPA, Mycophenolate mofetil (MMF) started to be used against acute rejection [45, 46].

10.3.2 Ciclosporin A (CsA)

Another milestone in transplantation is the discovery and application of CsA. The initial purpose to extract CsA was to take it as a potential anti-fungi drug, which did not work. However, CsA was proved to be a powerful immunosuppressive drug as in 1978, it was reported that CsA strikingly increased the survival rates of kidney transplantation and bone marrow transplantation. Later, the immunosuppressive effect of CsA was further confirmed in the transplantation of other organs [47]. Since then, the golden standard of immunosuppressive strategy has formed: triple-drug immunosuppression, which utilizes the combination of three kinds of drugs: CsA, Azathioprine, and glucocorticoid. Thanks to CsA, the early 1980s witnessed the rapid development of transplantation. Mechanistically, CsA is a calcineurin inhibitor, which blocks IL-2 signaling pathway to inhibit the proliferation and function of T lymphocytes as well as to prevent the production and effect of T memory cells. The major side effects of CsA include kidney toxicity, liver toxicity, and nervous system toxicity. Therefore, the concentration of CsA and the functions of related organs need to be closely monitored. The discovery of CsA as an immunosuppressive drug not only improved the survival rate of transplantation by inhibiting graft rejection but also deepened the understanding of the mechanisms of rejection and facilitated the study on how to inhibit rejection as well as how to induce tolerance [48].

10.3.3 Tacrolimus (FK506)

FK506 was first applied in liver transplantation in 1987 by Dr. Starzl, which yielded a satisfactory outcome. In the 1990s, FK506 was brought to market first in Japan, then in other countries, such as the USA, England, and China. Nowadays, FK506 is the most widely used immunosuppressive drug in the clinic. Mechanistically, FK506, which is also a calcineurin inhibitor, functions similarly to CsA. However, FK506 has many advantages over CsA. In terms of effectiveness, FK506 is 50–100 times more efficient than CsA, indicating FK506 functions at a much lower dose, hence has fewer side effects and better outcomes. Currently, one of the routine immunosuppressive strategies is to combinedly use glucocorticoid, FK506 and MMF.

In addition to the immunosuppressive drugs mentioned above, there are many other ones, such as mTOR targeting drugs (sirolimus), monoclonal antibodies (anti-CD3, anti-CD25, anti-CD52), and polyclonal antibodies (anti-lymphocytic globulin, anti-thymocyte globulin). Different combinations of immunosuppressive drugs should be used case by case. For example, due to the feature of nephrotoxicity of calcineurin inhibitors (CNI), there are CNI free immunosuppressive protocols in renal transplantation.

10.4 Comparison of the Outcomes for Transplantation Between DBD and DCD

Donors from cardiac death (DCD) are classified into two groups: uncontrolled DCD (uDCD) and controlled DCD (cDCD). Currently, worldwide, most DCD transplants are with organs from controlled DCD. Compared to DBD, organs from cDCD suffer a longer time of ischemia, which has raised concerns about organ quality. As in renal transplantation, the incidence of delayed graft function (DGF) is strikingly higher in DCD transplantation than that in DBD transplantation. However, the long-term patient survival is comparable [5, 6, 49]. Data from several transplant centers in different countries also demonstrate that the overall outcome of lung transplant and pancreas/islet transplant with organs/tissues from DCD or DBD is comparable [50, 51]. Early results on the outcomes for DCD heart transplantation are also encouraging [52, 53]. However, the outcomes for DCD liver transplantation are not satisfactory due to higher complication rates, particularly biliary complications [54–58]. Still, increased use of organs from DCD is a promising way to expand the donor pool. However, DCD organ transplantation has to be more standardized in terms of donor/recipient selection, organ procurement, organ storage (perfusion protocol), and immunosuppressive therapy [59].

10.5 Updates on Immunosuppressive Protocols in DCD Transplantation

The incidence rate of DGF is significantly higher in DCD renal transplantation than that in DBD renal transplantation. DGF requires dialysis intervention and is associated with higher rates of acute rejection and shorter graft survival. Therefore, it is assumed that enhanced immunosuppression is needed post-transplantation in DCD renal transplantation. It has been demonstrated that enhanced immunosuppressive protocols improve graft function in the early post-transplant phase in the porcine renal transplant model using donors after cardiac death. In the large animal study, as expected, a significant increase in creatinine levels was observed in the DCD group compared to the non-DCD group. Enhanced immunosuppression promoted the recovery of renal functions and inhibited inflammation as well as acute rejection [60]. On the other hand, to minimize nephrotoxicity, CNI free immunosuppressive protocols were proposed, such as the combination of sirolimus, MMF, and basiliximab [45, 61]. However, CNI free immunosuppressive protocols were ineffective according to results from clinical trials (either no obvious advantage or even worse outcome). Therefore, delayed CNI free therapy after induction and CNI minimization are the most frequently used strategies. Currently, DCD donation is usually ruled out or constitutes a very small proportion in all kinds of randomized clinical trials, leading to missing information on the outcomes of various immunosuppressive protocols in transplantation using donors after cardiac death.

10.6 Conclusion

Even though DCD donation should not be taken as an equally acceptable alternative to DBD donation due to compromised graft quality caused by longer warm ischemia time, using organs from donors after cardiac death has been proved to be an effective way to expand the donor pool. It is essential to further explore the potential of DCD donation, particularly the long-term outcomes of transplantation with such donation. Moreover, the development and implementation of uniform guidelines will be of great importance for the appropriate use of such donation pools in the clinic, which include ethical concerns, donor/patient selection, organ procurement, organ storage, immunosuppressive therapies, etc. Research in the porcine renal transplant model has provided evidences that enhanced immunosuppressive protocols improve early allograft function with donors after cardiac death. However, well-designed clinical trials to evaluate different immunosuppressive protocols in transplantation using donors from cardiac death are needed to find the optimal strategy of immunosuppressive therapy.

References

1. Le Moine A, Goldman M, Abramowicz D. Multiple pathways to allograft rejection. Transplantation. 2002;73(9):1373–81.
2. Alegre ML, Florquin S, Goldman M. Cellular mechanisms underlying acute graft rejection: time for reassessment. Curr Opin Immunol. 2007;19(5):563–8.
3. Libby P, Pober JS. Chronic rejection. Immunity. 2001;14(4):387–97.
4. Christians U, Klawitter J, Klawitter J, Brunner N, Schmitz V. Biomarkers of immunosuppressant organ toxicity after transplantation: status, concepts and misconceptions. Expert Opin Drug Metab Toxicol. 2011;7(2):175–200.
5. Gavriilidis P, Inston NG. Recipient and allograft survival following donation after circulatory death versus donation after brain death for renal transplantation: a systematic review and meta-analysis. Transplant Rev (Orlando). 2020:100563.
6. Nankivell BJ, Alexander SI. Rejection of the kidney allograft. N Engl J Med. 2010;363(15):1451–62.
7. Adams AB, Williams MA, Jones TR, Shirasugi N, Durham MM, Kaech SM, et al. Heterologous immunity provides a potent barrier to transplantation tolerance. J Clin Invest. 2003;111(12):1887–95.
8. Chaplin DD. Overview of the human immune response. J Allergy Clin Immunol. 2006;117(2 Suppl Mini-Primer):S430–5.
9. Moreau A, Varey E, Anegon I, Cuturi MC. Effector mechanisms of rejection. Cold Spring Harb Perspect Med. 2013;3(11).
10. Terasaki PI, Cai J. Humoral theory of transplantation: further evidence. Curr Opin Immunol. 2005;17(5):541–5.
11. von Andrian UH, Mackay CR. T-cell function and migration. Two sides of the same coin. N Engl J Med. 2000;343(14):1020–34.
12. Wang D, Matsumoto R, You Y, Che T, Lin XY, Gaffen SL, et al. CD3/CD28 costimulation-induced NF-kappaB activation is mediated by recruitment of protein kinase C-theta, Bcl10, and IkappaB kinase beta to the immunological synapse through CARMA1. Mol Cell Biol. 2004;24(1):164–71.
13. Bromley SK, Iaboni A, Davis SJ, Whitty A, Green JM, Shaw AS, et al. The immunological synapse and CD28-CD80 interactions. Nat Immunol. 2001;2(12):1159–66.
14. Okimura K, Maeta K, Kobayashi N, Goto M, Kano N, Ishihara T, et al. Characterization of ASKP1240, a fully human antibody targeting human CD40 with potent immunosuppressive effects. Am J Transplant. 2014;14(6):1290–9.
15. Josefowicz SZ, Lu LF, Rudensky AY. Regulatory T cells: mechanisms of differentiation and function. Annu Rev Immunol. 2012;30:531–64.
16. Wood KJ, Sakaguchi S. Regulatory T cells in transplantation tolerance. Nat Rev Immunol. 2003;3(3):199–210.
17. Knechtle SJ, Pirsch JDH, Fechner JJ, Becker BN, Friedl A, Colvin RB, et al. Campath-1H induction plus rapamycin monotherapy for renal transplantation: results of a pilot study. Am J Transplant. 2003;3(6):722–30.
18. Borel JF, Feurer C, Gubler HU, Stahelin H. Biological effects of cyclosporin A: a new antilymphocytic agent. Agents Actions. 1976;6(4):468–75.
19. Cobbold SP, Graca L, Lin CY, Adams E, Waldmann H. Regulatory T cells in the induction and maintenance of peripheral transplantation tolerance. Transpl Int. 2003;16(2):66–75.
20. Graca L, Cobbold SP, Waldmann H. Identification of regulatory T cells in tolerated allografts. J Exp Med. 2002;195(12):1641–6.
21. Zheng XX, Sanchez-Fueyo A, Sho M, Domenig C, Sayegh MH, Strom TB. Favorably tipping the balance between cytopathic and regulatory T cells to create transplantation tolerance. Immunity. 2003;19(4):503–14.
22. Dong C, Temann UA, Flavell RA. Cutting edge: critical role of inducible costimulator in germinal center reactions. J Immunol. 2001;166(6):3659–62.
23. Jacquot S. CD27/CD70 interactions regulate T dependent B cell differentiation. Immunol Res. 2000;21(1):23–30.
24. Karahan GE, Claas FH, Heidt S. B cell immunity in solid organ transplantation. Front Immunol. 2016;7:686.
25. Pallier A, Hillion S, Danger R, Giral M, Racape M, Degauque N, et al. Patients with drug-free long-term graft function display increased numbers of peripheral B cells with a memory and inhibitory phenotype. Kidney Int. 2010;78(5):503–13.
26. Li Z, Wang M, Yao X, Li H, Li S, Liu L, et al. Development of novel anti-CD19 antibody-drug conjugates for B-cell lymphoma treatment. Int Immunopharmacol. 2018;62:299–308.
27. Callaghan CJ, Rouhani FJ, Negus MC, Curry AJ, Bolton EM, Bradley JA, et al. Abrogation of antibody-mediated allograft rejection by regulatory CD4 T cells with indirect allospecificity. J Immunol. 2007;178(4):2221–8.
28. He H, Stone JR, Perkins DL. Analysis of robust innate immune response after transplantation in the absence of adaptive immunity. Transplantation. 2002;73(6):853–61.
29. Iwasaki A, Medzhitov R. Regulation of adaptive immunity by the innate immune system. Science. 2010;327(5963):291–5.
30. Gordon S, Martinez FO. Alternative activation of macrophages: mechanism and functions. Immunity. 2010;32(5):593–604.

31. Mosser DM, Edwards JP. Exploring the full spectrum of macrophage activation. Nat Rev Immunol. 2008;8(12):958–69.
32. Jetten N, Verbruggen S, Gijbels MJ, Post MJ, De Winther MP, Donners MM. Anti-inflammatory M2, but not pro-inflammatory M1 macrophages promote angiogenesis in vivo. Angiogenesis. 2014;17(1):109–18.
33. Mantovani A, Biswas SK, Galdiero MR, Sica A, Locati M. Macrophage plasticity and polarization in tissue repair and remodelling. J Pathol. 2013;229(2):176–85.
34. Kitchens WH, Chase CM, Uehara S, Cornell LD, Colvin RB, Russell PS, et al. Macrophage depletion suppresses cardiac allograft vasculopathy in mice. Am J Transplant. 2007;7(12):2675–82.
35. Degli-Esposti MA, Smyth MJ. Close encounters of different kinds: dendritic cells and NK cells take centre stage. Nat Rev Immunol. 2005;5(2):112–24.
36. Cobbold SP, Nolan KF, Graca L, Castejon R, Le Moine A, Frewin M, et al. Regulatory T cells and dendritic cells in transplantation tolerance: molecular markers and mechanisms. Immunol Rev. 2003;196:109–24.
37. Morelli AE, Thomson AW. Tolerogenic dendritic cells and the quest for transplant tolerance. Nat Rev Immunol. 2007;7(8):610–21.
38. Turnquist HR, Thomson AW. Taming the lions: manipulating dendritic cells for use as negative cellular vaccines in organ transplantation. Curr Opin Organ Transplant. 2008;13(4):350–7.
39. Turnquist HR, Raimondi G, Zahorchak AF, Fischer RT, Wang Z, Thomson AW. Rapamycin-conditioned dendritic cells are poor stimulators of allogeneic CD4+ T cells, but enrich for antigen-specific Foxp3+ T regulatory cells and promote organ transplant tolerance. J Immunol. 2007;178(11):7018–31.
40. Gill RG. NK cells: elusive participants in transplantation immunity and tolerance. Curr Opin Immunol. 2010;22(5):649–54.
41. Laffont S, Seillet C, Ortaldo J, Coudert JD, Guery JC. Natural killer cells recruited into lymph nodes inhibit alloreactive T-cell activation through perforin-mediated killing of donor allogeneic dendritic cells. Blood. 2008;112(3):661–71.
42. Roy S, Barnes PF, Garg A, Wu S, Cosman D, Vankayalapati R. NK cells lyse T regulatory cells that expand in response to an intracellular pathogen. J Immunol. 2008;180(3):1729–36.
43. Yu G, Xu X, Vu MD, Kilpatrick ED, Li XC. NK cells promote transplant tolerance by killing donor antigen-presenting cells. J Exp Med. 2006;203(8):1851–8.
44. Halloran PF. Immunosuppressive drugs for kidney transplantation. N Engl J Med. 2004;351(26):2715–29.
45. Kreis H, Cisterne JM, Land W, Wramner L, Squifflet JP, Abramowicz D, et al. Sirolimus in association with mycophenolate mofetil induction for the prevention of acute graft rejection in renal allograft recipients. Transplantation. 2000;69(7):1252–60.
46. Meier-Kriesche HU, Steffen BJ, Hochberg AM, Gordon RD, Liebman MN, Morris JA, et al. Long-term use of mycophenolate mofetil is associated with a reduction in the incidence and risk of late rejection. Am J Transplant. 2003;3(1):68–73.
47. Saburi M, Kohashi S, Kato J, Koda Y, Sakurai M, Toyama T, et al. Effects of calcineurin inhibitors on sodium excretion in recipients of allogeneic hematopoietic stem cell transplantation. Int J Hematol. 2017;106(3):431–5.
48. Bram RJ, Hung DT, Martin PK, Schreiber SL, Crabtree GR. Identification of the immunophilins capable of mediating inhibition of signal transduction by cyclosporin A and FK506: roles of calcineurin binding and cellular location. Mol Cell Biol. 1993;13(8):4760–9.
49. Lamb KE, Lodhi S, Meier-Kriesche HU. Long-term renal allograft survival in the United States: a critical reappraisal. Am J Transplant. 2011;11(3):450–62.
50. Snell G, Levvey B, Paraskeva M, Whitford H, Levin K, Williams T, et al. Controlled donation after circulatory death (DCD) donors: a focus on the utilization of pediatric donors and outcomes after lung transplantation. J Heart Lung Transplant. 2019;38(10):1089–96.
51. Berney T, Boffa C, Augustine T, Badet L, de Koning E, Pratschke J, et al. Utilization of organs from donors after circulatory death for vascularized pancreas and islet of Langerhans transplantation: recommendations from an expert group. Transpl Int. 2016;29(7):798–806.
52. Macdonald P, Dhital K. Heart transplantation from donation-after-circulatory-death (DCD) donors: back to the future-evolving trends in heart transplantation from DCD donors. J Heart Lung Transplant. 2019;38(6):599–600.
53. Quader M, Toldo S, Chen Q, Hundley G, Kasirajan V. Heart transplantation from donation after circulatory death donors: present and future. J Card Surg. 2020;35(4):875–85.
54. Bath NM, Leverson G, Al-Adra DP, D'Alessandro AM, Mezrich JD, Foley DP. Microsteatosis in livers from donation after circulatory death donors is associated with inferior outcomes following liver transplantation. Liver Transpl. 2020;26(9):1127–37.
55. Brol MJ, Trebicka J. Changing dogma in donation after circulatory death liver transplantation? The role of microsteatosis and macrosteatosis in allografts. Liver Transpl. 2020;26(9):1085–7.
56. Cascales-Campos PA, Ferreras D, Alconchel F, Febrero B, Royo-Villanova M, Martinez M, et al. Controlled donation after circulatory death up to 80 years for liver transplantation: pushing the limit again. Am J Transplant. 2020;20(1):204–12.
57. Lazzeri C, Bonizzoli M, Marra F, Muiesan P, Ghinolfi D, De Simone P, et al. Uncontrolled donation after circulatory death and liver transplantation: evidence and unresolved issues. Minerva Anestesiol. 2020;86(2):196–204.
58. Nostedt JJ, Shapiro J, Freed DH, Bigam DL. Addressing organ shortages: progress in donation after circulatory death for liver transplantation. Can J Surg. 2020;63(2):E135–E41.

59. Foley DP. Simultaneous liver and kidney transplantation using organs from donation after circulatory death donors in the contemporary era: we are getting better! Liver Transpl. 2020;26(3):327–9.
60. Xu M, Garcia-Aroz S, Banan B, Wang X, Rabe BJ, Zhou F, et al. Enhanced immunosuppression improves early allograft function in a porcine kidney transplant model of donation after circulatory death. Am J Transplant. 2019;19(3):713–23.
61. Johnson RW, Kreis H, Oberbauer R, Brattstrom C, Claesson K, Eris J. Sirolimus allows early cyclosporine withdrawal in renal transplantation resulting in improved renal function and lower blood pressure. Transplantation. 2001;72(5):777–86.

Ischemia and Reperfusion Injury in Organ Transplantation from Cardiac Death Donors

11

Longshan Liu and Xirui Li

Abstract

The maintenance of normal functions of tissues and organs depends on good blood circulation. When the blood supply stops or drops, the nutrition and oxygen supply of the tissue cannot meet the needs, resulting in hypoxia of the tissue. However, when blood flow is restored, with the improvement of nutrition and oxygen supply, it leads to more serious tissue damage and inflammatory reaction. This kind of tissue injury caused by blood flow restoration is called reperfusion injury. Ischemia-reperfusion injury is common in the clinic, such as ischemia-reperfusion injury of various organs (heart, brain, liver, etc.) caused by thrombolytic therapy after thrombosis, ischemia-reperfusion injury of multiple organs caused by resuscitation after cardiogenic or ischemic shock, and ischemia-reperfusion injury of grafts caused by blood reflow after organ acquisition and transplantation. Although the pathological features of ischemia-reperfusion injury are similar, there are great differences among different organs, different degrees of ischemia and different ranges of ischemia. There are different characteristics between systemic ischemia-reperfusion and local ischemia-reperfusion. Even in the same organ, the pathophysiological process of warm ischemia and cold ischemia (in vitro protection process of transplanted donor organs) is also obviously different. Also, ischemia-reperfusion injury of local organs can cause injury of other organs and even multiple organs of the whole body through inflammatory reaction.

L. Liu (✉) · X. Li
Organ Transplant Center, The First Affiliated Hospital of Sun Yat-sen University,
Guangzhou, Guangdong, China

11.1 Overview

11.1.1 Definition of Ischemia-Reperfusion Injury (IRI)

Ischemia-reperfusion injury (IRI) is defined as a series of organ and tissue injuries following the restoration of blood flow to previously hypoxic-ischemic damage, which mostly occurs after shock, vascular recanalization, cardiopulmonary bypass, cardiopulmonary resuscitation, and organ transplantation.

The phenomenon of cardiac ischemia-reperfusion was first reported by Sewell in 1955. In 1960, Jennings proposed the concept of IRI for the first time and confirmed that reperfusion injury could cause irreversible myocardial damage [1]. Since then, there have been reports of IRI in the brain, liver, kidney, lungs, and the small intestine, demonstrating that IRI can cause dam-

X. He (ed.), *Organ Donation and Transplantation after Cardiac Death in China*,
https://doi.org/10.1007/978-981-16-0815-5_11

age to almost all organs and tissues. IRI is affected by multiple factors, including the ischemic duration (a prolonged duration of ischemia results in organ necrosis; development of collateral circulation, tolerance to hypoxia, reperfusion conditions (high pressure, high temperature, high PH) and so on [2].

Organ or tissue IRI is a pathological process involving multi-system (graft microcirculatory disorder, immune activation-inhibition imbalance, etc.), multiple cells (including T lymphocytes, neutrophils, tissue-specific macrophages, vascular endothelial cells, etc.) and molecules (oxygen free radicals-reactive oxygen species, endothelin, NO, adhesion molecules, chemokines, platelet-activating factor, etc.).

11.1.2 Impact of IRI on the Graft and IRI Features in DCD Donors

The donor organ inevitably experiences ischemic injury from the moment it is separated from donor blood. The injury initiates during the removal of the donor organ, which is related to a warm ischemic period caused by a temporary surgical procedure. Subsequently, it is followed by a relatively long period of cold ischemia in the cryopreservation solution. Finally, a short warm ischemic period appears during graft implantation. When the graft is revascularized, the blood of the ischemic organ reflows and induces a series of events that aggravate the graft injury, including oxygen free radical activation, calcium overload, etc. This pathological injury, described as IRI during organ transplantation, is commonly seen in transplantation surgery and largely inevitable. IRI during organ transplantation can induce cytokine storm, aggravates rejection and seriously affects the recovery of graft function.

11.1.2.1 Impact of IRI on Renal Transplantation

Early IRI in the donor's kidney triggers nonspecific inflammatory response, impairs graft renal function, induces graft vascular injury and chronic hypoxia, promotes fibrosis, and ultimately leads to graft dysfunction or even renal failure. In addition, IRI is also closely related to the occurrence of acute immune rejection and reduces graft survival [3]. In clinical practice, renal replacement therapy is required within 1 week after renal transplantation if postoperative renal dysfunction occurs early, which is called delayed graft function (DGF). Clinical evidence has proved that the risk of postoperative DGF in the transplanted kidney increases with the prolongation of ischemia time, and the prolongation of cold ischemia time is an independent risk factor for delayed graft function recovery. Long-term cold ischemia will greatly increase the occurrence of DGF and acute immune rejection and shorten the survival time of the graft [4]. Previous cohort study also showed that DCD donors did not differ significantly from DBD donors in the 5-year graft survival rate. However, the incidence of delayed graft function recovery of DCD grafts was significantly higher than that of DBD grafts [5].

11.1.2.2 Impact of IRI on Liver Transplantation

IRI is considered as an important risk factor for liver graft injury [6]. The liver graft encounters warm ischemia during harvesting, subsequent cold ischemia during preservation and a second hit of reperfusion injury during blood reflow. This process may induce mild graft dysfunction and even graft failure. Studies have shown that IRI is an important cause of liver failure after hepatectomy and early graft non-immunological incompetence after liver transplantation. It also increases the possibility of acute and chronic postoperative rejection, leading to late immunological incompetence [7].

The pathological process of IRI is briefly described as follows: ischemia and hypoxia cause cellular energy deficiency, transmembrane transport disorder, endothelial cell edema, vasoconstriction, sinusoidal stenosis, and leukocyte retention, aggravating sinusoidal microcirculation disorder and prolonging ischemia and hypoxia following blood reflow. Meanwhile, the retained leukocytes interact with endothelial cells, release inflammatory factors, further activate the Kupffer cells, and aggravate the inflammatory response. After reflowing, tissue reoxygenation leads to an abundant production of oxygen free radicals, further aggravates liver tissue injury [8–10].

11.1.2.3 Impact of IRI on Lung Transplantation

Oxygen can be obtained from the alveoli and dual blood supply system (pulmonary arteries, bronchial artery) for the lungs. The lungs, therefore, are more tolerable to ischemia compared to other organs. In lung transplantation, oxygen is inaccessible for the lungs due to a complete block of ventilation and blood flow. The damage related to lung transplantation is, therefore, more severe than ventilatory hypoxia-related injury (such as thrombotic diseases, etc.) [11].

When ischemia occurs, vascular endothelial cells are damaged, immune cells are activated, and adhesion molecules are up-regulated, resulting in increased microvascular resistance and permeability. Recanalization after reperfusion results in pulmonary edema, ventilation-perfusion mismatch, and gas exchange disorder [12]. In addition, alveolar macrophages release phospholipase A2, which degrades surfactant, resulting in decreased alveolar compliance and affecting lung function [13]. During reperfusion, the transplanted lung may experience a "no-reflow phenomenon" (no-reflow phenomenon), which means that microcirculatory blood flow cannot be restored although ventilation has been restored and blood vessels have opened. During the ischemic phase, pulmonary parenchymal cells release chemokines, causing a large number of inflammatory cells (e.g., macrophages, neutrophils, and T cells) to adhere and occlude the microcirculation [14]. This phenomenon may be responsible for delayed recovery of transplanted lung function or persistent functional abnormalities. It is of note that injury to the contralateral lung may occur after reperfusion, even with unilateral lung ischemia [15].

A DCD donor usually refers to a patient who has failed resuscitation or is awaiting cardiac death. The organs donated by DCD donors usually suffer a certain degree of hypoperfusion and hypoxic damage before acquisition because the vital signs (such as respiration, heartbeat, blood pressure, blood oxygen saturation, etc.) and the internal environment (including electrolytes, PH, etc.) experience great fluctuations in the final stage of life. DCD organs are associated with serious IRI injury [16].

11.2 Pathophysiological Mechanisms of IRI

11.2.1 Damage by Reactive Oxygen Species

Reactive oxygen species damage is the most important injury pathway after ischemia-hypoxia and blood reflow. Reactive oxygen species refer to chemically active oxygen-containing metabolites, including oxygen free radicals (such as superoxide anion and hydroxyl radical), hydrogen peroxide, singlet oxygen, lipid peroxides and their metabolites. The oxidative burst is related to various tissue damage. It causes lipid peroxidation of the cell membrane, destroys the membrane structure, reduces membrane fluidity and permeability, inducing intracellular calcium overload. At the same time, dysfunction of membrane protein, calcium pump and sodium pump result in intracellular calcium overload and cell swelling [17]. Oxygen free radicals also directly inhibit protein function. For example, they decrease muscle fibrin activity and reduce myocardial contractility. Sarcoplasmic reticulum calcium transport can be inhibited by oxygen free radicals, which end in abnormal intracellular calcium regulation. In addition, these excessive oxygen free radicals also impair nucleic acids and chromosomes [18, 19].

11.2.2 Calcium Overload

Calcium overload mediates tissue damage during ischemia-reperfusion. Calcium overload is a phenomenon manifested by cell injury and dysfunction due to increased intracellular calcium content (calcium paradox) with multiple causes.

The main causes of calcium overload during IRI include abnormal sodium-calcium exchange and biofilm damage. Ischemia and hypoxia cause ATP synthesis disorder and sodium pump activity to decrease, leading to high intracellular Na^+ levels. Meanwhile, ischemia induces acidosis. After reperfusion, the interstitial H^+ level decreases, but intracellular high H^+ level is maintained. The high Na^+ and H^+ levels activate the Na^+-Ca^{2+} exchanger and intracellular calcium overload. The highly activated intracellular protein kinase C can also indirectly activate the Na^+-Ca^{2+} exchanger. Increased cell membrane permeability and membrane protein dysfunction lead to calcium influx. Sarcoplasmic reticulum lipid peroxidation damage and insufficient ATP production both result in calcium pump dysfunction and reduced sarcoplasmic reticulum calcium intake. Mitochondrial membrane dysfunction, decreased ATP synthesis, and impaired intracellular antioxidant system result in increased oxygen free radicals.

Intracellular calcium overload contributes to increased generation of oxygen free radicals (activation of calcium-dependent proteolytic enzymes), aggravated acidosis and biofilm damage (ATPase activation, hydrolysis of high-energy phosphate, release of large amounts of H^+/activate phospholipases, decomposition of membrane structure), and mitochondrial dysfunction (calcium overload in mitochondria, inhibition of oxidative phosphorylation) [20].

11.2.3 Impact of Leukocyte

Ischemia induces endothelial cell injury, tissue swelling, capillary narrowing, leukocyte and platelet adhesion, thrombosis, and capillary injury. The No-reflow phenomenon is manifested by insufficient microvascular perfusion even if the blood flow is restored. This phenomenon further prolongs ischemia time and aggravates tissue damage.

During ischemia, the velocity of the local blood flow is reduced, endothelial cells are swollen, and the lumens are narrowed, which is conducive to leukocyte adhesion. Vascular endothelial injury and increased production of adhesion molecules and chemokines promote the recruitment, adhesion, and aggregation of leukocytes. Aggregated leukocytes release a large number of pro-inflammatory factors, such as free radicals and lysosomal enzymes, which further aggravate tissue and cellular injury [21].

11.3 Molecular Mechanisms Involved in IRI Regulation

11.3.1 Toll-Like Receptors Pathways

Toll-like receptors (TLR) are important transmembrane protein receptors involved in innate immunity and act as a bridge between non-specific and specific immunity. TLR mainly recognizes molecules with conserved structures derived from external microorganisms and activates the body to generate immune responses. In addition, TLR also responds to endogenous ligands and is activated under internal stress. Through downstream protein–protein interactions, endogenous, or exogenous pressure signals are transmitted to the nucleus, causing a series of downstream gene expression changes, including the up-regulation of pro-inflammatory factors and changes in the mitochondrial respiratory chain [22].

The Human Toll-like receptors (TLRs) family includes ten members. Ischemia significantly upregulates TLR2 and TLR4 expression and induces apoptosis. TLR2 and TLR4 show multivalent ligand-binding activity and can be activated by exogenous ligands (e.g., lipopolysaccharide) and endogenous ligands (e.g., heat shock protein, non-histone chromatin-binding protein high-mobility group box 1, and extracellular matrix components (hyaluronic acid, fibronectin, etc.)) [23, 24]. Hence, TLRs specifically recognize exogenous mediators (such as pathogens, etc.) or endogenous mediators and activate the innate and adaptive immune systems. Ischemia-reperfusion of donor organs can activate the innate and adaptive immune systems through both exogenous and endogenous pathways and then activate the TLRs family to mediate graft injury. Additionally, TLRs are also involved in the process of acute and chronic immune rejection [25].

11.3.2 Heat Shock Protein (HSP) Pathway

HSP is a highly conserved protein molecule that exists widely in prokaryotic and eukaryotic organisms. HSP expression is up-regulated, and the body's self-protection mechanism is initiated once in a state of high temperature, nutrient deprivation, and oxidative stress [26]. HSP promotes proper protein folding and refolding and maintains protein structure stability mainly in the form of chaperones. HSP contains six families (HSP110, 90, 70, 60, 40, and small molecule HSP) and is involved in the development of multiple diseases [27].

It has been shown that induction of HSP70 expression can enhance myocardial antioxidant capacity, stabilize macromolecular protein structure, and reduce myocardial IRI [28]. Induction of HSP70 expression alleviates renal IRI injury as well. HSP72 reduces the stress response, protects glomerular endothelial cells, and mitigates apoptosis and necrosis [29]. HSP27 up-regulation attenuates hepatic IRI [30]. In summary, HSP as a protective protein has a protective effect on IRI in multiple organs and tissues.

11.3.3 Hypoxia-Inducible Factor (HIF) Pathway

HIF pathway is a protective response following hypoxia, which is characterized by the up-regulation of some specific genes. The key regulator of this pathway is HIF, a transcription factor regulating metabolic adaptation, angiogenesis, red blood cell production, cell growth, survival, and apoptosis. HIF is also engaged in physiological hypoxia, regulating stem cell microenvironment, embryonic development, and tumor metastasis [31].

HIF consists of two subunits: the oxygen-sensitive HIF-α and the constitutively expressed HIF-β subunit [32]. HIF-1α is hydroxylated and involved in the formation of HIF-1α/PvHL/ubiquitin ligase complex, which is responsible for ubiquitinated degradation of HIF-1α to maintain low concentrations under normoxic conditions [33]. Under hypoxia, hydroxylation is inhibited. The HIF-α subunit dimerizes with HIF-1β without ubiquitinated degradation and then enters the nucleus to regulate the gene expression. These gene products participate in normal physiological responses and adaptive cell survival [34].

Many studies have proved the protective effect of HIF-1α in IRI [35, 36]. Previous studies demonstrated that HIF-2α mitigates myocardial IRI by inducing the expression of epithelial growth factor biregulin (AREG) and enhancing myocardial tolerance to ischemia [37]. Up-regulation of HIF and HIF pathway activation initiate the body's self-protection mechanism and mitigate IRI.

11.3.4 Autophagy and IRI

Autophagy is an evolutionarily conserved lysosome-dependent cellular degradation program. It is an important process for maintaining homeostasis by degrading damaged organelles, proteins and other macromolecules under stress conditions. Self-digestion of hepatocytes was firstly discovered in 1962 [38]. The degradation of the cell contents isolated in autophagic vesicles depends on lysosomes [39]. Autophagy is normally a self-protective mechanism after tissue and cell damage. However, excessively prolonged or strong stress stimuli lead to excessive autophagy and cell death [40].

Autophagy is commonly referred to as macro-autophagy. Damaged components in the cytoplasm (including damaged organelles and proteins, etc.) are membrane wrapped and transported into lysosomes to form autophagic lysosomes for degradation and recycling. This process roughly includes phagocytic vesicle formation, phagocytic vesicles derived into autophagosomes, and autophagolysosome formation with autophagosome-lysosome fusion [41].

IRI triggers the autophagic response. As one of the important mediated pathways during IRI, the TLR pathway enhances autophagy through promoting the interaction of MyD88 or TRIF with Beclin1 and inhibiting its binding to Bcl-2 [42]. ROS regulates autophagy through the mTOR pathway [43]. ROS also promotes autophagy by inhibiting Atg4 activity and promotes the formation of LC3II [44].

Autophagy reduces IRI. A considerable amount of ROS, damaged organelles including mitochondria and damaged proteins accumulate during IRI. At this moment, the automatically activated autophagy promptly clears damaged organelles and proteins, maintains homeostasis, and protects cells' function [45]. Meanwhile, autophagy inhibits inflammation through the elimination of inflammatory complexes, damaged organelles and proteins [46].

However, excessive autophagy aggravates IRI while autophagy normally mitigates IRI. Autophagy plays a dual role in renal IRI depending on the duration of ischemia and different IRI stage [47].

11.3.5 Ferroptosis and IRI

Iron is an important essential trace element. Iron homeostasis is critical in the maintenance of cellular homeostasis. Ferroptosis is induced once iron homeostasis is broken. It is a unique iron-dependent programmed death process featured with the destruction of the antioxidant defense system, accumulation of lipid peroxidation products, mitochondrial shrinkage, and increased density of mitochondrial membranes [48]. Ferroptosis and cell apoptosis are closely related and mutually affected [49]. Ferroptosis is also closely related to a variety of pathophysiological processes, including tumors, tissue damage, IRI, etc. [50].

Studies have proved that ferroptosis is critical in the induction of IRI in isolated hearts. IRI can be reduced with the application of deferoxamine and ferroptosis inhibitors [48, 51]. During IRI, the occurrence of ferroptosis may be related to the ischemia-induced expression of HIF-1α and up-regulation of transferrin receptor (TFR) [52]. Ferroptosis causes endoplasmic reticulum stress (ERS) and further induces cell apoptosis [49]. Prolonged ERS may cause irreversible myocardial damage, although ERS in the early stage protects the myocardium to some extent.

11.4 Treatment of IRI

11.4.1 Clinical Guidelines for the Treatment of Donor Organs

Three aspects are involved in reducing IRI in DCD donor organs: (1) optimizing the evaluation and maintenance of the donor in ICU, (2) shortening the organ acquisition and transportation time, optimizing surgical procedures and organ preservation methods, (3) standardized management after surgery.

11.4.1.1 Optimize the Evaluation and Maintenance of Donors in ICU

DCD donors require a comprehensive evaluation to ensure the effectiveness of organ transplantation. Strict screening of DCD donors enhances the successfulness of liver transplantation with DCD donors, which may be equivalent to that of standard DBD donors [16].

The donor's basic physiological indicators (including respiration, heart rate, blood pressure, blood oxygen saturation, etc.) and laboratory tests (including routine blood test, electrolytes, liver, and kidney function, coagulation function, arterial blood gas analysis, etc.) should be measured in time for the maintenance of vital signs (including ventilator management, airway management, circulatory volume monitoring and supplement, application of vasoactive drugs, etc.). Particular tests such as biopsy should be performed based on the organ type. ECMO can be used to maintain circulation and oxygenation after cardiac arrest to protect organ functions to the maximum extent (see Chap. 4 for details).

11.4.1.2 Shorten the Organ Acquisition and Transportation Time, Optimize the Surgical Procedure and Organ Preservation Method

Shortening the duration of organ ischemia and restore blood flow as soon as possible can effectively reduce the degree of IRI. Measures include the establishment of a standardized organ acquisition process; shortening the operation time to reduce warm ischemia damage; shortening the organ transport time for a reduction in cold ischemia time; optimizing the composition of the organ preservation solution (low perfusion pressure, low calcium and low sodium) and temperature to reduce cold ischemic injury, etc. (see Chap. 5 for details).

In recent years, the technology of non-ischemic liver and kidney transplantation has realized non-ischemia in the process of transplantation by optimizing and improving the surgical methods, minimized the ischemia-reperfusion injury of the graft, improved the survival rate of the graft, and greatly reduced the incidence of postoperative complications and graft dysfunction [53].

11.4.1.3 Postoperative Patient Management

Effective postoperative management should be performed, which includes monitoring of transplanted organ function, timely measurement of physiological indicators and correct application of anti-rejection drugs, antioxidant drugs, calcium ion antagonists, neutrophil inhibitors and protective agents of cellular metabolism, etc. Many drugs such as calcium channel blockers, mannitol, adenosine, and *N*-acetylcysteine have shown protective effects on IRI in preclinical models. However, no drug so far appears to be effective in clinical trials [54].

11.4.2 Preclinical Research

11.4.2.1 Ischemic Preconditioning and IRI

Ischemic preconditioning refers to the ability of short periods of ischemia to make the organs or tissues more resistant to a subsequent ischemic insult. It was first discovered in myocardial injury. In 1986, Reimer et al. proved that transient ischemic treatment made the myocardium more resistance to ischemic damage and subsequently showed that this treatment was capable of reducing the infarct size, endothelial damage and incidence of arrhythmia. This protective phenomenon is called "ischemic preconditioning" [55].

"Ischemia preconditioning" reduces tissue damage through undergoing one or more short periods of ischemia and reperfusion. The concept of ischemic preconditioning has been expanded to "ischemic regulation," including pre-ischemic preconditioning, ischemic post-conditioning and remote ischemic conditioning [56, 57]. The protective effect of ischemic preconditioning is believed to be related to the up-regulation of HSP expression [58]. Extensive research on the protective strategies of ischemic preconditioning has been conducted in the clinical practice of acute myocardial infarction and coronary artery bypass grafting over the past 30 years. A large number of preclinical experiments have confirmed that transient ischemic preconditioning can increase the heart's resistance to subsequent ischemic attacks and significantly reduce the infarct size. The protective effects that occur within 24 h after the initial preconditioning stimulation include reducing infarct size, the occurrence of contractile dysfunction after ischemia, and endothelial damage [59].

The underlying protective mechanism of ischemic preconditioning may involve induction of heat stress effect, up-regulation of the antioxidant system, etc. [60]. This transient ischemic preconditioning is an effective stimulus to induce heat stress and promote the expression of HSP. HSP promotes protein synthesis, stabilizes newly formed proteins, and repair denatured proteins. In addition, ischemic preconditioning can activate antioxidant systems, such as superoxide dismutase or catalase, which directly leads to the reduction of oxygen-derived free radicals during reperfusion [61]. Some studies revealed that preconditioning could reduce myocardial energy requirements during ischemia, resulting in a decrease in the utilization of high-energy phosphate and anaerobic glycolysis rate, a promotion on adenosine triphosphate preservation and a reduced metabolic load, which explain the protective effect of preconditioning against ischemic cell death [62].

11.4.2.2 Protective Drugs of IRI

Drug therapies such as protease inhibitors and antioxidant drugs have been attempted based on the pathophysiological mechanism of IRI.

Inhibitors of apoptosis (protease inhibitors) are applicable because Inhibiting cell apoptosis can effectively reduce IRI. Reports have shown that apoptosis protease inhibitors (caspase3 inhibitors) can remarkably lower the level of apoptosis in mice undergoing renal ischemia-reperfusion by reducing the activation of caspase 3. Moreover, the efficacy of caspase 1 inhibitors outperformed that of caspase 3 and pan-caspase inhibitors [63]. Nafamostat mesylate inhibit the inflammatory response and cell apoptosis by inhibiting the complement system, which ultimately inhibits the ischemia-reperfusion injury of the heart, liver, small intestine, and kidney [64].

ROS plays an important role in IRI. The removal of ROS effectively decreases the level of tissue damage. Antioxidant drugs are mostly reductive and capable of reducing cell injury through redox reactions with ROS. Active oxygen scavengers include enzymes (SOD, catalase, glutathione peroxidase, etc.) and non-enzymatic antioxidants (vitamins A, C, E, etc.). Xanthine oxidase (XO) inhibitor febuxostat may effectively reduce oxidative stress damage [65]. Melatonin reduces IRI by resisting oxidative stress [66]. *N*-acetylcysteine as an antioxidant can also reduce oxidative stress [67].

In addition, leptin reduces kidney IRI by lowering tumor necrosis factor-α levels and increasing nitrite levels [68]. Levosimendan alone or combined with coustodiol protects renal IRI due to its antioxidant, anti-apoptotic, and survival-promoting function, which is dependent on the mitochondrial potassium channels and nitric oxide related mechanisms [69]. Verapamil and iloprost both have independent effects on warm IRI injury with a synergistic effect when combined. The cytoprotective mechanism may be related to the inhibition of lipid peroxidation [70]. Doxycycline may mitigate oxidative kidney damage and promote damage repair [71].

11.5 New Methods to Reduce IRI

At present, a variety of methods have been tried in the prevention and treatment of IRI, namely stem cell therapy, exosome therapy, immune cell therapy (such as regulatory T cells), signaling pathway regulators (such as inhibitors of TLR pathway and complement activation pathway, etc.) and therapeutic gases (hyperbaric oxygen, H_2S, etc.), etc.

11.5.1 Stem Cell Therapy and IRI

Stem cell therapy is a novel and promising method for the treatment of IRI [72]. As the most widely used cell type in the field of stem cell therapy, mesenchymal stem cells have advantages because they have a wide range of sources (isolated successfully from fat, bone marrow, umbilical cord and other tissues), well-established applications (many mesenchymal stem cells related clinical studies are ongoing currently), and a broad spectrum of treatments (IRI in kidney, liver, myocardium, and other tissues) [73].

Mesenchymal stem cells have immunomodulatory, anti-inflammatory, and tissue repair properties. They have the ability to differentiate into a variety of tissue cells of the mesoderm lineage, which mitigates ischemic tissue injury and accelerates tissue regeneration after IRI. Moreover, mesenchymal stem cells have the ability to migrate into injured sites and stimulate tissue repair through paracrine mechanisms [74]. Compared with other cell types, mesenchymal stem cells are easier to be genetically manipulated and more conducive to targeted genetic modification for maximizing therapeutic effects [75].

In the field of basic research, mesenchymal stem cells obtained from different human tissues have broad application prospects. Adipose-derived mesenchymal stem cell transplantation can significantly reduce the inflammatory response after ischemia-reperfusion and hemihepatectomy in pigs and promote liver regeneration [76]. These cells alleviate liver IRI and liver resection-related injury by regulating oxidative stress and autophagy. Level to reduce injury [77]. Mesenchymal stem cells derived from induced pluripotent stem cells also have the characteristics of classic mesenchymal stem cells and can effectively reduce acute renal IRI [78].

Mesenchymal stem cells perform well in immune regulation in addition to tissue repair. Therefore, treatment with bone marrow mesenchymal stem cells can not only alleviate IRI but effectively promote immune tolerance as well. Results from a large number of clinical trials have displayed good safety and efficacy in stem cell transplantation with autologous or allogeneic bone marrow mesenchymal stem cells. The use of bone marrow mesenchymal stem cells in kidney transplantation is associated with improved graft function, reduced rejection, reduced dependence and maintenance of immunosuppressive regimens, and less incidence of rejection events [79–81].

11.5.2 Exosomes and IRI

Stem cell-based therapy has become a promising therapeutic strategy for the treatment of ischemic diseases. However, stem cell transplantation also has some defects, such as immune rejection, tumorigenicity, and infusion-related toxicity. Increasing evidences have shown that the therapeutic effects of stem cells are mainly mediated through the secretion of paracrine factors.

It was discovered recently that transferrin receptor (TfR) could be released outside the cell in the process of reticulocytes turning into red blood cells. Gold particles labeled transferrin concentrates in endosomes with a diameter of about 50 nm and could be released by cells. Endosomal vesicles secreted by reticulocytes during maturation are called exosomes [82, 83].

Exosomes are microvesicles secreted by living cells that contain a variety of biologically active substances with a size of about 30–100 nm and a density of 1.13–1.19 g/ml. Exosomes have specific protein and lipid components and a lipid bilayer. Exosomes have important physiological functions in the signal transmission between cells. Many biologically active substances are contained in exosomes, such as nucleic acids (DNA, mRNA, miRNA, lncRNA, etc.), lipids, antigen-presentation molecules, signal transduction molecules, adhesion molecules, etc. The vesicle structure of exosomes can effectively protect these biologically active substances from degradation to exert benefits in target cells.

Exosomes derived from mesenchymal stem cells alleviate renal IRI by inhibiting inflammation and apoptosis [84]. Glomerular and tubular progenitor cells and their derived exosomes promote the recovery of acute kidney injury as well [85]. Exosomes derived from umbilical cord mesenchymal stem cells reduce liver IRI in rats via the inhibition of neutrophil-mediated inflammation and oxidative stress [86].

Cell-free therapy based on microRNAs encapsulated in stem cell exosomes is considered as a safe and effective alternative to stem cell therapy. Studies have shown that microribonucleic acid derived from stem cells or progenitor cells, including embryonic stem cells, induced pluripotent stem cells, mesenchymal stem cells and cardiac stem/progenitor cells, can be transferred from transplanted stem cells to recipients through exosomes. They regulate processes including cardiomyocyte proliferation, apoptosis, oxidative stress, differentiation, and angiogenesis. MiRNAs including miR-19a, miR-21, miR-21-5p, miR-21-a5p, miR-22, miR-24, miR-26a, miR-29, miR-125b-5p, miR-126, miR-201, miR-210, and miR-294 can enhance the cardiomyocyte survival, reduce cardiac fibrosis, and play a cardioprotective effect. MiR-126, miR-210, miR-21, miR-23a-3p, and miR-130a-3p exert cardioprotective effect by inducing the angiogenesis of the ischemic heart after myocardial infarction [87]. Extracellular microvesicles significantly alleviate renal IRI [88].

11.5.3 Autophagy Modulators and IRI

Autophagy affects IRI severity as one of the cellular protective mechanisms. The problem is whether regulating autophagy can mitigate IRI.

Studies have shown that urolithin A pretreatment can promote autophagy, reduce IRI-induced expression of pro-inflammatory cytokines including tumor necrosis factor-α, interleukin 1β, macrophage colony-stimulating factor 1α and macrophage colony-stimulating factor 2, and reduce kidney IRI [89]. Some studies demonstrated that spermine could reduce myocardial IRI by regulating autophagy. After pretreatment with spermine, the activity of target proteins in the mTOR pathway was significantly lowered while the autophagy-related proteins were upregulated. Therefore, spermine is considered a potential novel method to prevent IRI [90]. When everolimus was used to treat liver IRI in a mouse model, it was found that everolimus could decrease the expression of pro-apoptotic proteins, inhibit the release of pro-inflammatory cytokines (IL-6 and tumor necrosis factor-α), reduce elevated liver enzymes (aspartate aminotransferase, alanine aminotransferase and ammonia), reverse liver pathological changes and increase the level of autophagy. Everolimus was proved to alleviate liver IRI by autophagy activation [91]. Hence, IRI can be mitigated by regulating autophagy.

IRI in donated organs greatly affects the successfulness of transplantation. The reduction of oxidative stress after organ ischemia-reperfusion can not only ensure the quality of the transplant but also reduce the occurrence of immune rejection after transplantation. Further study on IRI-related molecular mechanisms may provide new strategies and targets for the prevention and treatment of IRI.

References

1. Jennings RB, Sommers HM, Smyth GA, et al. Myocardial necrosis induced by temporary occlusion of a coronary artery in the dog. Arch Pathol. 1960;70:68–78.
2. Eltzschig HK, Eckle T. Ischemia and reperfusion—from mechanism to translation. Nat Med. 2011;17(11):1391–401.
3. Zhao HL, Alam A, Soo AP, et al. Ischemia-reperfusion injury reduces long term renal graft survival: mechanism and beyond. Ebiomedicine. 2018;28:31–42.
4. Quiroga I, McShane P, Koo DDH, et al. Major effects of delayed graft function and cold ischaemia time on renal allograft survival. Nephrol Dial Transpl. 2006;21(6):1689–96.
5. Summers DM, Johnson RJ, Allen J, et al. Analysis of factors that affect outcome after transplantation of kidneys donated after cardiac death in the UK: a cohort study. Lancet. 2010;376(9749):1303–11.
6. Zhou J, Chen J, Wei Q, et al. The role of ischemia/reperfusion injury in early hepatic allograft dysfunction. Liver Transpl. 2020;26(8):1034–48.
7. Zhai Y, Petrowsky H, Hong JC, et al. Ischaemia-reperfusion injury in liver transplantation—from bench to bedside. Nat Rev Gastroenterol Hepatol. 2013;10(2):79–89.
8. Lemaster JJ, Thurman RG. Hypoxia and reperfusion injury to liver. Prog Liver Dis. 1993;11:85–114.
9. Van Golen RF, Van Gulik TM, Heger M. The sterile immune response during hepatic ischemia/reperfusion. Cytokine Growth Factor Rev. 2012;23(3):69–84.
10. Siniscalchi A, Gamberini L, Laici C, et al. Post reperfusion syndrome during liver transplantation: From pathophysiology to therapy and preventive strategies. World J Gastroenterol. 2016;22(4):1551–69.
11. Weyker PD, Webb CA, Kiamanesh D, et al. Lung ischemia reperfusion injury: a bench-to-bedside review. Semin Cardiothorac Vasc Anesth. 2013;17(1):28–43.
12. Ng CS, Wan S, Arifi AA, et al. Inflammatory response to pulmonary ischemia-reperfusion injury. Surg Today. 2006;36(3):205–14.
13. Matthay MA, Fukuda N, Frank J, et al. Alveolar epithelial barrier. Role in lung fluid balance in clinical lung injury. Clin Chest Med. 2000;21(3):477–90.
14. Kuhnle GE, Reichenspurner H, Lange T, et al. Microhemodynamics and leukocyte sequestration after pulmonary ischemia and reperfusion in rabbits. J Thorac Cardiovasc Surg. 1998;115(4):937–44.

15. Palazzo R, Hamvas A, Shuman T, et al. Injury in nonischemic lung after unilateral pulmonary ischemia with reperfusion. J Appl Physiol (1985). 1992;72(2):612–20.
16. Doyle MBM, Collins K, Vachharajani N, et al. Outcomes using grafts from donors after cardiac death. J Am Coll Surg. 2015;221(1):142–52.
17. McCord JM. Oxygen-derived free radicals in postischemic tissue injury. N Engl J Med. 1985;312(3):159–63.
18. Plotnikov E, Chupyrkina A, Vasileva A, et al. The role of reactive oxygen and nitrogen species in the pathogenesis of acute renal failure. BBA Bioenerg. 2008;1777:S58–S9.
19. Parks DA, Bulkley GB, Granger DN. Role of oxygen free radicals in shock, ischemia, and organ preservation. Surgery. 1983;94(3):428–32.
20. Nath KA, Norby SM. Reactive oxygen species and acute renal failure. Am J Med. 2000;109(8):665–78.
21. Lu L, Zhou H, Ni M, et al. Innate immune regulations and liver ischemia-reperfusion injury. Transplantation. 2016;100(12):2601–10.
22. Kawasaki T, Kawai T. Toll-like receptor signaling pathways. Front Immunol. 2014;5:461.
23. Rusai K, Sollinger D, Baumann M, et al. Toll-like receptors 2 and 4 in renal ischemia/reperfusion injury. Pediatr Nephrol. 2010;25(5):853–60.
24. Wu H, Chen G, Wyburn KR, et al. TLR4 activation mediates kidney ischemia/reperfusion injury. J Clin Invest. 2007;117(10):2847–59.
25. Smith SF, Hosgood SA, Nicholson ML. Ischemia-reperfusion injury in renal transplantation: 3 key signaling pathways in tubular epithelial cells. Kidney Int. 2019;95(1):50–6.
26. Moura CS, Lollo PCB, Morato PN, et al. Dietary nutrients and bioactive substances modulate heat shock protein (HSP) expression: a review. Nutrients. 2018;10(6).
27. Verghese J, Abrams J, Wang Y, et al. Biology of the heat shock response and protein chaperones: budding yeast (Saccharomyces cerevisiae) as a model system. Microbiol Mol Biol Rev. 2012;76(2):115–58.
28. Wright MA, Aprile FA, Bellaiche MMJ, et al. Cooperative assembly of Hsp70 subdomain clusters. Biochemistry. 2018;57(26):3641–9.
29. Rao SN. The role of heat shock proteins in kidney disease. J Transl Int Med. 2016;4(3):114–7.
30. Chen SW, Park SW, Kim M, et al. Human heat shock protein 27 overexpressing mice are protected against hepatic ischemia and reperfusion injury. Transplantation. 2009;87(10):1478–87.
31. Semenza GL. HIF-1: mediator of physiological and pathophysiological responses to hypoxia. J Appl Physiol (1985). 2000;88(4):1474–80.
32. Semenza GL. Regulation of oxygen homeostasis by hypoxia-inducible factor 1. Physiology (Bethesda). 2009;24:97–106.
33. Ivan M, Kondo K, Yang H, et al. HIFalpha targeted for VHL-mediated destruction by proline hydroxylation: implications for O2 sensing. Science. 2001;292(5516):464–8.
34. Andringa KK, Agarwal A. Role of hypoxia-inducible factors in acute kidney injury. Nephron Clin Pract. 2014;127(1-4):70–4.
35. Eltzschig HK, Bratton DL, Colgan SP. Targeting hypoxia signalling for the treatment of ischaemic and inflammatory diseases. Nat Rev Drug Discov. 2014;13(11):852–69.
36. Eckle T, Kohler D, Lehmann R, et al. Hypoxia-inducible factor-1 is central to cardioprotection—a new paradigm for ischemic preconditioning. Circulation. 2008;118(2):166–75.
37. Koeppen M, Lee JW, Seo SW, et al. Hypoxia-inducible factor 2-alpha-dependent induction of amphiregulin dampens myocardial ischemia-reperfusion injury. Nat Commun. 2018;9(1):816.
38. Ashford TP, Porter KR. Cytoplasmic components in hepatic cell lysosomes. J Cell Biol. 1962;12:198–202.
39. Deter RL, Baudhuin P, De Duve C. Participation of lysosomes in cellular autophagy induced in rat liver by glucagon. J Cell Biol. 1967;35(2):C11–6.
40. Liu Y, Levine B. Autosis and autophagic cell death: the dark side of autophagy. Cell Death Differ. 2015;22(3):367–76.
41. Kaushal GP, Shah SV. Autophagy in acute kidney injury. Kidney Int. 2016;89(4):779–91.
42. Shi CS, Kehrl JH. MyD88 and Trif target Beclin 1 to trigger autophagy in macrophages. J BIOL CHEM. 2008;283(48):33175–82.
43. Wu C, Jing M, Yang L, et al. Alisol A 24-acetate ameliorates nonalcoholic steatohepatitis by inhibiting oxidative stress and stimulating autophagy through the AMPK/mTOR pathway. Chem Biol Interact. 2018;291:111–9.
44. Li LL, Tan J, Miao YY, et al. ROS and autophagy: interactions and molecular regulatory mechanisms. Cell Mol Neurobiol. 2015;35(5):615–21.
45. Malaviya R, Laskin JD, Laskin DL. Oxidative stress-induced autophagy: Role in pulmonary toxicity. Toxicol Appl Pharm. 2014;275(2):145–51.
46. Lapaquette P, Guzzo J, Bretillon L, et al. Cellular and molecular connections between autophagy and inflammation. Mediat Inflamm. 2015; https://doi.org/10.1155/2015/398483.
47. Decuypere JP, Ceulemans LJ, Agostinis P, et al. Autophagy and the kidney: implications for ischemia-reperfusion injury and therapy. Am J Kidney Dis. 2015;66(4):699–709.
48. Dixon SJ, Lemberg KM, Lamprecht MR, et al. Ferroptosis: an iron-dependent form of nonapoptotic cell death. Cell. 2012;149(5):1060–72.
49. Lee YS, Hong SH, Lee DH, et al. Molecular crosstalk between ferroptosis and apoptosis: Emerging role of ER stress-induced p53-independent PUMA expression. Cancer Res. 2018;78(13).

50. Stockwell BR, Angeli JPF, Bayir H, et al. Ferroptosis: a regulated cell death nexus linking metabolism, redox biology, and disease. Cell. 2017;171(2):273–85.
51. Gao MH, Monian P, Quadri N, et al. Glutaminolysis and transferrin regulate ferroptosis. Mol Cell. 2015;59(2):298–308.
52. Tacchini L, Bianchi L, Bernelli-Zazzera A, et al. Transferrin receptor induction by hypoxia—HIF-1-mediated transcriptional activation and cell-specific post-transcriptional regulation. J Biol Chem. 1999;274(34):24142–6.
53. He X, Guo Z, Zhao Q, et al. The first case of ischemia-free organ transplantation in humans: A proof of concept. Am J Transplant. 2018;18(3):737–44.
54. Sethi K, Rao K, Bolton D, et al. Targeting HIF-1alpha to prevent renal ischemia-reperfusion injury: does it work? Int J Cell Biol. 2018;2018:9852791.
55. Murry CE, Jennings RB, Reimer KA. Preconditioning with ischemia: a delay of lethal cell injury in ischemic myocardium. Circulation. 1986;74(5):1124–36.
56. Granfeldt A, Lefer DJ, Vinten-Johansen J. Protective ischaemia in patients: preconditioning and postconditioning. Cardiovasc Res. 2009;83(2):234–46.
57. Hausenloy DJ, Yellon DM. Preconditioning and postconditioning: underlying mechanisms and clinical application. Atherosclerosis. 2009;204(2):334–41.
58. Benjamin IJ, McMillan DR. Stress (heat shock) proteins: molecular chaperones in cardiovascular biology and disease. Circ Res. 1998;83(2):117–32.
59. Hausenloy DJ, Yellon DM. Ischaemic conditioning and reperfusion injury. Nat Rev Cardiol. 2016;13(4):193–209.
60. Hausenloy DJ. Signalling pathways in ischaemic postconditioning. Thromb Haemost. 2009;101(4):626–34.
61. Richard V, Kaeffer N, Thuillez C. Delayed protection of the ischemic heart—from pathophysiology to therapeutic applications. Fundam Clin Pharmacol. 1996;10(5):409–15.
62. Murry CE, Richard VJ, Reimer KA, et al. Ischemic preconditioning slows energy metabolism and delays ultrastructural damage during a sustained ischemic episode. Circ Res. 1990;66(4):913–31.
63. Chatterjee PK, Todorovic Z, Sivarajah A, et al. Differential effects of caspase inhibitors on the renal dysfunction and injury caused by ischemia-reperfusion of the rat kidney. Eur J Pharmacol. 2004;503(1-3):173–83.
64. Na KR, Choi H, Jeong JY, et al. Nafamostat mesilate attenuates ischemia-reperfusion-induced renal injury. Transpl P. 2016;48(6):2192–9.
65. Tsuda H, Kawada N, Kaimori J, et al. Febuxostat suppressed renal ischemia-reperfusion injury via reduced oxidative stress. Biochem Biophys Res Commun. 2012;427(2):266–72.
66. Qiao YF, Guo WJ, Li L, et al. Melatonin attenuates hypertension-induced renal injury partially through inhibiting oxidative stress in rats. Mol Med Rep. 2016;13(1):21–6.
67. D'Amico F, Vitale A, Piovan D, et al. Use of N-acetylcysteine during liver procurement: A prospective randomized controlled study. Liver Transpl. 2013;19(2):135–44.
68. Erkasap S, Erkasap N, Koken T, et al. Effect of leptin on renal ischemia-reperfusion damage in rats. J Physiol Biochem. 2004;60(2):79–84.
69. Grossini E, Molinari C, Pollesello P, et al. Levosimendan protection against kidney ischemia/reperfusion injuries in anesthetized pigs. J Pharmacol Exp Ther. 2012;342(2):376–88.
70. Dosluoglu HH, Aktan AO, Yegen C, et al. The cytoprotective effects of verapamil and iloprost (ZK 36374) on ischemia/reperfusion injury of kidneys. Transpl Int. 1993;6(3):138–42.
71. Kucuk A, Kabadere S, Tosun M, et al. Protective effects of doxycycline in ischemia/reperfusion injury on kidney. J Physiol Biochem. 2009;65(2):183–91.
72. Lee KH, Tseng WC, Yang CY, et al. The anti-inflammatory, anti-oxidative, and anti-apoptotic benefits of stem cells in acute ischemic kidney injury. Int J Mol Sci. 2019;20(14).
73. Mushahary D, Spittler A, Kasper C, et al. Isolation, cultivation, and characterization of human mesenchymal stem cells. Cytometry A. 2018;93(1):19–31.
74. Hu H, Zou C. Mesenchymal stem cells in renal ischemia-reperfusion injury: biological and therapeutic perspectives. Curr Stem Cell Res Ther. 2017;12(3):183–7.
75. Xu HB, Chen C, Hu LK, et al. Gene-modified mesenchymal stem cell-based therapy in renal ischemia-reperfusion injury. Curr Gene Ther. 2017;17(6):453–60.
76. Jiao ZH, Ma YJ, Liu XN, et al. Adipose-derived stem cell transplantation attenuates inflammation and promotes liver regeneration after ischemia-reperfusion and hemihepatectomy in swine. Stem Cells Int. 2019; https://doi.org/10.1155/2019/2489584.
77. Ge YS, Zhang QZ, Jiao ZH, et al. Adipose-derived stem cells reduce liver oxidative stress and autophagy induced by ischemia-reperfusion and hepatectomy injury in swine. Life Sci. 2018;214:62–9.
78. Ko SF, Chen YT, Wallace CG, et al. Inducible pluripotent stem cell-derived mesenchymal stem cell therapy effectively protected kidney from acute ischemia-reperfusion injury. Am J Transl Res. 2018;10(10):3053–67.
79. Pileggi A, Xu X, Tan J, et al. Mesenchymal stromal (stem) cells to improve solid organ transplant outcome: lessons from the initial clinical trials. Curr Opin Organ Transplant. 2013;18(6):672–81.
80. English K, Wood KJ. Mesenchymal stromal cells in transplantation rejection and tolerance. Cold Spring Harb Perspect Med. 2013;3(5):a015560.
81. Casiraghi F, Perico N, Cortinovis M, et al. Mesenchymal stromal cells in renal transplantation: opportunities and challenges. Nat Rev Nephrol. 2016;12(4):241–53.
82. Harding C, Heuser J, Stahl P. Receptor-mediated endocytosis of transferrin and recycling of the

transferrin receptor in rat reticulocytes. J Cell Biol. 1983;97(2):329–39.

83. Johnstone RM, Adam M, Hammond JR, et al. Vesicle formation during reticulocyte maturation. Association of plasma membrane activities with released vesicles (exosomes). J Biol Chem. 1987;262(19):9412–20.
84. Li L, Wang R, Jia Y, et al. Exosomes derived from mesenchymal stem cells ameliorate renal ischemic-reperfusion injury through inhibiting inflammation and cell apoptosis. Front Med (Lausanne). 2019;6:269.
85. Ranghino A, Bruno S, Bussolati B, et al. The effects of glomerular and tubular renal progenitors and derived extracellular vesicles on recovery from acute kidney injury. Stem Cell Res Ther. 2017;8(1):24.
86. Yao J, Zheng J, Cai J, et al. Extracellular vesicles derived from human umbilical cord mesenchymal stem cells alleviate rat hepatic ischemia-reperfusion injury by suppressing oxidative stress and neutrophil inflammatory response. FASEB J. 2019;33(2):1695–710.
87. Moghaddam AS, Afshari JT, Esmaeili SA, et al. Cardioprotective microRNAs: Lessons from stem cell-derived exosomal microRNAs to treat cardiovascular disease. Atherosclerosis. 2019;285:1–9.
88. Farzamfar S, Hasanpour A, Nazeri N, et al. Extracellular micro/nanovesicles rescue kidney from ischemia-reperfusion injury. J Cell Physiol. 2019;234(8):12290–300.
89. Wang Y, Huang H, Jin Y, et al. Role of TFEB in autophagic modulation of ischemia reperfusion injury in mice kidney and protection by urolithin A. Food Chem Toxicol. 2019;131:110591.
90. Duan Q, Yang W, Jiang D, et al. Spermine ameliorates ischemia/reperfusion injury in cardiomyocytes via regulation of autophagy. Am J Transl Res. 2016;8(9):3976–85.
91. Lee SC, Kim KH, Kim OH, et al. Activation of autophagy by everolimus confers hepatoprotection against ischemia-reperfusion injury. Am J Transplant. 2016;16(7):2042–54.

Imaging Related to Transplantation from Cardiac Death Donors

12

Yan Wang

Abstract

Transplantation is the treatment of choice for end-stage organ failure. Up to now, the most common transplantation procedures performed in the abdomen mainly involve the liver and renal transplantations. Following organ transplantation, ultrasound, or radiology imaging is often used to monitor the transplanted allograft and assess the presence of possible complications, on account of clinical or biochemical assessments is often nonspecific and unreliable. Knowledge and early recognition of the imaging appearances can help to rapid and accurate diagnosis and timely and appropriate treatment, which can improve long-term graft survival. Ultrasonography (US) is the first-line imaging method for the evaluation of allografts due to its easy availability, cost-effective, lack of radiation and nephrotoxicity, and high sensitivity in the detection of complications. However, US is limited by the availability of suitable acoustic windows and the experience of operator. Other radiology imaging includes Computed Tomography (CT) and Magnetic Resonance Imaging (MRI). Both contrast-enhanced CT and MRI are limited by exposure of the patient to ionizing radiation and the potential nephrotoxicity of contrast media. US, including the gray-scale US with color, spectral Doppler imaging and Contrast-enhanced ultrasound (CEUS), plays an important role in the transplantation. This chapter mainly depicts the spectrum of US findings involving normal allograft imaging and post-transplantation complications in liver and renal transplant recipients. The complications after liver transplant include (a) vascular complications, including the hepatic artery (HA), portal vein (PV), hepatic veins (HV), and inferior vena cava (IVC); (b) biliary complications; (c) parenchymal complications; (d) perihepatic complications; and (e) neoplastic complications. The common complications after renal transplant include (a) vascular complications; (b) renal allograft parenchymal complications; (c) perinephric fluid collections (hematoma, urinoma, abscess, and lymphocele); (d) obstructive urologic complications; and (e) infectious complications (Polyomavirus nephropathy).

12.1 Liver Transplantation

In order to treat various benign and malignant diseases of the liver and biliary system, liver transplantation is becoming an increasingly rou-

Y. Wang (✉)
Department of Medical Ultrasonics, The First Affiliated Hospital, Institute of Diagnostic and Interventional Ultrasound, Sun Yat-Sen University, Guangzhou, China

X. He (ed.), *Organ Donation and Transplantation after Cardiac Death in China*, https://doi.org/10.1007/978-981-16-0815-5_12

tine surgical operation [1]. US is the preliminary imaging method for the evaluation of liver graft, including liver parenchyma, biliary tree, and vasculature. Early detection of posttransplant abnormalities will help to reduce mortality and may prolong graft survival time [2]. The most common complications after liver transplant are (a) vascular complications, including HA, PV, HV, and IVC; (b) biliary complications; (c) parenchymal complications; (d) perihepatic complications; and (e) neoplastic complications [3].

12.1.1 Vascular Complications

Vascular complications of liver transplantation include HA thrombosis-stenosis, pseudoaneurysm, PV thrombosis-stenosis, and IVC or hepatic vein stenosis-thrombosis. Vascular complications are the main factors affecting the graft function and survival rate. Vascular complications can occur immediately or several months and years later after vascular anastomosis. The earlier the complications, the greater impact on liver function occurs. After liver transplantation, hemodynamic parameters have great variation. There is a mutual transformation process between normal, abnormal hemodynamics and vascular complications. Not all hemodynamic abnormalities will lead to vascular complications. Therefore, it is necessary to observe closely and increase the frequency of examination when hemodynamic abnormalities occur. Ultrasound contrast agent is a kind of intravascular tracer; therefore CEUS can clearly show the vessels. In addition to vascular patency, CEUS can also improve the depiction of parenchymal perfusion. CEUS can increase the confidence of diagnosis and has proven to be an important tool in liver transplantation, and it may obviate CT and angiography [3, 4].

12.1.1.1 Hepatic Artery

The diameter of HA is smaller than that of PV. It is difficult to clearly show the lumen of HA by gray-scale ultrasound. CDFI can show the blood flow of normal HA and spectral Doppler can detect the characteristic fluctuation spectrum. The velocity of normal HA is about 25–120 cm/s, and the resistive index (RI) is 0.50–0.80, and acceleration time (the interval from end-diastole to the first systolic peak) is less than 80 ms. The frequency spectrum was characterized by a rapid systolic upstroke in the early systole and continuous flow in the diastole. In some patients, immediate postoperative Doppler US shows RI increased, which may be related to edema of the anastomosis [3, 5].

CEUS can clearly show HA and its branches (Fig. 12.1).

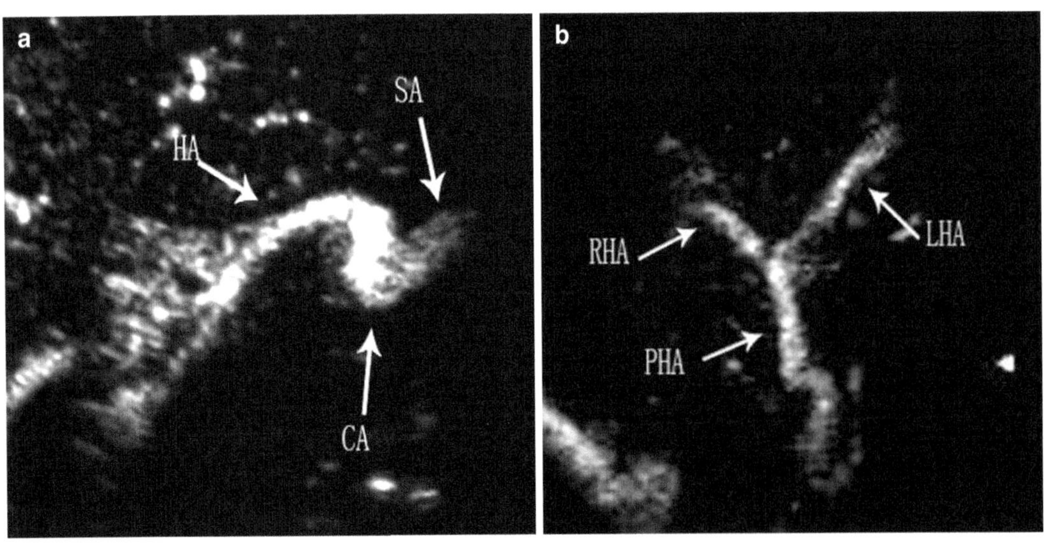

Fig. 12.1 CEUS of liver transplant artery. CA, celiac artery; SA, splenic artery; HA, hepatic artery; PHA, proper hepatic artery; RHA, right hepatic artery; LHA, left hepatic artery

Hepatic Artery Thrombosis

HA thrombosis is one of the most serious vascular complications of liver transplantation, and it is often associated with graft failure. It is reported that its incidence is about 2–12% and the time of occurrence is 15–132 days after transplantation [2]. HA thrombosis occurs more frequently in children than in adults, probably because the blood vessels are smaller, and it often occurs in the early stage in children [3]. Risk factors of HA thrombosis include rejection, end-to-end anastomosis, short warm ischemia time, ABO incompatibility and pediatric transplantation. HA thrombosis can occur suddenly or progress gradually, which results in reduced blood flow and a flattened Doppler spectrum [3].

HA thrombosis is very difficult to make an accurate diagnosis by gray-scale ultrasound. The color Doppler US shows that the blood flow signal of HA and intrahepatic branches disappeared, and CEUS shows that there was no contrast agent in the HA and intrahepatic branches (Fig. 12.2).

Doppler US has high sensitivity and specificity in the diagnosis of HA thrombosis. There are false-positive results in the diagnosis of HA thrombosis by the disappearance of flow signal in HA. Some factors can affect the display of HA, such as obesity, gastrointestinal flatulence, early anastomotic edema, hepatic artery displacement, high-grade HA stenosis, systemic hypotension, and insufficient sensitivity of the instrument [3, 4]. HA hypoperfusion state, whether secondary

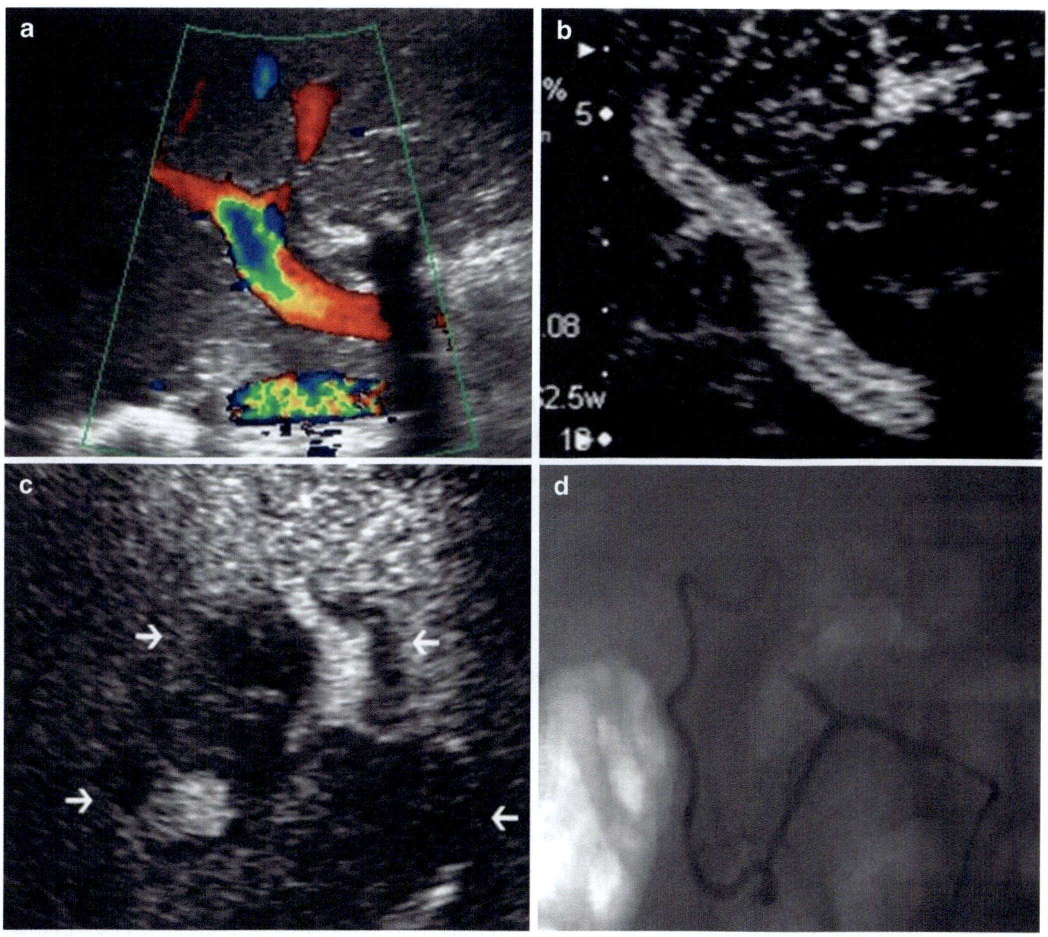

Fig. 12.2 Hepatic artery thrombosis in a 50-year-old male patient 13 days after he had undergone liver transplantation. (**a**) Color Doppler US does not show hepatic artery blood flow; (**b**) CEUS shows enhancement in portal vein, but without hepatic artery; (**c**) CEUS shows liver parenchyma ischemic necrosis (arrow); and (**d**) DSA confirms hepatic artery thrombosis

to HA spasm or to low cardiac output, can also result in nonvisualization of HA flow at Doppler US. On the other hand, if there are arterial collateral vessels, false-negative results are a possibility, which may occur from within the first month to several years after liver transplant [3].

When HA thrombosis is suspected by color Doppler US, CEUS is recommended, because CEUS can depict the patency of HA (Fig. 12.3). The accuracy of CEUS in the diagnosis of HA thrombosis is comparable to that of CT angiography.

Other complications may be secondary to HA complications, including hepatic infarct and biliary ischemia, which lead to bile leaks or strictures of the bile ducts, because the HA is exclusively blood supply to the bile duct in grafts. Biliary ischemia may lead to biloma [1–3]. When HA thrombosis accompanies intrahepatic infarction, biloma, intrahepatic bile duct dilatation or liver abscess, gray-scale ultrasound can show irregular hypoechoic, anechoic, or mixed echo areas in liver parenchyma and no blood flow signal or strip blood flow signal at Doppler US. The CEUS findings of biloma or abscess are regular or irregular non-perfusion area or peripheral enhancement with center liquefactive necrosis.

Hepatic Artery Stenosis

The incidence of HA stenosis after liver transplantation is 2–11%, and the median time is 100 days. Allograft rejection, poor surgical technique, and clamp injury are risk factors of HA stenosis [2]. HA stenosis is mostly anastomotic stenosis. Improper management of HA stenosis can lead to HA thrombosis, but it is difficult to determine the probability of its development into HA thrombosis in clinical cases. Intraoperative gray-scale ultrasound can show HA anastomosis, but gray-scale ultrasound examination after closing the abdomen is difficult to show the location and extent of stenosis. The color Doppler US features of HA stenosis is turbulent flow at artery stenosis. The spectral Doppler US features of HA stenosis include local increased peak systolic velocity (more than 200 cm/s, or an increase of more than two to three times) at HA stenosis and typical tardus parvus waveform at the distal end of stenosis, characterized by a low resistive index (less than 0.5) and a long systolic acceleration time (more than 80 ms) [2, 3, 6] (Fig. 12.4).

In patients with chronic HA thrombosis, collateral vessels may also show this tardus parvus waveform, which is similar to HA stenosis. It is difficult to detection of low-grade HA stenosis at

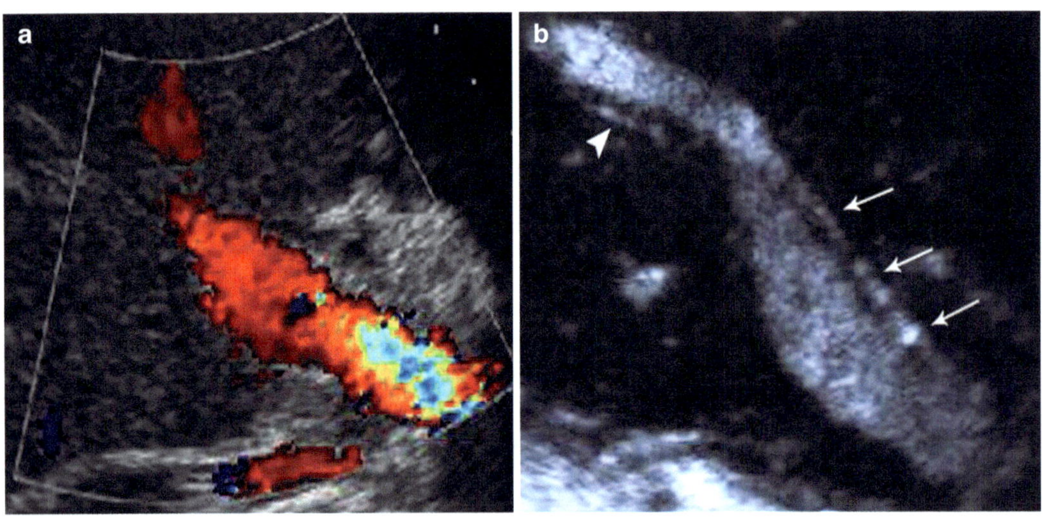

Fig. 12.3 CEUS of hepatic artery. (**a**) In a suspicious, color Doppler US cannot detect hepatic artery blood flow. (**b**) CEUS depicts the hepatic artery (arrow) accompanied by portal vein

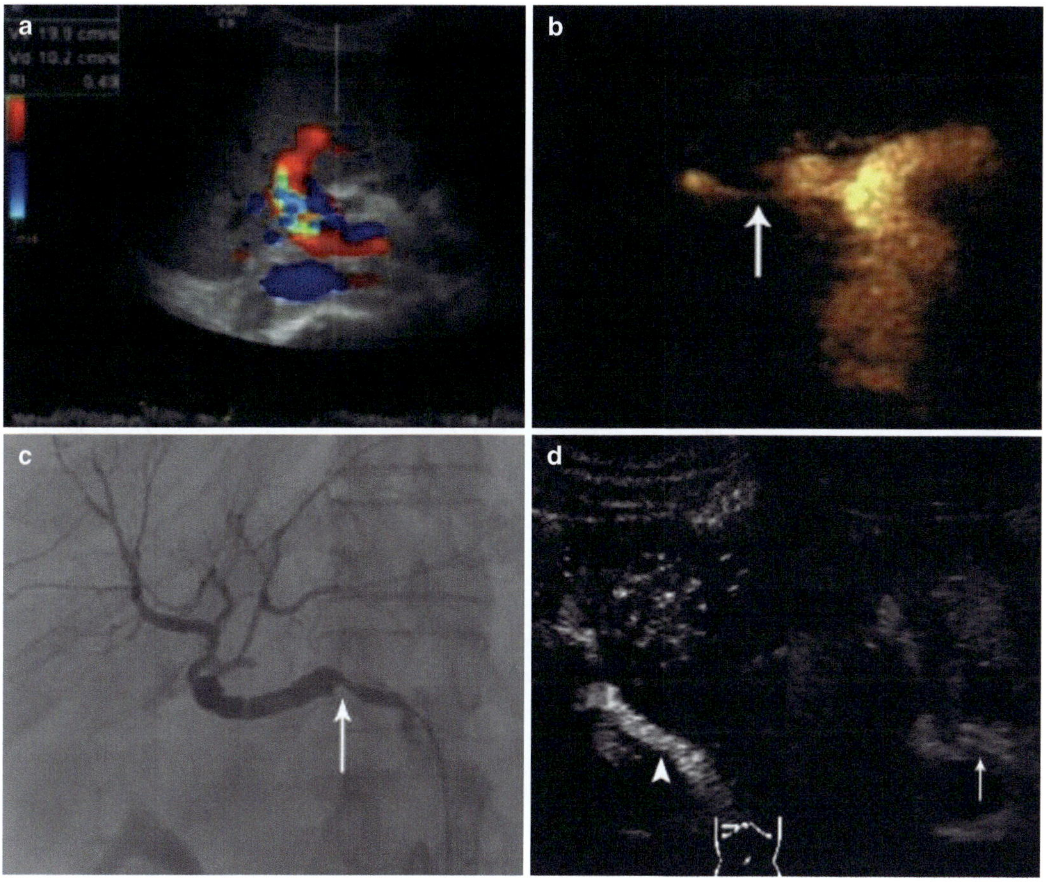

Fig 12.4 Hepatic artery stenosis in a 45-year-old male patient 9 days after he had undergone liver transplantation. (**a**) Doppler US shows tardus-parvus waveform distal to the stenosis (PSV 19.9 cm/s, RI 0. 49, sat > 0.08). (**b**, **c**) CEUS and DSA show severe stenosis of the anastomotic site (arrow). (**d**) US shows stent echo (arrow) and anastomotic site without stenosis at CEUS (arrowhead) after stent implantation

Doppler US. In suspicious cases, CEUS is recommended, and it can describe the size and shape of the hepatic artery. CEUS can show the focal narrowing and extent of stenosis (Fig. 12.4). It has important clinical value in the diagnosis of HA complications.

Early postoperative hepatic artery spasm and edema can lead to abnormal waveform spectrum of HA, including increased peak velocity, increased or decreased RI, which usually returns to normal within a few days [2, 3]. In addition, anastomotic edema may also cause arterial abnormal waveform similar to stenosis, which is reversible [3]. Close imaging follow-up is important for these patients. The RI of the intrahepatic artery can be less than 0.5 during and early period after the operation (within 24 h), so low RI should be treated differently. If the Doppler examination of HA is normal in the early postoperative period, and then the SAT is prolonged, the diagnostic significance is greater.

Hepatic Artery Pseudoaneurysm

HA pseudoaneurysm is an uncommon complication, which can be divided into extrahepatic pseudoaneurysm and intrahepatic pseudoaneurysm. Extrahepatic pseudoaneurysms most often occur at HA anastomosis or secondary to angioplasty. On the other hand, intrahepatic pseudoaneurysm may be associated with graft biopsy, biliary surgery, or infection [2, 3]. Generally, the patient of HA pseudoaneurysm has no conscious symptoms. However, if the pseudoaneurysm ruptures into the abdominal cavity, it may appear the manifestations of acute shock caused by acute blood loss [3].

The gray-scale ultrasonographic feature of pseudoaneurysms is the cystic structure or mixed mass abutting the vessel in hepatic hilum or within liver parenchyma, and a disorganized, turbulent, bidirectional flow pattern could be observed in cystic structures by color Doppler. The blood flow in the pseudoaneurysm cavity is slow. The typical feature of pseudoaneurysm is the yin-yang sign at color Doppler US and the to-and-fro pattern at pulsed Doppler US [3]. CEUS demonstrates a focal lesion with hyperenhancement in the arterial phase that is synchronous with the HA.

Doppler US and CEUS are very helpful in the diagnosis of pseudoaneurysm. When gray-scale ultrasound shows cystic structure near the artery anastomosis, further evaluation with Doppler US is required, and CEUS should be recommended if necessary to exclude pseudoaneurysm.

12.1.1.2 Portal Vein

In liver transplantation patients, PV anastomosis is the most common end-to-end. The diameter of PV is about 0.7–1.3 cm. The normal PV is anechoic lumen at the gray-scale ultrasound. A focal narrowing at the anastomotic site of PV may be observed, but it does not indicate stenosis. Color Doppler US of normal PV shows continuous flow toward the liver. Pulsed Doppler US shows continuous and monophasic flow spectrum, which is fluctuated with respiration. However, in the early postoperative period, the turbulent flow of PV may be normal [3–5]. Early postoperative PV velocity difference is large. The velocity range is 20–110 cm/s, and the average velocity is about 46 cm/s, gradually decreased with the time after the operation.

When the PV lumen is not clearly displayed on gray-scale ultrasound, CEUS can clearly display it.

PV complications are relatively rare and occur in about 1–13% of transplant patients [2]. The incidence of PV complications in patients of split and reduced-size transplants is higher than that in patients of orthotopic liver transplants. High-risk factors include faulty surgical technique, inconsistent portal vein caliber between donor and recipient, decreased PV inflow and previous PV surgery or thrombosis. PV complications may lead to portal hypertension associated with splenomegaly and ascites, hepatic failure, and lower extremity edema [2, 3].

Portal Vein Thrombosis

In liver transplantation, the incidence of PV thrombosis is about 3%, and it usually occurs in the extrahepatic PV in the first month after transplantation [2].

US imaging of PV thrombosis is an echogenic luminal thrombus without blood flow, mostly hypoechoic [3] (Fig. 12.5). The images of partial

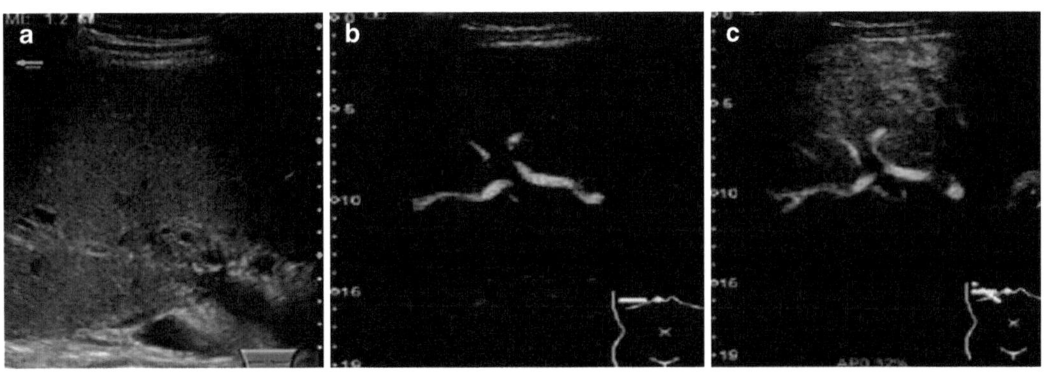

Fig. 12.5 PV thrombosis in a 56-year-old male patient 10 days after he had undergone liver transplantation. (**a**) US shows an echogenic luminal thrombus in PV. (**b, c**) CEUS shows PV without enhancement

thrombosis , which can be treated non-surgically, include hypoechoic or mixed echo emboli and vessel narrowing. Color Doppler findings include intraluminal filling defect at the site of thrombosis and thinner blood flow at the non-thrombotic sites. CEUS shows narrowed PV and non-enhancement thrombosis.

When the thrombus completely fills the portal vein (complete thrombosis), the PV blood flow signal disappears, and there is no contrast agent perfusion in the PV on CEUS (Fig. 12.5). Complete thrombosis requires timely treatment.

Portal Vein Stenosis

PV stenosis mostly occurs at the PV anastomosis. Color Doppler US imaging findings include the narrow lumen and focal high-speed (more than 125 cm/s) disorder flow in portal vein stenosis and dilated PV lumen post-anastomotic segment. The difference of velocity between the anastomotic site and the preanastomotic segment measured by spectral Doppler can be three to four times, and portal hypertension is also present [2, 3]. PV anastomotic narrowing that due to a size discrepancy between the recipient and donor PV is relatively common. A PV anastomotic narrowing may simply represent this discrepancy sometimes. The variation of PV diameter is very big, so the standard of PV anastomosis is not uniform.

The focal narrowing can be depicted with CEUS; therefore CEUS has important clinical value.

12.1.1.3 Inferior Vena Cava and Hepatic Vein

The diameter of IVC and HV changes with respiratory movement and cardiac cycle. The blood flow velocity ranges widely. The spectrum Doppler of normal IVC and HV shows multiphasic waveform based on the respiratory cycle. However, some patients can manifest monophasic waveform. HV and IVC complications occur in only 1–2% of liver transplantations, and they are less frequent than other vascular complications. The incidence in children is higher than that in adults [2, 3].

Inferior Vena Cava Stenosis and Thrombosis

The reasons of IVC stenosis include anastomotic narrowing and extrinsic compression secondary to allograft swelling, perihepatic effusion, or perihepatic hematoma. Clinical manifestations of IVC stenosis include liver congestion, hepatomegaly, ascites, and pleural effusion, which are usually nonspecific.

The ultrasonographic changes of the stenosis of IVC are similar to imaging findings of Budd Chiari syndrome, including focal increased peak velocity associated color Doppler aliasing, dilatation of the HV with loss of phasicity of Doppler waveform, and reverse PV flow, poststenotic dilatation of IVC, hepatomegaly, and ascites [2, 3, 7]. If we can directly see the narrow lumen and the increased velocity at the anastomotic site, the diagnosis will be more confident. CEUS can clearly demonstrate focal narrow lumen of the IVC. The diagnosis of IVC stenosis needs to be combined with clinical symptoms, such as lower limb edema and scrotal edema.

The main risk factors of IVC thrombosis include hypercoagulable state, surgical factors, and use of intravascular catheters. The US findings of IVC thrombosis is an intraluminal hypoechoic thrombus. CEUS can demonstrate focal narrowing of the IVC (partial thrombosis) or absence of ultrasound contrast agent at the site of thrombosis (complete thrombosis) [2].

Hepatic Vein Stenosis and Thrombosis

Because the donor HV is anastomosed to the recipient IVC in living donor liver transplantation, HV stenosis occurs mostly in those patients [2]. The ultrasonographic appearance of HV stenosis can be monophasic HV waveform, but it is nonspecific [2].

HV thrombosis manifests as an intraluminal hypoechoic thrombus in HV and a lack of blood flow at Doppler US. CEUS can demonstrate thrombus without enhancement.

12.1.2 Biliary Complications

In liver transplantation, the incidence of biliary complications is about 5–15%, which usually occurs in the early postoperative period (the first 3 months after surgery). Biliary complications include bile duct obstruction, biliary strictures (anastomotic or non-anastomotic), stones, bile leak, biloma, biliary necrosis, and cholangitis. Magnetic resonance cholangiopancreatography (MRCP) is the best noninvasive imaging method to evaluate the biliary tract in liver transplantation. If there is T tube in situ, T tube cholangiography is better. The US can easily detect bile duct dilatation. However, the sensitivity of US to other biliary complications is low (54%) [1–3].

12.1.2.1 Biliary Strictures

Biliary stricture can be classified as anastomotic stricture or non-anastomotic stricture. Most biliary strictures are anastomotic strictures (extrahepatic strictures), which may be related to anastomotic scar formation. Non-anastomotic biliary stricture is often caused by biliary ischemia and cholangitis. The influencing factors of ischemia include HA thrombosis or stenosis. Patients usually have no clinical symptoms, but some patients may have jaundice. However, laboratory results are often abnormal, including elevated levels of bilirubin and/or transaminase [1, 2].

Anastomotic stricture is often accompanied by dilated bile duct upstream of anastomosis. US can demonstrate dilated bile duct and focal stricture at the anastomosis. US is an ideal screening tool for detecting upstream dilatation. Despite severe anastomotic stricture, bile duct dilatation may not occur in liver transplantation. Therefore, the absence of bile duct dilatation does not mean the absence of anastomotic stenosis. MRCP has high sensitivity, specificity, and accuracy in depicting anastomotic strictures [1].

At US, non-anastomotic stenosis may show multifocal stenosis, often accompanied by related biliary dilated areas. Non-anastomotic stricture is often associated with HA complications or cholangitis, therefore, in the patients with non-anastomotic strictures, the presence of HA thrombosis or stenosis should be carefully evaluated [1]. In the literature, CEUS can observe the microvascular perfusion of the bile duct wall, which may play an important role in the diagnosis and prognosis evaluation of non-anastomotic strictures. At CEUS, normal bile duct wall after liver transplantation shows hyper- or iso-enhancement compares with surrounding liver parenchyma in arterial phase, iso- or hypoenhancement in portal vein phase and delayed phase. When there was no blood perfusion in the bile duct wall, it shows non-enhancement of the bile duct wall at all stages. Hypoenhancement in the arterial phase and portal phase indicates poor perfusion of the bile duct wall [8].

It should be noted that a donor-recipient biliary diameter mismatch may cause misdiagnosis. Not all focal stenosis or dilatation at US imaging have clinical symptoms or significance [1].

12.1.2.2 Biliary Obstruction

Biliary obstruction is often secondary to anastomotic stricture or choledocholithiasis. At US, the indirect sign of biliary obstruction is dilatation of bile duct upstream of obstruction. In patients with obstruction secondary to bile duct stones, US may show the stones in the obstruction. MRCP is very useful in the evaluation of biliary obstruction. US is less reliable, especially in the detection of mild intrahepatic bile duct obstruction and common bile duct stones. MRCP is recommended if the biliary obstruction is suspected, but no abnormality is found by US [1–3].

12.1.2.3 Biliary Stones

At US, Stones demonstrate iso-echoic or hyperechoic lesion, with or without posterior acoustic shadow. Sometimes US may detect biliary dilatation upstream of the stone. US is less reliable in the detection of choledocholithiasis when the stone is not hyperechoic [1–3].

12.1.2.4 Biliary Leak

Bile leaks occur in 4.3% of liver transplantations, most commonly at the biliary anastomosis, cystic duct remnant, or the T tube exit site. Bile leak usually occurs in the first few months after surgery. Patient may have no symptoms in the early process. Bile leaks are often caused by anastomotic dehiscence. US of bile leaks can demonstrate irregular or round hypoechoic fluid collections. It is difficult to distinguish bile leaks from nonbiliary postoperative effusion such as ascites, abscess, and hematoma by US [1–3]. CEUS of bile leakage shows no enhanced bile.

12.1.2.5 Biloma

Most of bilomas occur within the first year after liver transplantation. The risk factors include HA complications and hepaticojejunostomy. HV thrombosis or stenosis can result in biliary ischemia with biloma formation [1, 2].

The ultrasonographic features of intrahepatic bilomas are similar to cysts. The features include round hypoechoic or anechoic structures, often with posterior acoustic enhancement. CEUS of bilomas shows no enhancement and no contrast medium (there is no contrast agent in bilomas) [1–3].

12.1.3 Parenchymal Complications

12.1.3.1 Hepatic Infarction

Hepatic infarction is mainly secondary to decreased flow in the HA (arterial thrombosis or severe arterial stenosis). The early manifestation of hepatic ischemia is an irregular, poorly defined hypoechoic area. If the ischemia is improved, the echo can return to normal. If the ischemia worsens further, it will become a real infarction, which is characterized as irregular, hypoechoic, or heterogeneous echo lesion, with non-enhancement at CEUS [1, 2] (Fig. 12.2c).

12.1.3.2 Intrahepatic Abscess

Intrahepatic abscess after liver transplantation is an uncommon complication with an incidence of 1–3%, and it is often secondary to hepatic ischemia or hepatic infarction. Biliary complication and hepatic parenchymal ischemia caused by HA complications are risk factors. Immunosuppressive therapy after liver transplantation increases the probability of liver abscess. The clinical manifestation of abscess is different, but it often includes fever, chills, abdominal discomfort, and pain [1–3].

The imaging features of hepatic abscess in the transplanted liver are similar to those in the native liver. The ultrasonographic feature of hepatic abscess is round or irregular, poorly defined, hypoechoic, or inhomogeneous lesion. They usually contain liquefaction areas inside, which are anechoic. Hepatic abscess may contain gases that appear hyperechoic. At US, a mixed fluid collection with air-liquid level suggests a possible abscess. The typical CEUS manifestation of hepatic abscess is perilesional hyper-enhancement in the arterial phase, which indicates inflammation and hyperemia, and it will become hypo-enhanced or iso-enhanced in the portal venous phase and delayed phase. There is no blood perfusion; therefore, liquefied areas appear non-enhancement [1–3].

12.1.3.3 Fatty Liver or Recurrent Liver Cirrhosis

The ultrasonographic features of chronic liver cirrhosis are the same as those in pre-transplant patients, including liver atrophy, left lobe hypertrophy, widened hepatic fissure. Chronic liver cirrhosis may accompany by portal hypertension, splenomegaly, ascites, and so on [1].

The US features of fatty liver include enlargement of liver volume, hyperechoic liver parenchyma with partial posterior attenuation. In severe fatty liver cases, blood vessels are unclear because of sound attenuation [1].

12.1.4 Hepatocellular Cancer

Liver transplantation is considered as a treatment for hepatocellular cancer (HCC). Unfortunately, tumor recurrence is another complication in liver transplantation. The incidence of HCC recurrence after liver transplantation is about 8–26%. It is reported that the average time is about 2 years, with a range of 9 months to 6 years [1, 9]. The high-risk factors for recurrence include large volume of primary hepatic tumor, vascular invasion, portal vein tumor thrombus and poorly differentiated tumor. Recurrent tumors can be single lesion, multiple lesions, or extrahepatic metastasis [9].

US imaging finds of recurrent HCC are similar to those of primary HCC. The ultrasonographic features of intrahepatic HCC are hypoechoic lesions with round or irregular shape, clear or unclear boundary and sparse or abundant blood supply. The typical CEUS findings of HCC are hyper-enhancement in the arterial phase, with washout in portal phase or delayed phase [9].

12.1.5 Perihepatic Fluid Collections

In the early postoperative period, a small amount of perihepatic fluid collections is common and can be absorbed spontaneously. Perihepatic fluid collections may be loculated ascites, seromas, hematomas, and so on. At US, fluid collections are hypoechoic or heterogeneous areas with irregular shapes. On CEUS, fluid collections show no enhancement. Differentiation among fluid collections is difficult by imaging. US-guided aspiration and drainage is a good method of diagnosis and treatment [1–3].

12.1.6 Posttransplantation Lymphoproliferative Disorder

Posttransplantation lymphoproliferative disorder (PTLD) is related to immunosuppressive therapy after transplantation and may be related to Epstein-Barr viral infection. The incidence is higher in children than in adults. The imaging finds of PTLD are very different. At US, PTLD may manifest as enlargement or other abnormalities of lymph nodes, periportal hypoechoic mass or mass involving any abdominal organ [1, 3, 10].

12.1.7 Rejection

Rejection is a common cause of allograft failure. Clinical manifestation and image features of rejection are nonspecific. When liver function is abnormal and vascular and biliary complications are excluded by imaging examination, rejection is possible. The gold standard diagnosis of rejection is biopsy. The role of the US is to exclude other complications, such as vascular and biliary complications, that can clinically mimic rejection and to guide graft biopsy, if indicated [2, 3].

12.2 Renal Transplantation

The renal transplantation is the most common solid organ transplantation. The graft is often placed in the right iliac fossa. End-to-side anastomosis is usually used. En bloc transplantation of two smaller pediatric kidneys may also be performed [11]. It is very suitable for ultrasound examination because of its superficial position and little influence on respiration. Vascular anastomosis, especially arterial anastomosis, is an important part of ultrasound observation.

12.2.1 The Normal Renal Allograft

The US features of a normal renal allograft are similar to those of a native normal kidney. The renal allograft is usually located in the iliac fossa, so it is easier to detect by US and its imaging is more clearly because of its more superficial location and little influence of respiration. It is suggested that the low-frequency probe (1–4 MHz) combined with the high-frequency probe (5–12 MHz) should be used to scan the renal allograft. High-frequency probe can display the structure of renal allograft more clearly (Fig. 12.6).

The size of the normal graft is similar to that of the donor allograft, sometimes with compensatory enlargement such as pediatric donors. The allograft cortex is iso-echoic, with clear differentiation from the medullary pyramid, which is more hypoechoic. Located centrally, hyperechoic fat-containing renal sinus is surrounded by the renal pelvis. There is no existence of hydronephrosis in the normal graft, sometimes no more than 1–2 mm of anechoic fluid can be detected in renal pelvis when the bladder is full. According to the presence or absence of color blood flow signals, color Doppler US can well distinguish the hydronephrosis and renal vessels.

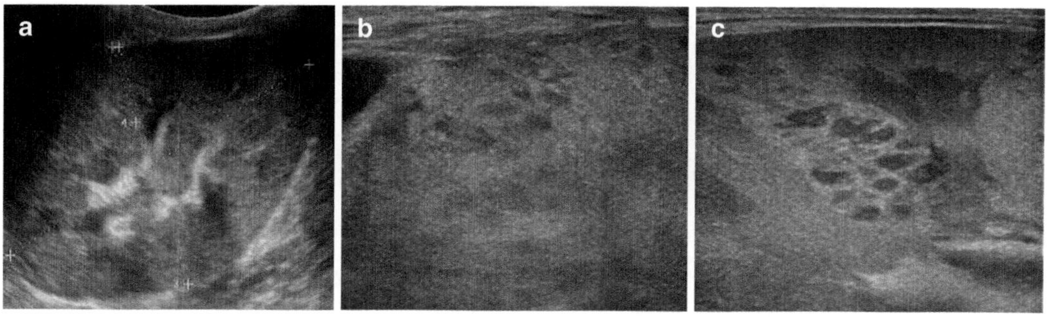

Fig. 12.6 The imagings of low-frequency probe and high-frequency probe in a 35-year-old male patient who had fever after renal transplantation. (**a**) US with low-frequency probe shows no abnormality of renal parenchyma. (**b**, **c**) At US with high-frequency probe, the parenchyma of the transplanted kidney is not uniform, and small hypoechoic areas are found in the renal parenchyma, which are small abscesses confirmed by pathology

Color Doppler US can observe the abundant renal flow. From the hilum to the cortex, blood vessels are uniformly distributed like coral throughout the whole allograft. The spectrum of the internal renal artery (segmental artery, interlobar artery and arcuate artery) is similar to that of the native kidney. Determination of peak systolic velocity and resistive index (RI) of renal artery is routine. The peak velocity varies greatly. The normal RI ranged from 0.5 to 0.8. At the early stage after transplantation, the peak systolic velocity of renal artery at the anastomotic site may be increased because of perianastomotic edema with functional anastomotic narrowing. The decrease of peak velocity downstream of anastomotic narrowing may lead to the decrease of RI. On the other hand, RI may increase due to diffuse graft edema and reduced diastolic blood flow. These findings usually improve or normalize within the first day after transplantation, and close observation is usually required if transient postoperative symptoms are suspected [11, 12] (Fig. 12.7).

At CEUS, iliac artery, renal artery, segmental artery, interlobar artery, arcuate artery and interlobular artery are successively enhanced after US contrast agent injection. The enhancement of the cortex increased rapidly from inside to outside. The medulla usually begins to image slightly later than the renal cortex. The contrast agent infuses from the edge of the renal pyramid and gradually flows to the center. The transplanted kidney is homogeneously enhanced and showed like a fireball. CEUS can display the renal microcirculation and transplant vascular, especially the transplanted renal artery (Fig. 12.8).

12.2.2 Vascular Complications

Vascular complications include renal artery (renal artery stenosis or thrombosis, arteriovenous fistula and pseudoaneurysm) and vein thrombosis. May occur at any time after transplantation, vascular complications are particularly important in the early postoperative period., Vascular complications are an important cause of graft dysfunction, although seen in less than 10% of renal transplant recipients.

12.2.2.1 Renal Artery Thrombosis (RAT)

RAT is an uncommon but very serious complication, occurring in approximately 0.4% of renal transplants, which can result in graft loss. Arterial thrombosis typically occurs in the early postoperative period (within minutes to days). The risk of RAT includes anastomotic occlusion, hyperacute rejection, kinking of renal artery, and pediatric transplant recipients, especially babies weighing less than 7 kg because of thin arterial caliber. RAT occurs in 3–4% of pediatric renal transplants overall. The main clinical symptoms include sudden anuria and worsening hypertension. Renal infarction can be segmental or sys-

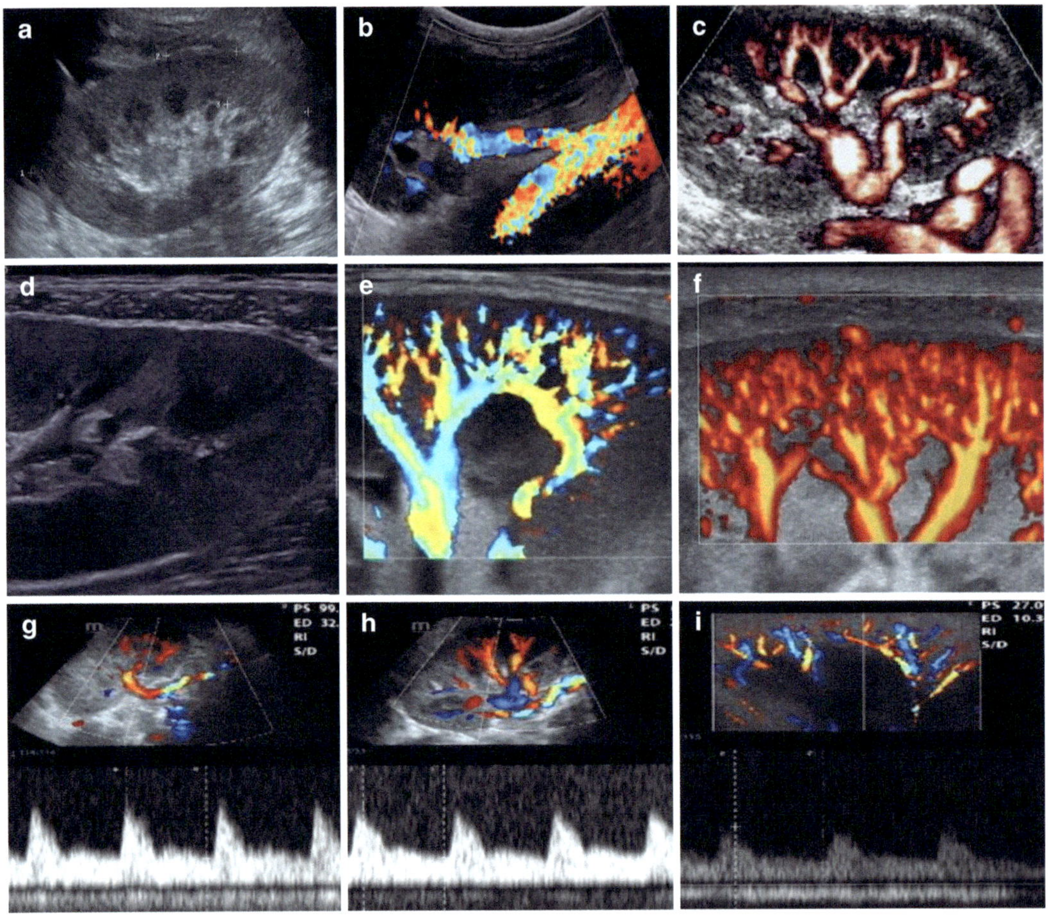

Fig. 12.7 Normal images of renal allograft. (**a**) Grayscale ultrasound with low-frequency probe shows the morphology and feature of renal allograft similar to those of a native kidney. (**b**) Color Doppler US shows end-to-side anastomosis of the donor renal artery and recipient external iliac artery. (**c**) Power Doppler US shows dendritic blood flow in the allograft. (**d**) Grayscale ultrasound with high-frequency probe shows the cortex and medulla of allograft more clearly. (**e**) Color Doppler ultrasound with high-frequency probe shows interlobular artery and arcuate artery clearly. (**f**) Power Doppler US imaging with high-frequency probe. (**g**–**i**) Spectrum Doppler ultrasound shows the spectrum of renal portal artery (**g**), segmental artery (**h**), and arcuate artery (**i**)

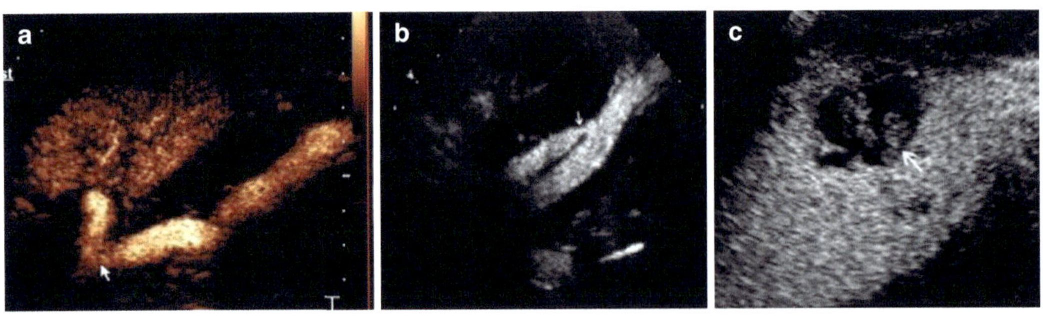

Fig. 12.8 The application of CEUS in renal transplantation. CEUS can clearly show the shape of renal artery trunk (**a**), the location and diameter of renal artery stenosis (**b**), and the focal infarct in the parenchyma of renal allograft (**c**)

temic. If the thrombus only involves one segment of the renal artery, the clinical prognosis is not so serious. According to the vascular grade of embolism, renal infarction can be divided into segmental or systemic. If the thrombosis only involves one segment of the renal artery, the clinical prognosis is less severe [11, 12].

Segmental infarct of US imaging findings will appear as hypoechoic wedge-shaped region without blood flow at color or power Doppler US (Fig. 12.9). Global infarct may demonstrate as diffuse hypoechoic renal parenchyma without blood flow throughout the graft at color Doppler US (Fig. 12.10). Color Doppler techniques fail to demonstrate intrarenal venous and arterial flow in the infarction portion. CEUS of infarct area shows contrast agent filling defect.

12.2.2.2 Transplant Renal Artery Stenosis

In renal transplantation, transplant renal artery stenosis (TRAS) is a common complication, occurring from 1 month to 3 years after the operation, with the first year being the most common. The main clinical manifestations are hypertension and vascular murmurs, with or without severe impairment of renal function [11].

Gray-scale US is difficult to show the stricture directly. Doppler US (color Doppler US and spectral Doppler US) has been proved to be an excellent noninvasive modality for evaluating the renal artery. Doppler US features of significant TRAS include (a) aliasing and spectral broadening of narrowing site due to marked turbulence. (b) elevated peak systolic velocity (PSV) at narrowing renal artery. PSV usually exceeds 250 cm/s; (c) elevated ratio of PSV in the narrowing renal artery to ipsilateral external iliac artery (EIA) PSV (measured near the anastomotic site), which is often greater than 1.8. (d) Indirect signs of distal or downstream to the stenosis site: reduced PSV, reduced RI and prolonged acceleration time (tardus parvus waveform) [11] (Fig. 12.11).

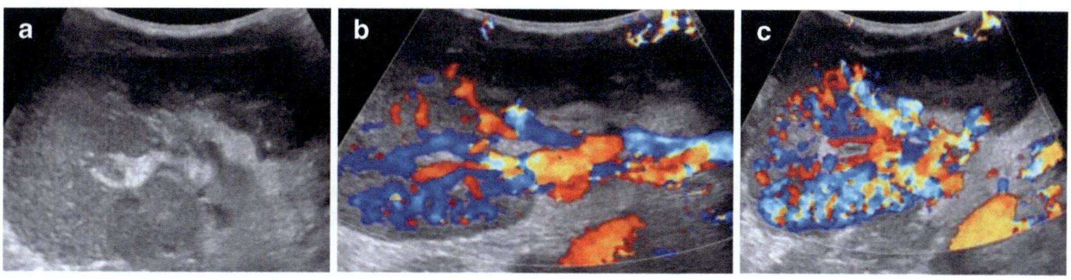

Fig. 12.9 Segmental renal artery thrombosis in a 29-year-old male patient who underwent transplantation. (**a**) Longitudinal grayscale US image shows hypoechoic renal parenchyma in the lower pole. (**b**, **c**) Color Doppler image confirms absent flow in the lower pole

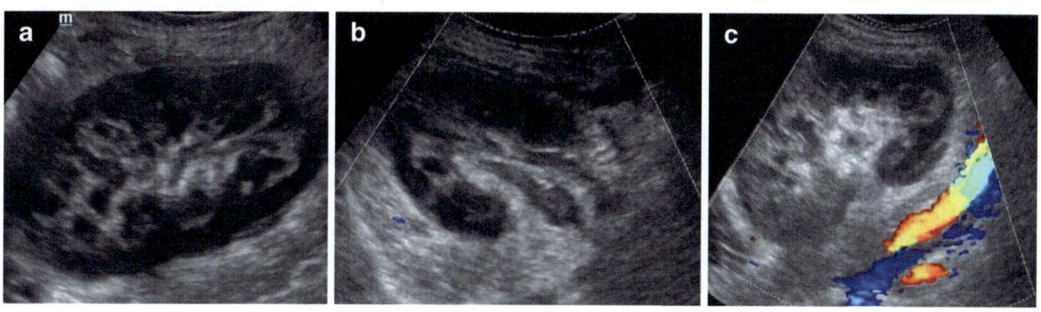

Fig. 12.10 Renal artery thrombosis in a 60-year-old female patient who underwent transplantation. Global infarct manifests as diffuse hypoechoic renal parenchyma (**a**) which is absence of blood flow throughout the graft (**b**, **c**)

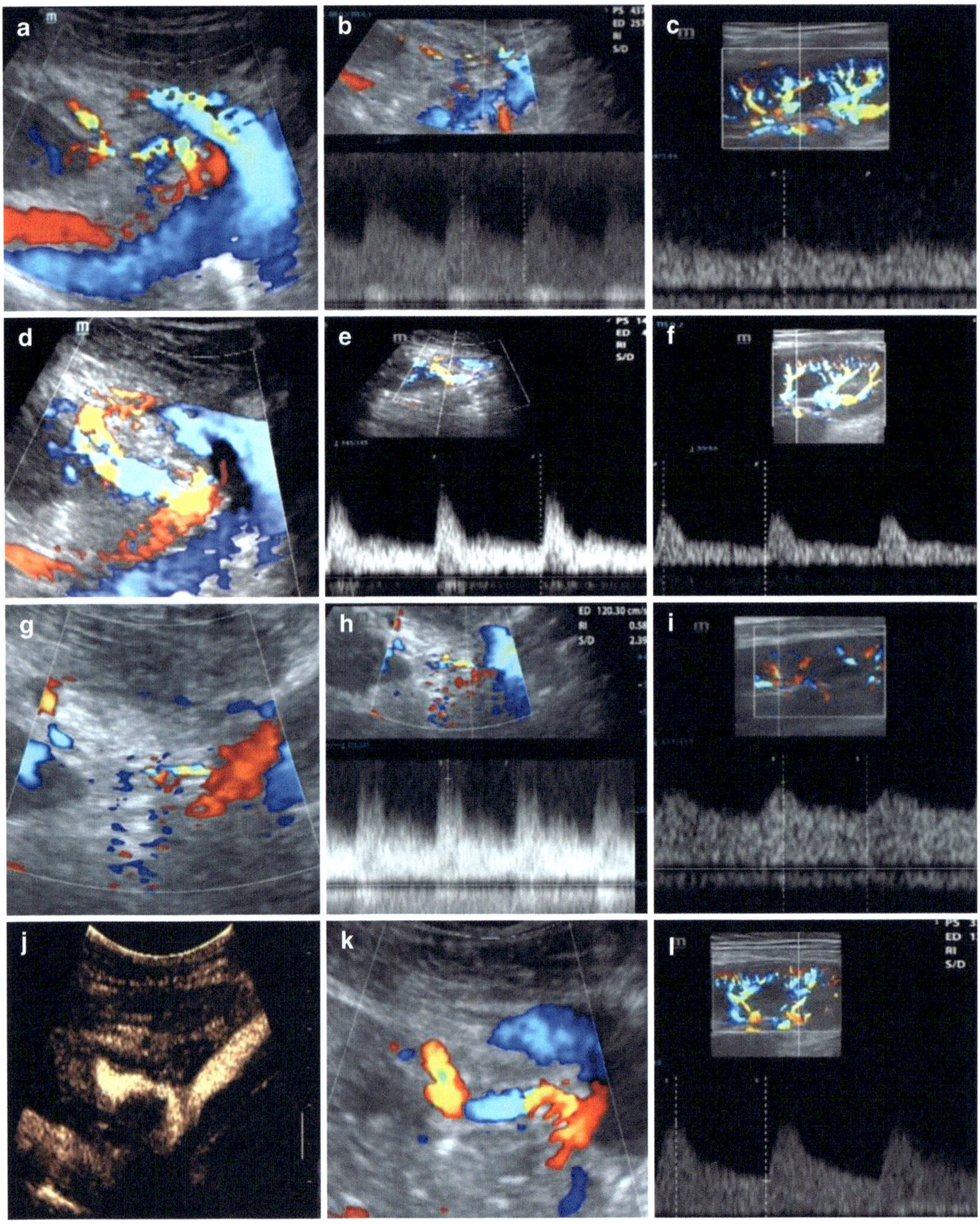

Fig. 12.11 Renal artery stenosis in a 35-year-old male patient who underwent transplantation. (**a–c**) US imaging of 6 months after transplantation. Color Doppler ultrasound shows that the main renal artery was thin (**a**). Elevated peak systolic velocity (437 cm/s) is seen at the site of narrowing (**b**). Tardus-parvus waveform (PSV = 12.6 cm/s, RI = 0.42, the systolic acceleration time > 0.08 s) is seen distal or downstream to the site of stenosis (**c**). (**d–f**) After stent placement, Color and spectral Doppler ultrasound imaging findings include the main renal artery without local stenosis (**d**), normal PSV of the main renal artery (142 cm/s) (**e**), and normal spectrum of intrarenal arcuate artery (PSV = 25 cm/s, RI = 0.67) (**f**). (**g–j**) After 8 months of stent implantation, Color Doppler ultrasound shows that the blood flow at renal artery stent is fine and aliasing (**g**). Elevated peak systolic velocity (287 cm/s) is seen at the site of stent (**h**). Tardus-parvus waveform (PSV = 9.1 cm/s, RI = 0.37, the systolic acceleration time > 0.08 s) is seen distal to the site of stent (**i**). CEUS shows transplant renal artery local stenosis at the site of stent (**j**). According to the clinical features, stent thrombosis is considered. (**k, l**) After interventional thrombolytic therapy, Color Doppler ultrasound shows no local stenosis of renal artery (**k**). The spectrum of intrarenal interlobar artery is normal (PSV = 35.6 cm/s, RI = 0.61) (**l**)

However, in the early postoperative period, Doppler US may lead to false-positive diagnoses of TRAS. In the postoperative period, isolated elevated PSV in the main renal artery may be related to edema or spasm of the arteries. Short-term follow-up Doppler US is recommended. Therefore, PSV and spectrum waveform of the main renal artery, RIs intrarenal renal artery and clinical symptoms of patients should be considered together when the patient is suspected of TRAS [11].

CEUS is superior to gray-scale and Doppler US for it can show the stenosis directly and improve specificity in diagnosis (Figs. 12.8 and 12.11j). Digital subtraction angiography (DSA) is the gold standard for diagnosing TRAS after renal transplantation.

12.2.2.3 Renal Vein Thrombosis

Renal vein thrombosis generally occurs in the early stage after renal transplantation with an incidence of less than 5%, which usually occurs within the first 5 days after transplantation. The symptoms of thrombosis include allograft swelling, tenderness, oliguria, hemoglobinuria, and proteinuria [11].

The US findings of renal vein thrombosis may include enlarged allograft because of graft edema, loss of corticomedullary differentiation, thickened cortex, and perinephric fluid. The main trunk of the renal vein is obviously dilated, sometimes hypo- or iso-echoic thrombus without enhancement on CEUS can be seen, which fill in the renal vein. When diastolic blood flow reversion occurs in the transplant renal artery at spectral Doppler US, it is highly suggestive of renal vein thrombosis, but it may also be seen with other abnormal conditions such as graft torsion, severe allograft rejection, and acute tubular necrosis (ATN). When reversed diastolic flow in the transplant artery is identified, the renal vein should be carefully assessed [11]. CEUS shows that the contrast agent is filled in the artery, and there is no contrast agent in renal parenchyma or renal sinus.

Early accurate diagnosis of renal vein thrombosis is critical for graft salvage.

12.2.2.4 Arteriovenous Fistula

An arteriovenous fistula (AVF) is the most common result of vascular trauma during the percutaneous biopsy, occurring in approximately 8% of biopsy patients. Most of AVFs are entirely asymptomatic, and more than 75% will dissolve spontaneously. Large AVF may cause graft ischemia and dysfunction, so it should be effectively treated with embolization [11].

AVFs of gray-scale US imaging is an anechoic structure similar to a cyst. When AVF is very small, it cannot be displayed on gray-scale US. Doppler US can show internal blood flow signal, which is different from the cyst. Therefore, CDFI can easily distinguish AVF from cyst [11]. AVF can display hyper-enhancement at CEUS.

12.2.2.5 Transplanted Renal Artery Pseudoaneurysm

Pseudoaneurysms may be caused by infection, surgery, percutaneous interventional procedures such as biopsy. Small intrarenal pseudoaneurysms are often asymptomatic. Pseudoaneurysm of the main renal artery or progressive enlargement should prompt treatment [11].

Pseudoaneurysm is closely related to the renal vessels. Pseudoaneurysms can be divided into intrarenal and extrarenal pseudoaneurysms. At US, an intrarenal pseudoaneurysm is depicted as a cystic structure, similar to AVF or cyst. Extrarenal pseudoaneurysms are anechoic structure, too. Therefore, color Doppler US must be recommended for all anechoic cystic structures identified at gray-scale US. Doppler US reveals a cystic structure with a disorganized, turbulent, aliased, bidirectional, or even slow monophasic flow pattern. The typical color Doppler US finding of pseudoaneurysm is the yin-yang sign. CEUS can show a blood pool hyper-enhancement in the pseudoaneurysm next to the artery [11] (Fig. 12.12).

12.2.3 Renal Allograft Parenchymal Complications

Renal allograft parenchymal complications may include delayed graft function (DGF), allograft

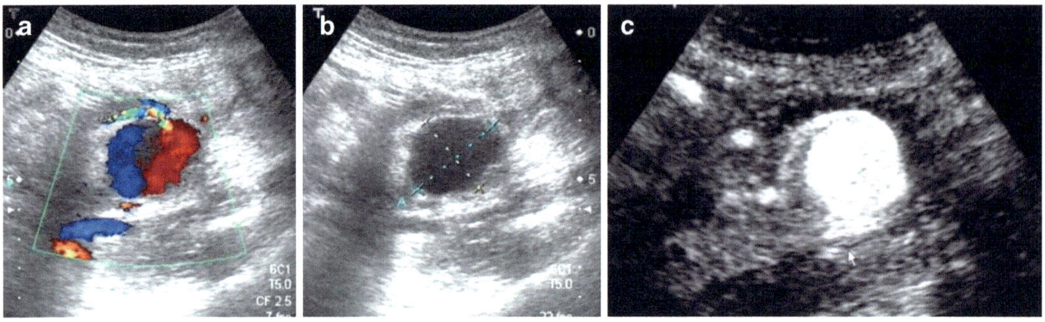

Fig. 12.12 Renal artery pseudoaneurysm in a 41-year-old female patient who underwent transplantation. (**a**, **b**) A pseudoaneurysm is depicted as cystic structure that is closely related to the renal vessels. Doppler US reveals a cystic structure with a disorganized, turbulent flow. (**c**) CEUS shows a blood pool hyperenhancement in the pseudoaneurysm next to the artery

rejection, acute tubular necrosis (ATN), and drug-related nephrotoxic effects.

The imaging findings of rejection are nonspecific. US findings of rejection included edematous cortical thickening, loss of corticomedullary differentiation, diminished cortical blood flow and increased renal parenchymal RI. Secondary segmental cortical infarction may occur. Elevated RI does not necessarily represent rejection. It can also occur in ATN, ureteral obstruction, nephrotoxicity to some immunosuppressants (such as tacrolimus or cyclosporine) and mass effect on allografts (such as extrinsic compression of perirenal effusion). It is also helpful for us to evaluate renal transplantation in combination with clinical diseases. At CEUS, delayed cortical perfusion may be observed in acute rejection [11].

The causes of ATN, an important cause of early renal allograft dysfunction, include prolonged ischemia (cold or warm) and reperfusion injury. The US appearance of ATN is nonspecific and variable, varying from its severity. In ATN, increased RI may be observed.

At US, It is a great challenge to identify the causes of graft dysfunction, such as DGF, rejection, ATN, drug-related nephrotoxic effects, recurrence of underlying disease. Ultrasound-guided percutaneous biopsy is still the gold standard for a definite diagnosis.

12.2.4 Perinephric Fluid Collections

Perinephric fluid collection often occurs after renal transplantation, which mainly includes hematoma, abscess, urinoma, and lymphocele. It can be detected by US. Imaging findings at gray-scale US may overlap; therefore it is necessary to combine color Doppler US with clinical information. Postoperative interval is important clinical information for differential diagnosis.

12.2.4.1 Perinephric Hematoma

Perinephric hematomas often occur in the immediate postoperative period, and they can also occur after biopsy or trauma. Small perinephric hematoma is often asymptomatic and can be resolved spontaneously. Larger hematomas that cause significant mass effects on the graft require surgery or puncture drainage.

Perinephric hematomas may appear anechoic, hypoechoic, or hyperechoic mass, varying according to the time of hematoma progression. Acute fresh hemorrhage may be anechoic or heterogeneously hyperechoic mass. Over time, it can become heterogeneous central hypoechoic mass. In the end, it could become cystlike areas with scattered internal thin septa [11]. Color Doppler US shows no blood flow signal in the hematoma.

12.2.4.2 Urinoma

Urinoma is the leakage of urine from the renal pelvis, ureter, or ureterovesical anastomosis site, most often between the graft and bladder. At US, urinoma appears as a simple hypoechoic fluid collection [11].

12.2.4.3 Perinephric Abscess

Perinephric abscess can be caused by infection of graft infection or adjacent abdominopelvic organs. Clinical information may include fever and leukocytosis.

The ultrasonographic feature of perinephric abscess is irregular thick-walled heterogeneously hypoechoic fluid collection with the prominent septum and internal hyperechoic debris. Gas can be seen in some abscesses. In color Doppler US, blood flow signals may be detected at the thickened wall and septa. At CEUS, it shows a rim-enhancing fluid collection, which may be related to peripheral hyperemia and inflammatory. But these characteristics are nonspecific. Ultrasound-guided percutaneous drainage can be used as a mean of diagnosis and treatment [11].

12.2.4.4 Lymphocele

Lymphoceles most commonly occur between 4 weeks and 6 months after transplantation. The cause of lymphocele is considered to be the destruction of normal lymphatic channels or hilar lymphatics. Most lymphoceles are asymptomatic, but large lymphoceles can cause mass effects. The US features of lymphocele are well-defined, anechoic, sometimes containing thin internal septa. CEUS of lymphocele shows no enhancement [11].

12.2.5 Obstructive Urologic Complications

Urinary tract obstruction most often occurs within 1–6 months after surgery. It is related to ischemic anastomotic stricture or scar tissue, extrinsic compression, or less commonly intraluminal abnormalities such as renal calculi and blood clots. Urinary tract obstruction can present as hydronephrosis on US imaging. US may demonstrate dilated calices and urinary tract [11] .

12.2.6 Infectious Complications: Polyomavirus Nephropathy

BK virus is a polyomavirus that is latent in an estimated 75% of the adult population. But in transplantation patients with low immunity, BK virus can affect renal allograft, leading to polyomavirus nephropathy. Polyomavirus nephropathy is an important factor in declining renal function or graft loss. The virus is often activated within the first 3 months after surgical operation, causing tubulointerstitial inflammatory changes which are similar to acute cellular rejection.

The imaging appearance of BK virus nephropathy is investigated in the literature. It is reported that the streaky pattern of alternating hypoechoic bands at gray-scale US is suggestive of polyomavirus nephropathy. In some patients with BK virus nephropathy, mild hydronephrosis can be seen in US. At present, the gold standard method for the diagnosis of BK virus-associated nephropathy is biopsy [11].

12.3 Conclusions

Multiple complications can be observed after transplantation. US, including gray-scale US with color, spectral Doppler US and Contrast-enhanced ultrasound (CEUS), plays an important role in monitoring complications, especially vascular complications.

References

1. Camacho JC, Coursey Moreno C, Telleria JC, et al. Nonvascular post-liver transplantation complications: from US screening to cross-sectional and interventional imaging. Radiographics. 2015;35(1):87–104.
2. Singh AK, Nachiappan AC, Verma HA, et al. Postoperative imaging in liver transplantation: what radiologists should know. Radiographics. 2010;30(2):339–51.

3. Horvat N, Marcelino ASZ, Horvat JV, et al. Pediatric liver transplant: techniques and complications. Radiographics. 2017;37(6):1612–31.
4. García-Criado A, Gilabert R, Bianchi L, et al. Impact of contrast-enhanced ultrasound in the study of hepatic artery hypoperfusion shortly after liver transplantation: contribution to the diagnosis of artery steal syndrome. Eur Radiol. 2015;25(1):196–202.
5. Crossin JD, Muradali D, Wilson SR. US of liver transplants: normal and abnormal. Radiographics. 2003;23(5):1093–114.
6. Caiado AH, Blasbalg R, Marcelino AS, et al. Complications of liver transplantation: multimodality imaging approach. Radiographics. 2007;27(5):1401–17.
7. Quiroga S, Sebastià MC, Margarit C, et al. Complications of orthotopic liver transplantation: spectrum of findings with helical CT. Radiographics. 2001;21(5):1085–102.
8. Ren J, Zheng BW, Wang P, et al. Revealing impaired blood supply to the bile ducts on contrast-enhanced ultrasound: a novel diagnosis method to ischemic-type biliary lesions after orthotropic liver transplantation. Ultrasound Med Biol. 2013;39(5):753–60.
9. Lee CH, Brubaker LM, Gerber DA, et al. MRI findings of recurrent hepatocellular carcinoma after liver transplantation: preliminary results. J Magn Reson Imaging. 2011;33(6):1399–405.
10. Dhillon MS, Rai JK, Gunson BK, et al. Posttransplant lymphoproliferative disease in liver transplantation. Br J Radiol. 2007;80(953):337–46.
11. Sugi MD, Joshi G, Maddu KK, et al. Imaging of renal transplant complications throughout the life of the allograft: comprehensive multimodality review. Radiographics. 2019;39(5):1327–55.
12. Nixon JN, Biyyam DR, Stanescu L, et al. Imaging of pediatric renal transplants and their complications: a pictorial review. Radiographics. 2013;33(5):1227–51.

13 Pathological Evaluation of DCD Donor Organs

Bing Liao and Wenfang Chen

Abstract

Although the overall amount of organ donations after decease is increasing in recent years with people's gradual recognition of organ donation, there is still an absolute shortage of donated organs, especially kidney and liver, because of the increasingly rising of the waiting list in China. A considerable proportion of the donated organs are from extended criteria donors (ECD) who are older than 60 years or have basic diseases such as hypertension, diabetes, and hepatitis. Precise evaluation of the quality of these ECD organs can help select the potentially suitable organs and reduce the risk of inappropriate transplantation. Pathological evaluation is one of the most essential components of the comprehensive evaluation of ECD organs. Effective pathological evaluation can help maximize the efficiency of organ allocation and utilization. In this chapter, we mainly focus on the pathological techniques, biopsy time points, and common pathological changes of donor liver and kidney.

B. Liao · W. Chen (✉)
Department of Pathology, The First Affiliated Hospital of Sun Yat-sen University, Guanghzou, China
e-mail: liaob@mail.sysu.edu.cn; chwfang@mail.sysu.edu.cn

13.1 Pathological Evaluation of DCD Donor Liver

13.1.1 Significance of DCD Liver Biopsy

DCD donor liver has become an important source for liver transplantation. Although DCD liver may carry more risk factors and result in primary nonfunction (PNF) and ischemic cholangiopathy, numerous studies in recent years have found that the strictly selected DCD donor's liver has a comparable prognosis compared with DBD donor liver [1–3]. Pathological evaluation of DCD donor livers is one of the important components of DCD donor evaluation and selection. DCD donor liver biopsy at the time of procurement/harvest can identify preexisting diseases and help to evaluate the suitability for transplantation. Time-zero biopsy can identify not only preexisting lesions but also changes related to organ preservation and reperfusion.

13.1.2 Time Points for Biopsy and Technical Considerations

The common indications for pathological evaluation of donor livers from deceased donors are listed in Table 13.1 [4].

Biopsy may be performed at three different time points, including procurement/harvest

X. He (ed.), *Organ Donation and Transplantation after Cardiac Death in China*,
https://doi.org/10.1007/978-981-16-0815-5_13

Table 13.1 Indications for pathological evaluation of donor liver

Liver biopsy from a deceased donor
Elevation of liver tests
Transaminases, bilirubin
High gamma-glutamyltransferase (>200 IU/L)
Suspicion of fatty liver disease
History of diabetes, obesity
Fatty (yellow) liver at procurement
History of alcohol use
Positive serologies for viral hepatitis
Anti-HCV antibody
Anti-HBc antibody
Findings during organ procurement
Abnormal liver contour or color
Suspicion of advanced fibrosis
Focal liver lesion

biopsy, preimplantation biopsy, and time-zero biopsy. Procurement biopsy and preimplantation biopsy mainly aim to assess the organ suitability for transplantation. The size, color, texture, and contour of the donor's liver should be carefully examined macroscopically. Biopsy is strongly recommended to be performed at the time of organ procurement/harvest from DCD donor liver, which is suspected of inferior quality such as unexplained focal lesions or steatosis. The pathological report should be made before transplantation. So procurement biopsy evaluation is time limited. It is often performed through frozen section immediatetly. Due to the disadvantages of frozen sections such as edematous artifacts, a rapid paraffin section is recommended in some centers. Time-zero biopsy refers to biopsy performed during the surgery before or after the graft got reperfusion. It is mainly used as a baseline assessment to detect preexisting diseases in the donor's liver and to identify changes related to organ preservation and reperfusion. There is relatively enough time for pathologists to perform zero-time biopsy evaluation. It can be performed as a routine liver biopsy using paraffin sections for hematoxylin and eosin (H&E), histochemistry, and immunohistochemistry staining.

Both needle biopsy and wedge biopsy can be used to obtain specimens from donor livers, the latter is preferred. Two cores, respectively from the right lobe and the left lobe, are recommended for assessment, and there are no preferred sites in the right and left lobes for obtaining these biopsies [5]. Wedge biopsies without accompanying needle biopsies are not appropriate enough for donor liver evaluation, because it mainly obtains subcapsular area tissue, and may lead to overestimation of fibrosis and preserve-reperfusion injury. Adequate specimens should contain two cores each of which is 1.5 cm at least in length. The liver biopsies containing at least ten intact portal areas and six central veins as well are required for pathological evaluation. Specimens contain four or less portal areas are considered unsatisfactory, and five to nine portal areas are accecptable. It should be stated in the donor liver biopsy report whether the specimens are satisfactory for pathological evaluation. Inadequate specimens will affect the reliability and accuracy of pathological evaluation.

13.1.3 Evaluation of Procurement/Harvest Biopsy

Pathological evaluation of procurement/harvest biopsy and pre-implantation biopsy aims to determine the suitability of the donor liver for transplantation through identification the underlying diseases and the extent of injury. The most important significant factors that affect the quality of a donor liver for transplantation are steatosis, necrosis, inflammation, fibrosis, and tumor. According to Expert Consensus on Evaluation and Application of Organ Donated after Cardiac Death in China [6], DCD donor liver with malignant tumor, severe hepatic macrovesicular steatosis (>60%), or cirrhosis is absolutely contraindications for transplantation. But it should be noted that except these absolute contraindications, pathological evaluation is not the exclusive determinant of whether to use the organ or not. Furthermore, there is no accredited consensus and criteria for pathological evaluation until now.

13.1.3.1 Steatosis

There are two different types of steatosis, macrovesicular and microvesicular steatoses.

Macrovesicular steatosis is the most common type and is divided into large droplet and small droplet (Figs. 13.1 and 13.2). Large droplet macrovesicular steatosis indicates one large lipid vacuole occupying nearly the whole cytoplasm of hepatocyte, pushing the nucleus to the periphery area. Small droplet macrovesicular steatosis is defined as lipid vacuoles smaller than half of the cell and do not displace the nucleus. The term microvesicular steatosis is used when the cytoplasm is filled with innumerable fine lipid vesicles without nuclear displacement [7], which sometimes may cause confusion with small droplet macrovesicular steatosis. The extent of steatosis is estimated as the percentage of liver parenchyma area that is involved (Figs. 13.3, 13.4, and 13.5). In our experience, this can be done in routine H&E staining in a frozen section without oil red O or Sudan III staining.

Macrovesicular steatosis is a common finding in donor liver biopsies with prevalence ranging from 13 to 50% [8, 9]. Steatosis donor liver is more susceptible to ischemia–reperfusion injury. Large droplet macrovesicular steatosis is a well-recognized risk factor for reduced short-term graft survival [10, 11]. It is recommended by Expert Consensus on Evaluation and Application of Organ Donated after Cardiac Death in China that frozen section of liver biopsy should be performed to identify the extent and type of steatosis when BMI of DCD donor is greater than 25 kg/m^2 [6].

Several studies reported the affect of macrovesicular steatosis/macrosteatosis on the outcome of

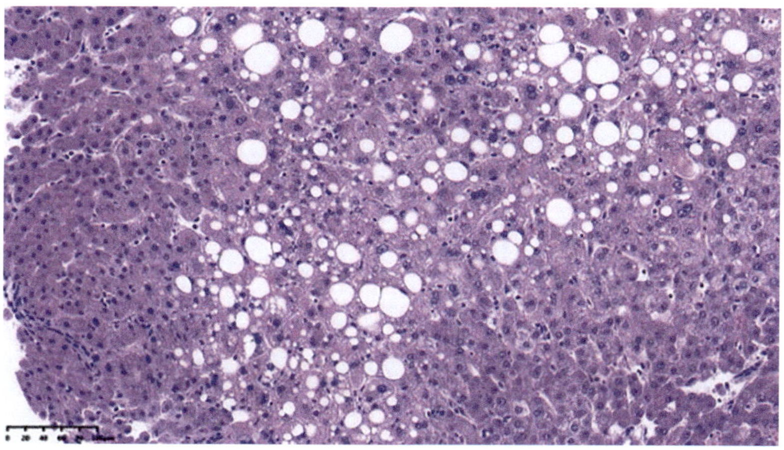

Fig. 13.1 Large droplet macrovesicular steatosis

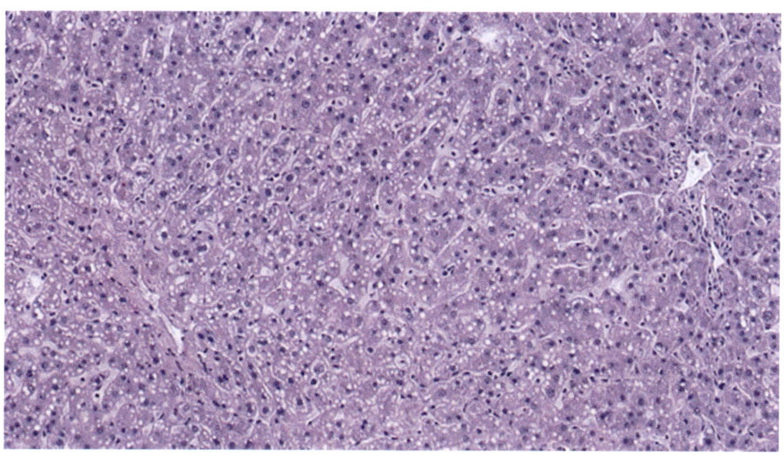

Fig. 13.2 Small droplet macrovesicular steatosis

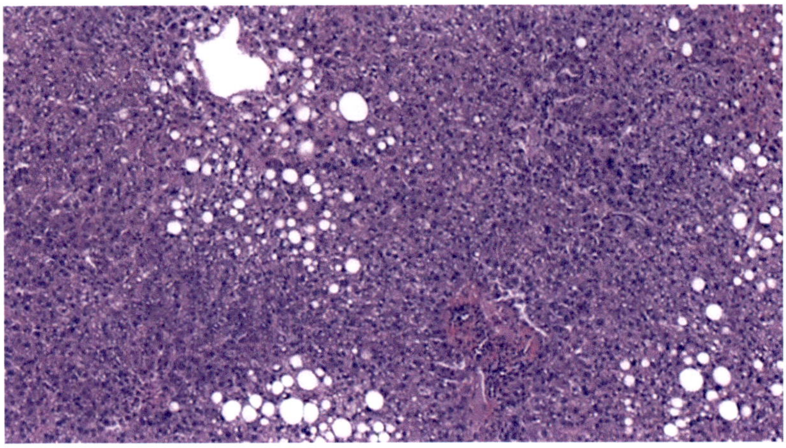

Fig. 13.3 Mild macrovesicular steatosis

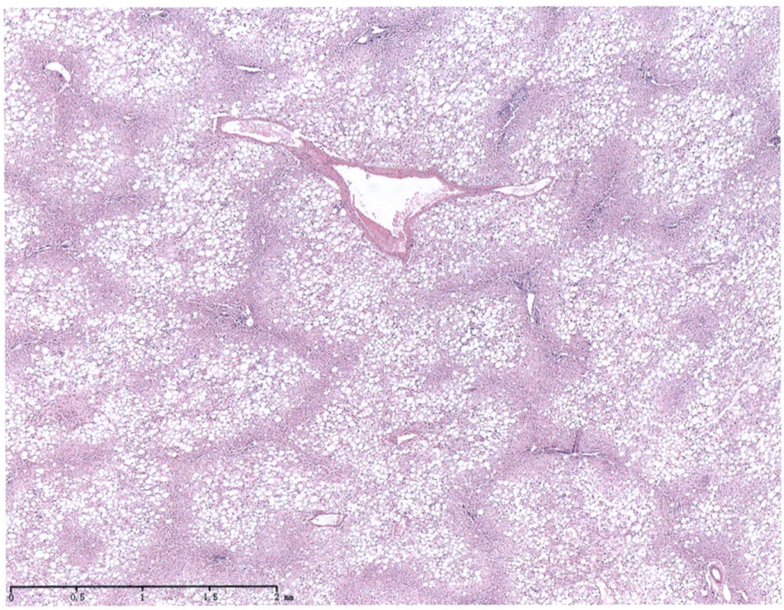

Fig. 13.4 Severe large droplet macrovesicular steatosis

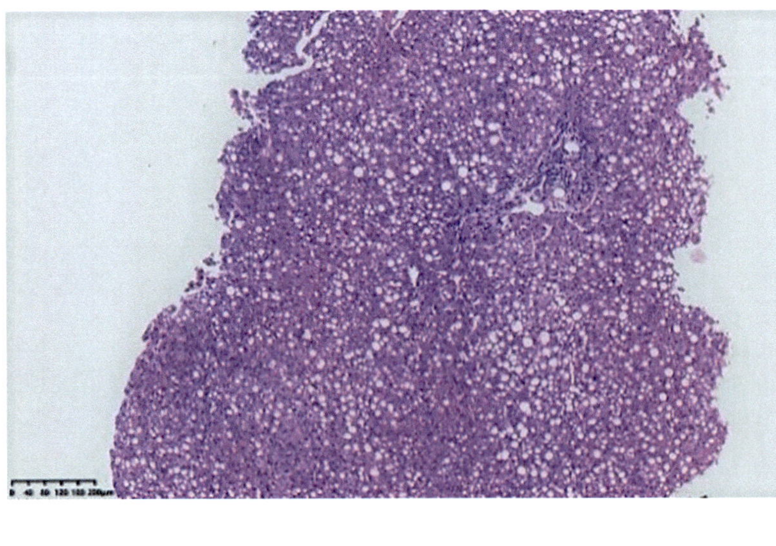

Fig. 13.5 Diffuse macrovesicular steatosis

DCD liver transplantation [12–15]. The common conclusion of these studies is that the more serious steatosis of the DCD donor liver is, the more likely it may have adverse effects on the survival of the organ. However, there is no consensus on the threshold beyond which the DCD donor liver must not be used, although different thresholds ranging from 15 to 30% are reported [12–15]. According to Clinical Technical Practice for Pathology of organ transplantation (2019 Edition) [16], DCD donor livers with mild (<20%) and moderate (20–30%) macrovesicular steatosis are relatively safe for transplantation. However, when accompanied by risk factors such as elderly donors (>70 years old), prolonged warm ischemia time (>30 min), or cold ischemia time (>11 h), donor liver with moderate (20–30%) macrovesicular steatosis is regarded as a marginal donor liver which may have an increasing risk of primary graft dysfunction (PGD) [17]. Severe macrosteatosis/macrovesicular steatosis (>30%) is an independent risk factor for PGD [9]. While according to Expert Consensus on Evaluation and Application of Organ Donated after Cardiac Death in China (2014 edition) [6], macrosteatosis/macrovesicular steatosis less than 15% is a condition for an ideal DCD liver donor; mild macrovesicular steatosis (15–30%) are relatively safe for transplantation; while livers with moderate macrovesicular steatosis (30–60%) should be utilized only in case of emergency, and severe macrovesicular steatosis (>60%) is contraindication for transplantation because of high risk of PNF.

It is prevailingly recognized that microsteatosis/microvesicular steatosis is a mild, reversible lesion and does not have significant impact on graft survival, because ischemia-reperfusion injury occurs less frequently and tend to be mild. However, several reports have suggested that it increased risk for early hepatic dysfunction [14, 18, 19]. Different extent of microvesicular steatosis ranging from 10 to 60% are reported to be used [14, 18, 19]. But there is no consensus on the threshold of this lesion beyond which the DCD donor liver must not be used. Thus, it is suggested that a donor liver with severe and exclusive microvesicular steatosis should not be used for transplantation, especially in patients who may have demonstrated signs and symptoms of an energy utilization depletion syndrome [4].

Briefly, DCD donor liver with severe hepatic macrovesicular steatosis (>60%) is contraindication for liver transplantation. However, the acceptable threshold for these lesions remains unknown. Actually, evaluation of suitability of DCD liver donors depends on multiple factors of both donors and recipients. Therefore, pathologists should describe in detail the actual extent, type of steatosis and other findings, avoiding an arbitrary decision on the suitability only based on histology.

13.1.3.2 Tumors

Donor liver with small benign lesions such as hemangioma and focal nodular hyperplasia (FNH) can be successfully transplanted [20]. Both primary and metastatic malignant tumors in donor livers are absolutely contraindication for transplantation, such as hepatocellular carcinoma, intrahepatic cholangiocarcinoma and metastatic adenocarcinoma. Malignant tumor transmission through liver transplantation rarely occurs, but it may result in disastrous consequences. It is reported that the most frequently transmitted malignancies by the way of liver transplantation are lymphoma, malignant melanoma, and neuroendocrine tumor [21–23]. Donor liver from patients with malignant melanoma, invasive breast carcinoma, colon carcinoma, lung cancer, malignant melanoma, and leukemia, are not suitable for transplantation because of high risks of transmission [4], even these malignancies are not found in the donor liver before or during the operation. Livers from donors with low-grade central nervous system tumors and small renal cell carcinoma may be used with caution due to extremely low risk of tumor transmission [4, 47, 48].

In brief, donor livers with primary and metastatic malignancies and livers from donors with various types of malignancies elsewhere are contraindication for liver transplantation. Once liver tumor is suspected, rapid frozen section diagnosis is required before transplantation.

13.1.3.3 Necrosis, Inflammation, and Fibrosis

Presence and the grade of interface and lobular active inflammation, the degree of necrosis, and the stage of fibrosis in donor liver should be evaluated. These lesions usually occur in DCD donors with positive hepatitis B and hepatitis C serologies, which liver biopsy is recommended [4]. Livers from HBsAg or anti-HBc or anti-HCV positive donors are recommended to have a comprehensive assessment of the risks and benefits before transplantation [24, 25]. HCV viremic donors older than 35 years with chronic infection should undertake liver biopsy to identify the extent of fibrosis. Livers with advanced fibrosis (F3 or F4) are not recommended to be used, while F0 to F2 fibrosis is acceptable for transplantation [24]. Biopsy findings that would exclude a donor liver for transplant include: (1) necrosis involving >10% of hepatocytes, (2) >50% macrovesicular steatosis, (3) moderate or severe atherosclerosis of intrahepatic arteries, and (4) advanced fibrosis (Ishak >F3; METAVIR >F2) [25].

In brief, necrosis, inflammation, and fibrosis should be evaluated, especially in livers from donors with hepatitis B or hepatitis C. Donor liver showing cirrhosis is a contraindication for transplantation [6, 24].

13.1.3.4 Other Pre-existing Changes

Additional changes may be found in a donor liver such as abnormalities of bile duct, granuloma, amyloidosis. Siderosis can be resulted from genetic and secondary hemochromatosis. The donor liver with siderosis grossly looks slightly dark and it may raise a doubt on the suitability of the organ. Liver biopsy shows large amount of hemosiderin deposition. It is reported that several cases of donor livers with genetic hemochromatosis are used for transplant. Hemosiderin may diminish gradually or persist for many years after transplantation, with normal or abnormal liver function [26, 27]. A similar case showing severe hepatocellular hemosiderosis by H&E staining and Prussian blue staining was also utilized for transplantation in our transplantation center (Figs. 13.6 and 13.7). The liver function of the recipient recovered back to normal within three weeks after transplantation, and maintained stable in the following one year (data unpublished).

13.1.4 Evaluation of Time-Zero Biopsy

The main purpose of time-zero biopsy is to detect the pre-existing lesions and identify changes related to donor liver preservation and reperfusion. It can provide not only baseline changes to compare with posttransplant biopsy for differentiated diagnosis, but also pathological information to predict prognosis. There are two time points of time-zero biopsy including pre-reperfusion biopsy and post-reperfusion biopsy. Both are performed routinely in our transplantation center. Pre-existing lesions found in time-zero biopsy are similar to those found in procurement biopsy as discussed above. The

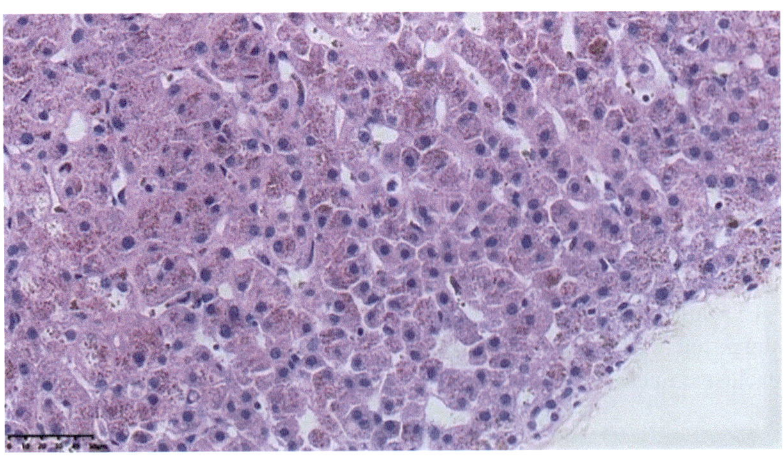

Fig. 13.6 Hemosiderin deposition mainly in hepatocytes, H&E staining

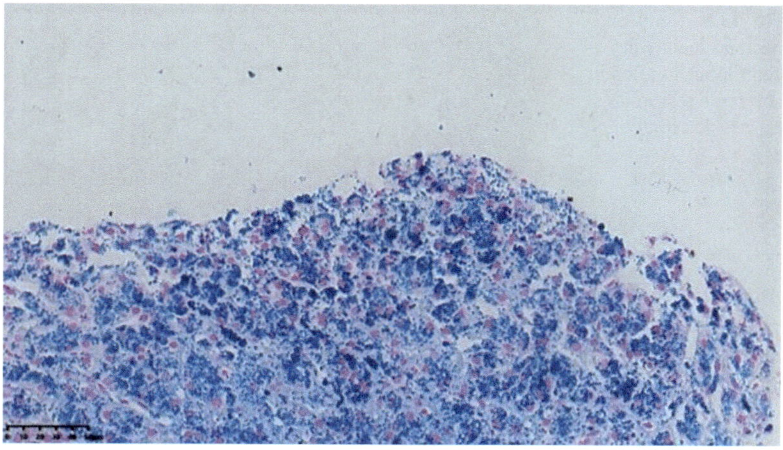

Fig. 13.7 Hemosiderin deposition mainly in hepatocytes, Prussian blue staining

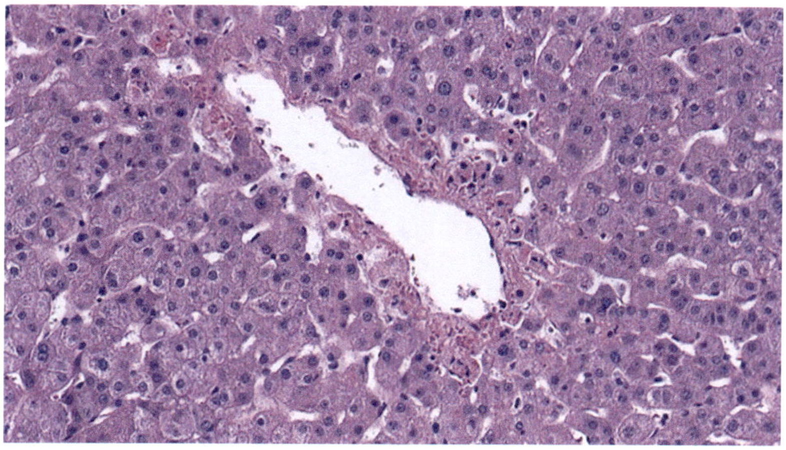

Fig. 13.8 Necrosis or apoptosis of several single hepatocytes around lobule central vein in mild preservation-reperfusion injury

pathological changes of preservation–reperfusion injury in post-reperfusion biopsy are generally severer than in pre-reperfusion biopsy.

Preservation-reperfusion injury is an important change found in time-zero biopsy. It refers to damage of the liver allograft caused by physiologic stress such as ischemia, preservation, reperfusion, and reimplantation. The histologic changes are generally mild and mainly in centrilobular region, including hepatocyte ballooning, detachment, necrosis, apoptosis, cholestasis, and neutrophil aggregation in the lobule (Fig. 13.8). Mild changes are reversible over several weeks. Prominent and large area of confluent necrosis can be seen in severe cases (Fig. 13.9). Necrosis may be more predominant in subcapsular parenchyma, but it is not always representative of the whole liver (Fig. 13.10). Steatosis livers are more sensitive to reperfusion damage. Fat droplets from damaged hepatocytes may subsequently be released into the extracellular space, mostly in Disse space and occasionally in sinusoid, resulting in the formation of cystic lesions named lipopeliosis [28]. Although fatty change is mainly considered to be a preexisting lesion, some studies indicate that graft ischemia and reperfusion injury may result in the development of microvesicular steatosis in the early posttransplant period [29, 30]. Histologic changes mentioned above are not characteristic of preservation-reperfusion injury, so we should pay attention to differential diagnosis in a particular case. Histologic changes of the post-reperfusion biopsy are usually related to the recovery of liver function in the early postoperative period.

In conclusion, pathological evaluation of DCD donor liver plays an important role to pre-

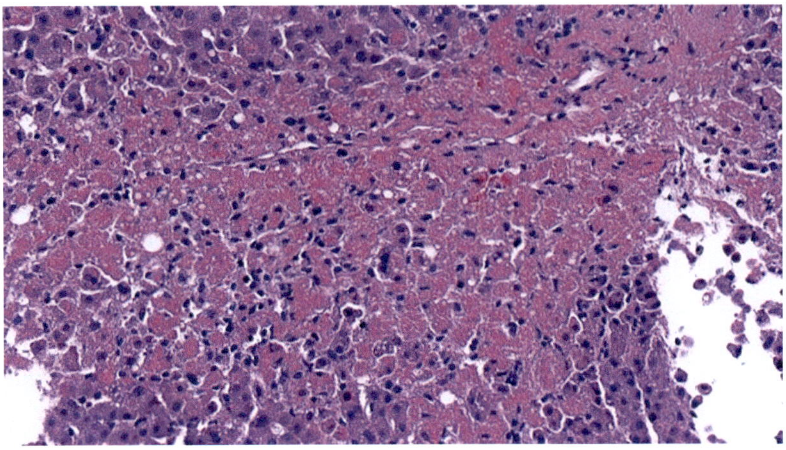

Fig. 13.9 Confluent necrosis mainly in centrilobular region in severe preservation-reperfusion injury

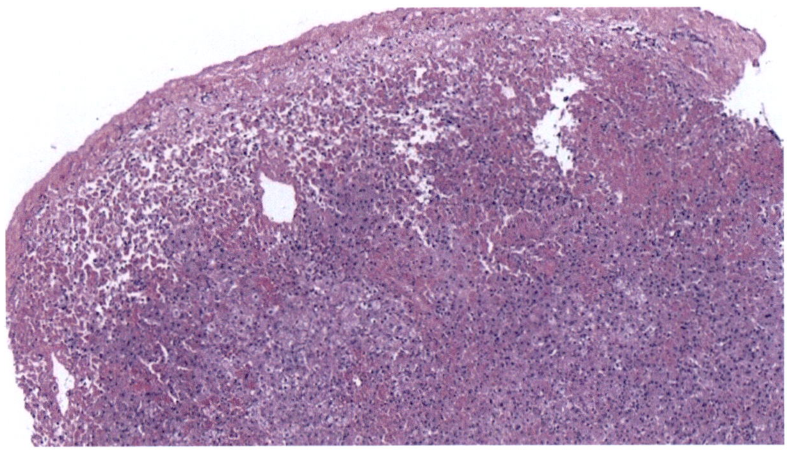

Fig. 13.10 Necrosis resulting from preservation-reperfusion injury is more obvious in subcapsular liver parenchyma

vent inappropriate transplantation. But besides histologic changes discussed above, there are lots of other pathological changes and variable clinical backgrounds. What the pathologist should do is to describe the presence and extent of reversible or irreversible lesions in detail. The pathological report should be interpreted based on clinical background by pathologists and clinicians to make a reasonable decision [31].

13.2 Evaluation of DCD Donor Kidney

13.2.1 Significance of DCD Kidney Biopsy

With the rapid development of organ transplantation in China, organs from DCD donors is becoming the most important source of kidney transplantation besides living-related donors since the year 2015 [32]. Although the pool of donors expanding every year, there is still an absolute shortage of organs resulting in the longer and longer waiting time for patients. Each organ has a pre-life and is affected by the conditions of the donor. Compared with the living-related donors, most of the DCD donors have underlying disease or died due to accidents and inevitably undergo hypotension, infection, and various drug exposures when treated in ICU, which may lead to kidney injury resulting in a high risk of DGF post-transplantation [33].

Glomeruli obsolescence increases with the age as well as the prevalence of hypertension, diabetes, and neoplasms. Biopsy at the time of procurement or implantation can help evaluate the degree of the organ affected by donors' diseases. Organs from marginal donors or ECD are used more widely than before leading to an increased risk of

PNF or DGF and making the evaluation of DCD organ very critical. It should be noted that evaluation of DCD donor is a complicated process and multiple factors of both the donor and the recipient should be considered including clinical history, gross appearance of the organ, and parameters of the organ perfusion supplement such as Lifeport [34]. Pathological evaluation is an essential component of the evaluation though it is not the only determinant to justify whether an organ should be transplanted or discarded.

13.2.2 Time Points for Biopsy and Technical Considerations

There are three different time points to do the biopsy which are procurement/harvest biopsy, preimplantation biopsy, and zero-hour implantation biopsy. Procurement biopsies and preimplantation biopsy are primarily performed to give information on the organ's suitability for transplantation. They are often evaluated on a rush basis with frozen sections by general pathologists during off-hours. Procurement biopsy is usually recorded under the donor's name because the kidney is not allocated until the biopsy and other clinical parameters show it is suitable for transplantation. Preimplantation biopsy can provide information on the organ suitability for transplantation and other pathological changes caused by the delivery and maintenance process as well. Zero-hour implantation biopsies provide insight into preexisting diseases relevant for comparative analyses for posttransplantation biopsies instead of evaluating the suitability for transplantation. So, zero-hour is performed with routine renal biopsy technique including paraffin sections, immunofluorescence, and electronic microscope.

There are two different methods of biopsy for donor kidneys including needle biopsy and wedge biopsy. Both have advantages and disadvantages. For needle aspiration, we can usually detect glomeruli in the cortex and the juxtamedullary nephron while in wedge biopsy mainly get the superficial cortex in the subcapsular area which easily develop nonspecific sclerosis leading to overestimation of the percentage of glomerular sclerosis, interstitial fibrosis, and underscore of vascular damage [35, 36] (Fig. 13.11). Immunofluorescence staining for IgG, IgM, IgA, complement C3 and C1q are tested to detect whether there is immune complex-mediated glomerulonephritis. Electronic microscope is aimed at the ultrastructure changes, especially when there is glomerulonephritis.

13.2.3 Evaluation of Procurement/Harvest Biopsy

The main purpose of preimplantation biopsy is to make a decision whether the DCD donor kidney is suitable for transplantation. Pathologists are required to give a very prompt evaluation with a frozen section so that the kidney can move to the allocation step. Due to the distorted structure, an inevitable drawback of frozen section, edematous artifact may easily be mistaken for interstitial

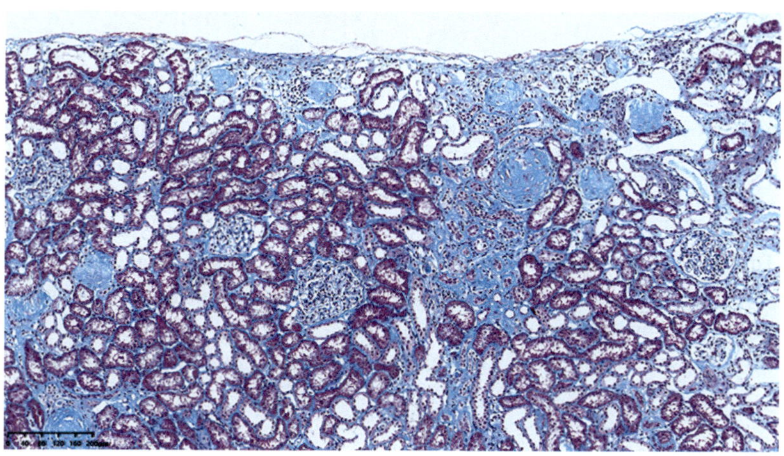

Fig. 13.11 Nonspecific scar in subcapsular area and aggregation of glomerulosclerosis (Masson ×100)

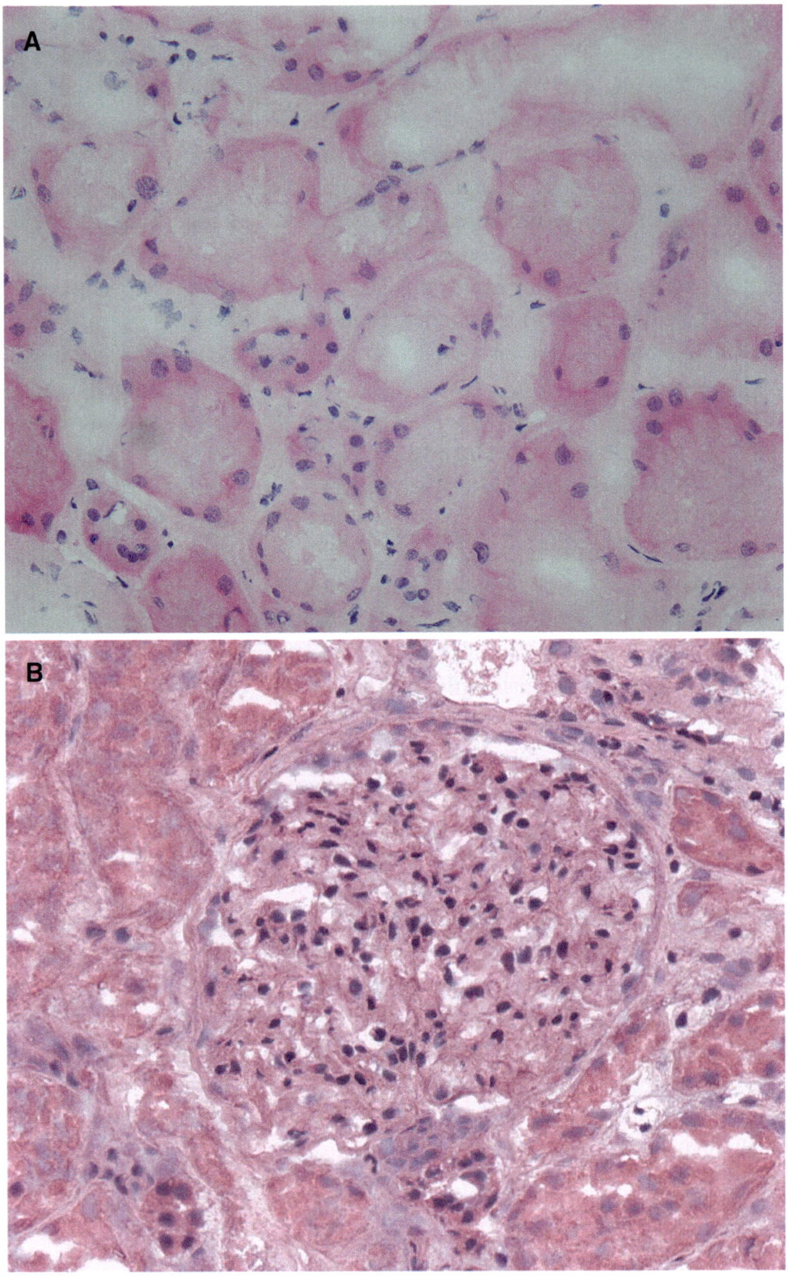

Fig. 13.12 **A**. Edematous artifact in the frozen section, which should not be mistaken for interstitial edema (frozen section HE ×200) **B**. Glomeruli appears hypercelluar

edema which is hard to distinguished from fibrosis in frozen section. Glomerular disease is difficult to evaluate because glomeuli tend to appear hypercellular in frozen section (Fig. 13.12). Tubules appear retracted and can be misinterpreted as atrophy or injury. We know that in some Chinese transplantation centers, rapid paraffin which is relatively time consuming but have much better morphology compared with frozen section is strongly recommended.

It should be noted that until now, an absolute, validated standard for donor kidney has not been established. So the threshold of glomerular sclerosis, IFTA (interstitial fibrosis and tubular atrophy), or arteriosclerosis beyond which a donor kidney must not be used has not been verified.

Sometimes it is not easy to answer whether a kidney is suitable for transplantation. In general, we need to evaluate the following elements: (1) The degree of chronic lesion in the DCD kidney including the percentage of glomerulosclerosis, proportion of IFTA area, and degree of artery thickening. These chronic lesions are relatively irreversible, when the severity reaches a certain degree might result in incomplete function or even PNF of the graft; (2) The presence of any active lesion such as acute tubular necrosis, fibroid necrosis of glomerular tuft, and interstitial inflammatory cell infiltration. These lesions are reversible but may lead to delayed graft function. The extent of these acute lesions can help predict the occurrence of DGF but may not affect the long-term prognosis of the graft. (3) The clinical significance of incidentally discovered neoplasms. Following are the most important changs which usually present in DCD donor kidneys.

13.2.3.1 Percentage of Glomerular Sclerosis

The percentage of glomerular sclerosis is one of the most important indexes in DCD donor kidney evaluation. It can represent to some degree the residue proportion of functional nephrons reflecting the reserved function of the kidney. The higher the percentage of glomerulosclerosis, the more likely to develop DGF and PNF in the short term and graft loss in the long term. But multivariate analysis shows that it is not an independent risk factor for the prognosis of the allograft [37]. Whether a certain percentage of glomerulosclerosis will affect the long-term survival of the graft correlates with the absolute numbers of functional nephrons and the basic metabolism rate of the recipient as well. Up to now, there is still no validated cut-off value that lower than which makes the kidney acceptable and beyond which leading to organ discard. One widely accepted cut-off value is 20%. In practical work whether a DCD kidney should be used or discarded when the sclerotic percentage is around 20%, several factors should be taken into account including age, body mass index, and the basic metabolic rate of both the donor and the recipient. Recipients with lower metabolism rate and less body surface area are preferred when there is a certain degree of loss of the glomeruli. With strict management of the patient blood pressure and body weight, graft function can remain stable for quite a long time. There is no controversy that once the percentage is more than 30%, the kidney should not be transplanted.

Physiological sclerosis is not uncommon in normal individuals even in children (usually less than 5%) and increases with the age after 40 years. A simple estimation of the percentage is age divided by 2 and then minors 10. For example, for patients of 60 years old the percentage is 60/2–10, which means glomerulosclerosis no more than 20% is acceptable in 60 years old person. If the biopsy shows more sclerosis, reasons other than age should be considered, in which the most frequent factors are hypertension and glomerulonephritis. In the following conditions, the percentage of sclerosis tends to be overestimated including (1) Presence of sclerotic foci in which numerous sclerotic glomeruli aggregating (Fig. 13.11). This is very common in superficial cortex, especially in subscapular area that might cause by occlusion of one small artery. In this circumstance, it is suggested that repeat biopsy in a different site should be done for re-evaluation. (2) Sample adequacy is very critical. Total numbers of glomeruli less than 15 tend to cause overestimation of the percentage of glomerular sclerosis. (3) The percentage of glomerular sclerosis is similar in bilateral kidneys when there is no autonomic abnormality. So, when there is a significant difference in the percentage of sclerosis, it is not necessarily reasonable to discard the one with a higher percentage. In this circumstance, multiple core biopsies or wedge biopsy should be done for overall evaluation.

There are several reasons that lead to loss of glomeruli, including physiological obsolescent, ischemic sclerosis, and glomerulonephritis usually manifested as proliferation of resident cells and matrix in glomeruli. So, it is necessary to identify the possible reason and figure out whether there is a possibility of glomerulonephritis. Due to the drawback of frozen section, it is not easy to diagnose glomerulonephritis in DCD donor evaluations when immunofluorescence and electronic microscope are not available. Only when there is presence of increased cell numbers and matrix, crescents formation, can a glomerulonephritis be suspected with frozen section. Confirmation and classification of glomerulonephritis should be based on the paraffin section with multiple staining combined with IF and EM.

13.2.3.2 Arterial and Arteriolar Lesions

The intimal of arteries undergo thickening and fibrosis with the increasing of age. Intimal fibrosis and arteriolar hyalinosis are frequently found in DCD donor kidneys, especially in ECD kidneys due to the presence of hypertension and diabetes which are very common underlying diseases in DCD donors. It is reported that more than half of the DCD kidney can be found with arterial intimal fibrosis and arteriolar hyalinosis. The percentage tends to be as high as 70% in living-related donors due to in most cases in China the donor is parents who donated to children. Evaluation of the extent of the arterial and arteriolar narrowing is a very important component of DCD donor kidney biopsy because the status of blood vessels correlated with the blood supply of the kidney after transplantation and may affect both the short- and the long-term survival of the graft [38–40].

Arteries that can be detected in renal biopsy include arcuate arteries that are located in the borderline of cortex and medulla, interlobular (cortical radiating) arteries, and arterioles (afferent and efferent arterioles). The most common lesion is arteriosclerosis (AS) (Fig. 13.13) and arteriolar hyalinosis (AH) (Fig. 13.14). In Banff

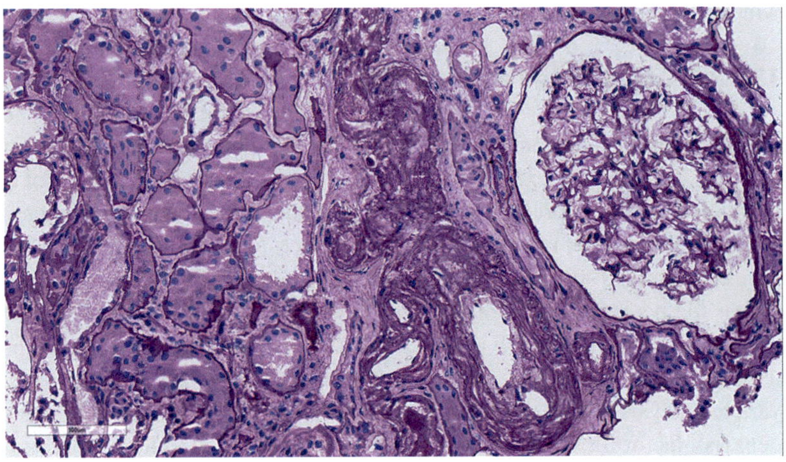

Fig. 13.13 Severe intimal fibrosis of the interlobular artery (frozen section PAS ×200)

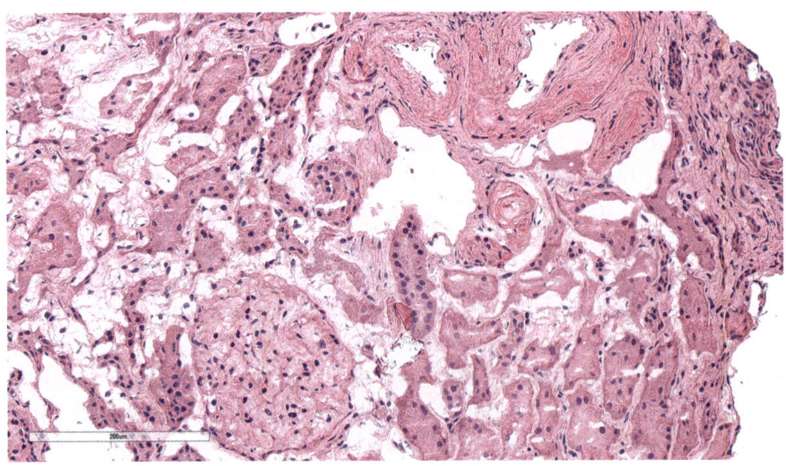

Fig. 13.14 Intimal fibrosis of the interlobular artery and arteriolar hyalinosis (arrow) (frozen section HE ×100)

Consensus for preimplantation kidney biopsies, vascular lesions are graded according to the extent of the narrowing and hyalinosis of the vessels [41]. Lesions lower than cv2 and ah2 will not have a significant impact on short-term creatinine levels post-transplantation and long-term survival of the graft. Clinical research proved that lesions grade higher than cv2 or ah3 usually occur in malignant hypertension (Fig. 13.15a, b) have higher risk of DGF and PNF compared with lower grade donor kidneys. So, lesions severer than cv2 or ah3 should be combined with the percentage of glomerulosclerosis, the extent of IFTA, and other clinical data for a reasonable decision.

Glomerular fibrin thrombi (GFT) are infrequent findings in DCD donors (Fig. 13.16). It is an acute injury and occurred in 3.5% DCD donor kidneys most correlated with higher blood coagulation associated with severe trauma, massive hemorrhage, cardiac arrest, or DIC. Glomerular fibrin thrombi cause occlusion of glomerular tuft and lead to increased risk of DGF. It is reported that the rate of DGF increased to 45% in the presence of GFT. Whether the grafts undergo DGF or not relates to the proportion of the involved glomerular tuft. GFT does not have significant impact on long term survival of the graft. But diffuse GFT will cause DGF inevitably. Focal GFT which means there are still a lot of glomerular tufts expired do not affect the survival of donor kidneys because the fibrinolytic system in the recipient will dissolve those thrombi [42]. Whether DCD donor kidneys should be discarded when there is diffuse GFT is controversial. Literature supports the opinion that most cases

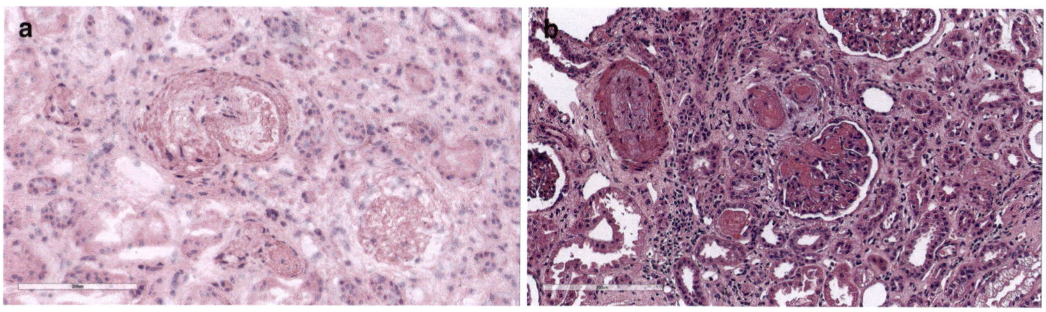

Fig. 13.15 (**a**) Severe thickening of the intimal leading to the obliteration of the arterial lumen in a malignant hypertension donor kidney (frozen section HE ×200). (**b**) Mucinous degeneration of the arterial intimal and arteriolar fibroid necrosis with fibrin thrombi in glomerular capillary in a malignant hypertension donor kidney (HE ×100)

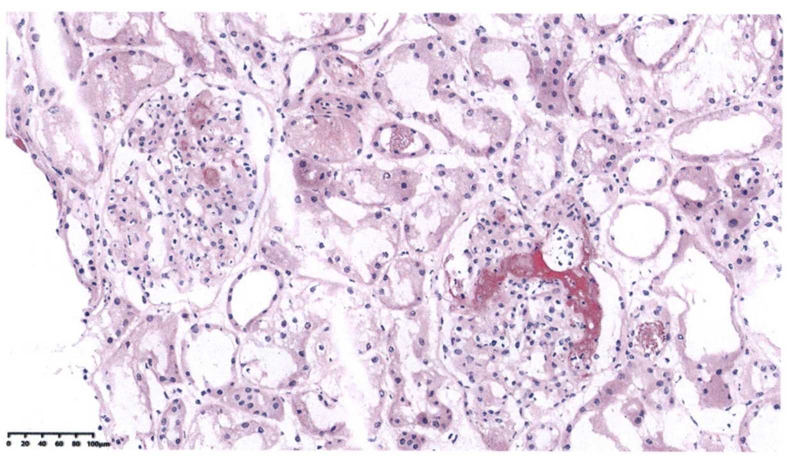

Fig. 13.16 Fibrin thrombi in the glomerular tufts (frozen section HE ×200)

are suitable for transplantation and do not have significance in the long-term survival of the graft [43]. It should be noted that those GFT caused by increased blood coagulation tend to have a good prognosis while those thrombi caused by endothelial injuries such as thrombotic microangiopathy or those thrombi involve larger arteries and result in focal infarction of renal cortex should be distinguished because the latter show high risk of PNF (Fig. 13.17).

13.2.3.3 Acute and Chronic Lesions of Tubules and Interstitium

DCD donor usually has various degrees of acute tubular injury (ATI) and even coagulative necrosis in severe cases. ATI is an important factor that correlated with the urine volume in the early post-transplantation period. Recipient may have normal or only slightly decreased urine volume when ATI is mild. Severe ATI or ATN causes oliguria or even anuria after transplantation. So, evaluation of the extent of ATI can help foresee the possibility of DGF and the duration of DGF, but do not affect the long-term survival of the graft [44, 45]. Tubular epithelial cells usually regenerate in 4–8 weeks as long as the tubular basement membrane is intact and urine increases gradually.

Banff divided ATI into three different grades according to the extent of the injury [41]. Mild ATI usually shows swollen or degeneration of tubular epithelial cells, losses of brush border resulting in flattening of the cells and dilation of the tubular lumen (Fig. 13.18). Mild ATI is very common in DCD donor kidneys caused by multi-factor including the ischemic procedure, hypo-

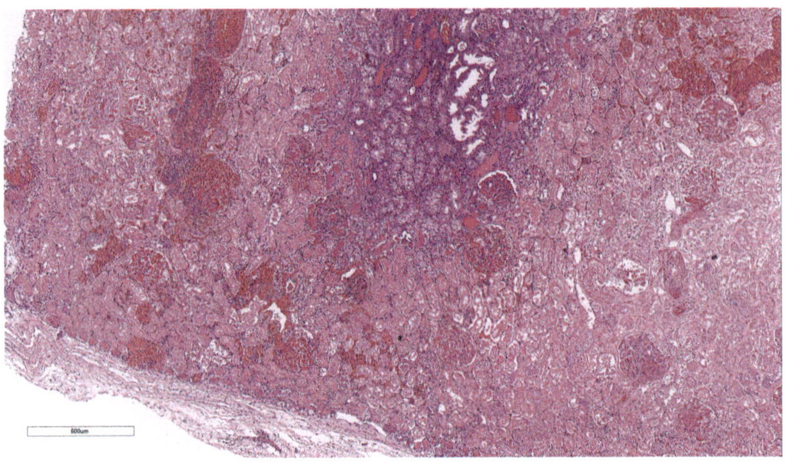

Fig. 13.17 Focal infarction of renal cortex in a patient with TMA (frozen section HE ×40)

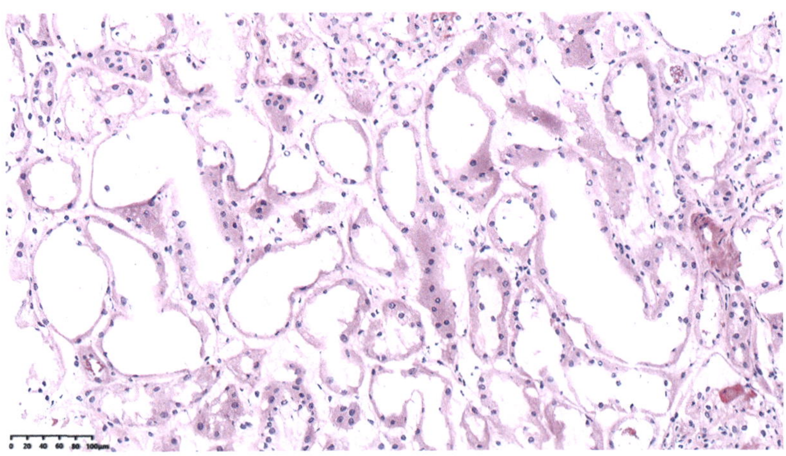

Fig. 13.18 Acute injury of renal tubule (frozen section HE ×200)

tension during the rescue process of the donor and drug, etc. Mild ATI will not affect the urine volume and the recovery of renal function thus creatinine usually decreases to normal in 1 week. The presence focal necrosis of tubular epithelial cells means moderate ATI (Fig. 13.19). When there is coagulative necrosis, it is critical to find out the etiology. Infectious disease, thrombosis, prolonged cold ischemic time are the common reasons and are not suggested to transplant. Necrosis caused by other reasons like trauma, injury got during the process of procurement and other mechanical factors might not affect the suitability for transplantation. Severe ATI manifests renal cortex infarction [41] (Fig. 13.17). Foci of infarction presenting in biopsy, often means there is thrombosis in larger arteries like arcuate arteries or even lobular arteries leading to larger area necrosis involving tubules and glomeruli. It is not suggested to be transplanted because necrosis often involves the total thickness of the cortex and there is a risk that the cortex might rupture after needle biopsy.

Except for ischemic and reperfusion injury, there are many other factors that can cause tubular injury including rhabdomyolysis caused by crush injury or drugs in which myoglobin cast occlude the tubular (Fig. 13.20). Recipients usually undergo DGF after transplantation, but long-term survival of the graft is not affected [46]. For DCD donor kidney, drug-induced tubular injury should also be considered because in most cases during the treatment in ICU, donors usually underwent numerous drugs exposure. Many drugs including antibiotics can cause tubular injury directly or indirectly and lead to ATN or

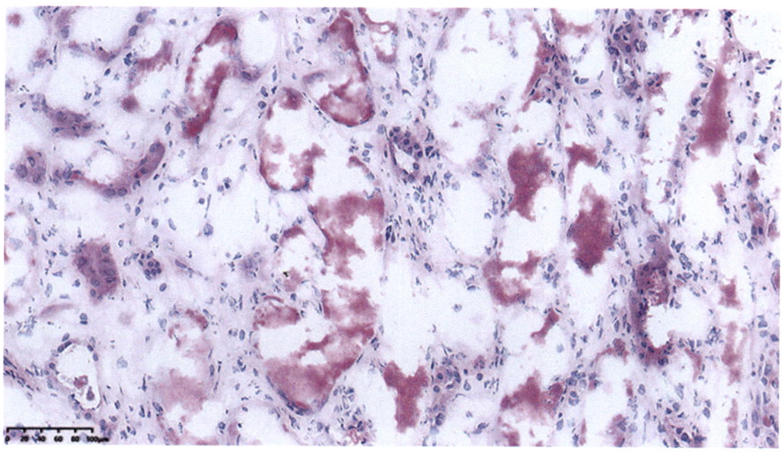

Fig. 13.19 Coagulative necrosis of proximal tubular epithelial cells (frozen section HE ×200)

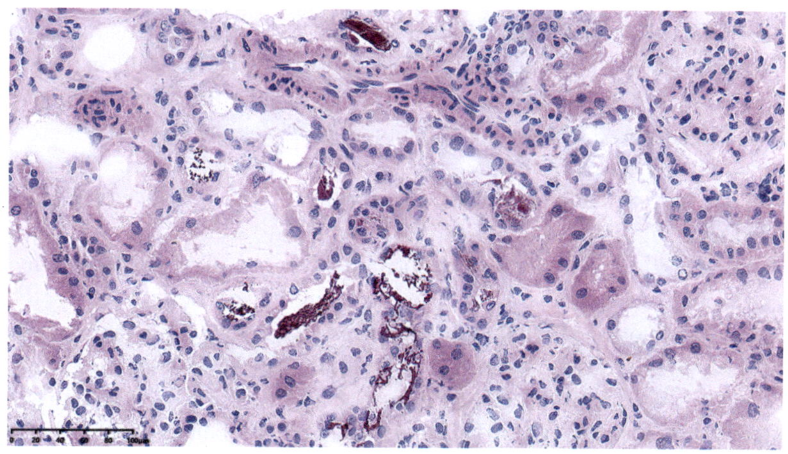

Fig. 13.20 Acuter tubular injuries with pigmented cast (myoglobin cast) in a donor with crush trauma (frozen section HE ×200)

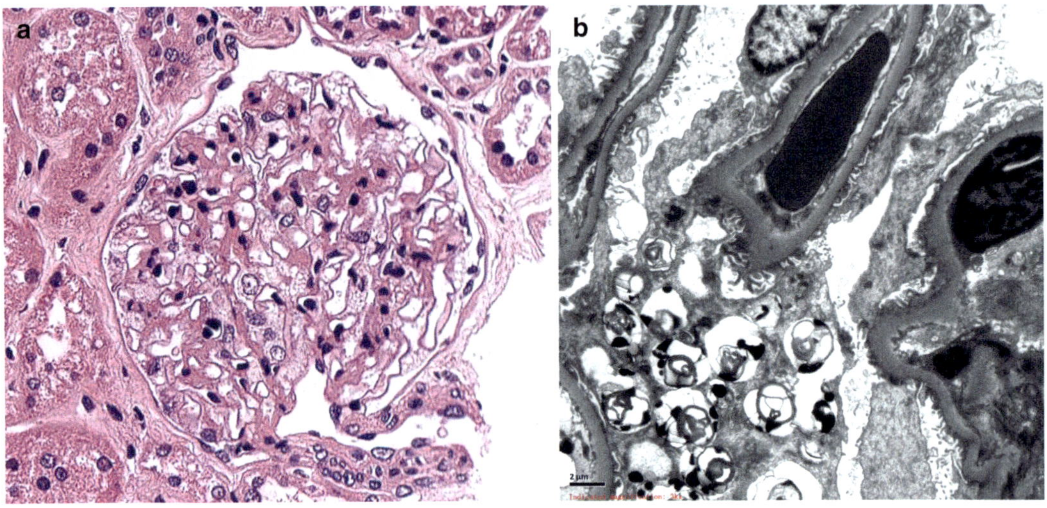

Fig. 13.21 (**a**) Vacuolar degeneration of the glomerular podocyte (HE ×400). (**b**) Numerous myeloid bodies in podocyte in a patient after Amiodarone treatment

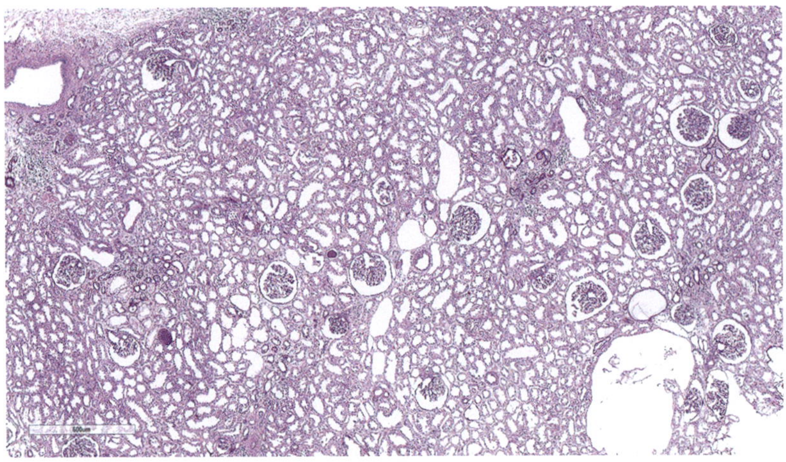

Fig. 13.22 Mild tubular atrophy and interstitial fibrosis (PAS ×40)

acute interstitial nephritis (AIN), or less frequently podocyte injury (Fig. 13.21a, b).

Acute lesions of interstitium usually manifest as edema and inflammatory cells infiltration. Interstitial edema is quite common in DCD donor kidneys due to ischemic process. The distance between tubules is widened and is loosened showing lightly stained in H&E and PAS staining (Fig. 13.12). It should be noted that frozen sections can cause artifacts that looks similar to edematous of the renal interstitium. This artifact should not be interpreted as significant change. Mild interstitial edema does not have significant impact in use of DCD donor kidney but severe edema causes significant increased internal tension which occasionally unfortunately results in rupture of the kidney. Interstitial infiltration is also very common in DCD donor kidneys. When there is inflammatory infiltrate, especially in the non-scar area, infection and drug-induced inflammation should be taken into account.

Chronic lesions include tubular atrophy and interstitial fibrosis (IFTA) (Fig. 13.22), both are very important components of DCD donor kidney evaluation. The extent of IFTA is categorized into four different grades in Banff criteria. For tubular atrophy, when less than 25%, 26–50%, or more than 50% of the cortical tubules are involved, it is defined as mild, moderate, and severe, respectively. Similarly, when interstitial fibrosis involved less than 10%, 10–25%, 26–50%, or more than 50% of cortex, they are defined as none, mild, moderate, and severe. IFTA is an important factor that predicts the survival of the graft [47]. DCD donor kidneys with severe IFTA (>50%) are not suggested to be transplanted.

13.2.3.4 Neoplasm of Donor Kidney

Space-occupying lesion is infrequent findings in DCD donor kidney. The most common benign tumors of the kidney are angiomyolipoma (PEcoma) (Fig. 13.23), which usually do not affect the survival of the graft. The most frequent malignancy is clear cell renal cell carcinoma. It is easy to identify a tumor in the frozen section but difficult to diagnose the specific classification. For example, clear cell renal cell carcinoma may be confused with epithelioid angiomyolipoma, intrarenal adrenals in frozen sections (Fig. 13.24). The detection of a renal cell carcinoma does not necessarily mean an absolute contraindication against transplantation. It is reported that small tumor (<1 cm) with low nuclear grade (ISUP grade 1–2) when completely removed has an estimated minimal risk of tumor transmission [48, 49]. But when the donor suffered from malignant tumor including invasive breast, neuroendocrine, colon carcinomas, malignant melanoma, leuke-

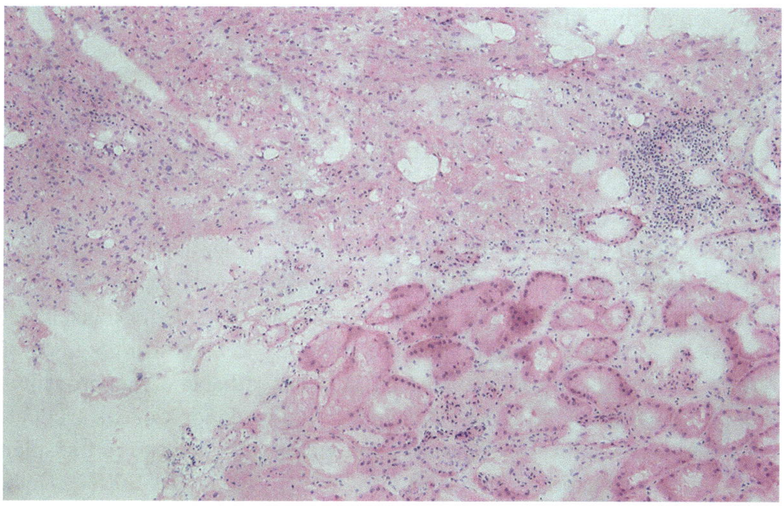

Fig. 13.23 Renal angiomyolipoma composed mainly of spindle tumor cells in the upper left area (frozen section HE ×100)

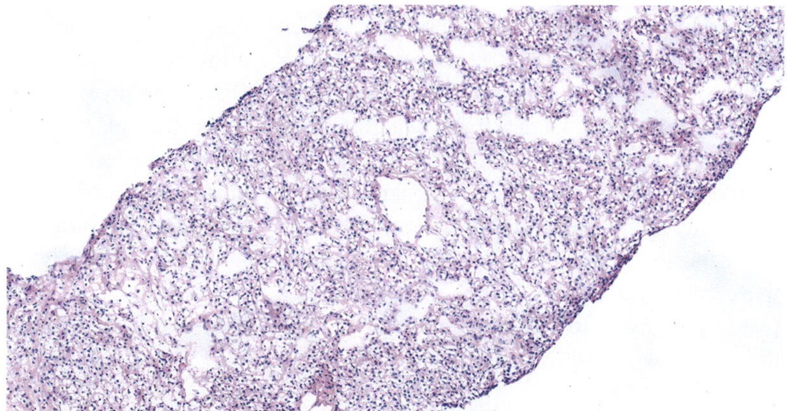

Fig. 13.24 Clear cell renal cell carcinoma (frozen section HE ×100)

mia, sarcomas, and lung cancer, organs from these donors carry a high risk (>10%) of disease transmission, and they should not be transplanted.

13.2.4 Evaluation of zero-Time Biopsy

Zero-time biopsy refers to biopsy performed during the surgery before or after the graft got reperfusion. At this time point, the kidney is undergoing transplantation, so the biopsy is not for making the decision whether or not to use the organ but to identify the baseline pathologic changes or the pre-exist lesions which can be of critical value in differential diagnosis in the future protocol and indicational biopsies. Zero-time biopsy is valuable for the prognosis of the graft long-term survival but is not critical, because for the long-term survival of the graft, rejection, infection, and recurrence of glomerulopathy are more important factors that influence the graft survival. The content of zero-time evaluation is similar with the procurement/harvest biopsy as discussed above. The difference is that there is enough time to do the multiple staining, immunofluorescence, and electronic microscope. It is suggested that when glomerular disease is suspected, zero-time biopsy should be done to have a detailed examination of the DCD donor kidney. Zero-time biopsies are valuable for clinical and translational research purposes, providing insight into risk factors for post-transplant events, and as baseline for comparison with post-transplant histology [50]. The most common pre-exist glomerulonephritis is IgA nephropathy which occurs in about 10% in DCD donor and higher incidence of IgA nephropathy was observed in living-related donor kidney transplantation compared with deceased donor kidney transplantation [51]. The lesion is relatively mild and in most cases only slight mesangial proliferation. Latent IgA deposition from the donor kidney, irrespective of mesangial expansion, does not affect transplant prognosis. In most of the cases, IgA deposition will resolve after several weeks or months post transplantation [52, 53]. But for those recipients whose primary disease is IgA nephropathy, latent IgA deposition from the donor kidney was one of the risk factors of recurrent IgAN and it would lead to the development of recurrent of IgAN. Moreover, recurrent IgAN will compromise graft survival, especially in cases with latent IgA deposition from the donor kidney [54]. Furthermore, other immune complex-mediated GN including membranous nephropathy [55] and lupus nephritis [56] is also reported to be transported successfully. Our transplantation centers have been successful in several pre-exist MN transplantations. Protocal biopsy showed the membranous change remain for quite a long time after the proteinuria disappeared and the intensity of IgG deposition and the thickness of GBM decreased gradually in the following several years. This finding indicates that after transplantation the etiology and mechanism of the donor kidney were interrupted leading to the ending of the progress of the disease, thus those reversible lesions such as immune complex deposition, GBM thickening, and resident cell proliferation will gradually recovered. So, for immune complex-mediated GN, as long as the percentage of sclerosis and IFTA is in acceptable range, they are suitable for transplantation.

Another common pre-exist glomerulopathy is diabetic nephropathy (Fig. 13.25). Diabetic donor kidneys account for a small but significant percentage of transplanted kidneys ranging from 3.5 to 6.5% [57]. Diabetic recipients had significantly higher risk of allograft failure and death than nondiabetic recipients and diabetic recipients of diabetic donor kidneys have even worse allograft survival compared to all other patients [58]. It is suggested kidney from donors with DM to be transplanted to nondiabetic recipients as long as the lesions is not severer than RPS classification IIa [59]. Recipients usually develop slight proteinuria at the early stage post-transplant and will gradually decrease. Protocol biopsy revealed that it takes several years for the expansion matrix and the thickened GBM to reverse back to normal. DCD with diabetic nephropathy

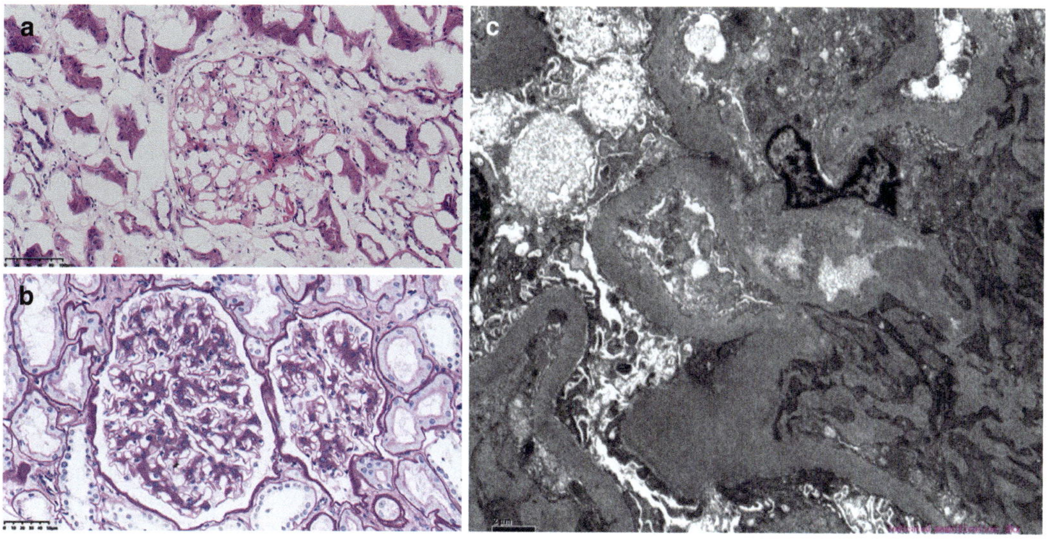

Fig. 13.25 (**a**) Enlarged glomerulus and the masangial area expanded with mainly matrix (frozen section HE ×400). (**b**) Enlarged glomerulus with masangial matrix expanding and GBM thickening (PAS ×400). (**c**) Diffuse GBM thickening in DN donor kidney

(DN) of class III or even IV should not be transplanted due to the high risk of unmanageable heavy proteinuria and PNF.

Due to the diverse basic conditions of the donor, various complications developed during the progression and therapy of the disease, different donors undergo different pathological changes, and the emphasis of evaluation may be different between DCD donors. Besides the points discussed above, there are numerous other conditions including abnormal gross appearance, unparalleled changes in bilateral kidneys. The precise evaluation should be based on the clinical background, gross appearance, and pathological changes to make a comprehensive and reasonable decision.

In conclusion, DCD donor biopsy can provide valuable information for the kidneys pre-life in the donor and compensate the shortcomings of evaluation based only on clinical data and gross examination. Precise evaluation of the DCD donor kidney can help decrease the risk of the occurrence of PNF, so that provide valuable information for the reasonable allocation and usage of the donor pool, especially in nowadays because we are facing an absolute shortage of donor kidneys [60].

References

1. Croome KP, Lee DD, Perry DK, et al. Comparison of long-term outcomes and quality of life in recipients of donation after cardiac death liver grafts with a propensity-matched cohort. Liver Transpl. 2017;23(3):342–51.
2. Kollmann D, Sapisochin G, Goldaracena N, et al. Expanding the donor pool: donation after circulatory death and living liver donation do not compromise the results of liver transplantation. Liver Transpl. 2018;24(6):779–89.
3. Mihaylov P, Mangus R, Ekser B, et al. Expanding the donor pool with the use of extended criteria donation after circulatory death livers. Liver Transpl. 2019;25(8):1198–208.
4. Saxena R, Fiel MI. Pathology of liver transplantation. In: Saxena R, editor. Practical hepatic pathology: a diagnostic approach, 2nd edn. Amsterdam: Elsevier; 2017. p. 629–62.
5. Frankel WL, Tranovich JG, Salter L, et al. The optimal number of donor biopsy sites to evaluate liver histology for transplantation. Liver Transpl. 2002;8:1044–50.
6. Chinese Society of Organ Transplantation. Expert consensus on evaluation and application of organ donated after cardiac death in China. Chin J Transplant (Electronic Edition). 2014;8(3):117–22. Chinese.
7. Naini BV, French SW. Liver transplant pathology. In: Wallace WD, Naini BV, editors. Practical atlas of transplant pathology. Cham: Springer; 2016. p. 111–31.

8. Markin RS, Wisecarver JL, Radio SJ,et al. Frozen section evaluation of donor livers before transplantation. Transplantation. 1993;56:1403–9.
9. Dutkowski P, Schlegel A, Slankamenac K, et al. The use of fatty liver grafts in modern allocation systems: risk assessment by the balance of risk (BAR) score. Ann Surg. 2012;256(5):861–8.
10. Todo S, Demetris AJ, Makowka L, et al. Primary nonfunction of hepatic allografts with preexisting fatty infiltration. Transplantation. 1989;47:903–5.
11. McCormack L, Dutkowski P, El-Badry AM, et al. Liver transplantation using fatty livers: always feasible? J Hepatol. 2011;54(5):1055–62.
12. Croome KP, Mathur AK, Mao S, et al. Perioperative and long-term outcomes of utilizing donation after circulatory death liver grafts with macrosteatosis: a multicenter analysis. Am J Transplant. 2020;20(9):2449–56.
13. Xia W, Ke Q, Wang Y, et al. Donation after cardiac death liver transplantation: graft quality evaluation based on pretransplant liver biopsy. Liver Transpl. 2015;21:838–46.
14. Bath NM, Leverson G, Al-Adra DP, et al. Microsteatosis in livers from donation after circulatory death donors is associated with inferior outcomes following liver transplantation. Liver Transpl. 2020;26(9):1127–37.
15. Zhang WJ, Xia WL, Pan HY, et al. Postreperfusion hyperkalemia in liver transplantation using donation after cardiac death grafts with pathological changes. Hepatobiliary Pancreat Dis Int. 2016;15(5):487–92.
16. Chinese Society of Organ Transplantation. Clinical technical practice for pathology of organ transplantation (2019 Edition). Organ Transplant. 2019;10(3):267–77. Chinese.
17. Spitzer AL, Lao OB, Dick AA, et al. The biopsied donor liver: incorporating macrosteatosis into high-risk donor assessment. Liver Transpl. 2010;16(7):874–84. https://doi.org/10.1002/lt.22085.
18. Yoong KF, Gunson BK, Neil DA, Mirza DF, et al. Impact of donor liver microvesicular steatosis on the outcome of liver retransplantation. Transplant Proc. 1999;31(1-2):550–1.
19. Croome KP, Lee DD, Croome S, et al. Does donor allograft microsteatosis matter? Comparison of outcomes in liver transplantation with a propensity-matched cohort. Liver Transpl. 2019;25(10):1533–40.
20. Tan M, Di Carlo A, Robinson P, et al. Successful outcome after transplantation of a donor liver with focal nodular hyperplasia. Liver Transpl. 2001;1:61–8.
21. Eccher A, Girolami I, Marletta S, et al. Donor-transmitted cancers in transplanted livers: analysis of clinical outcomes. Liver Transpl. 2021;27(1):55–66.
22. Pandanaboyana S, Longbotham D, Hostert L, et al. Transplantation of liver and kidney from donors with malignancy at the time of donation: an experience from a single centre. Transpl Int. 2016;29(1):73–80.
23. Sonbol MB, Halling KC, Douglas DD, et al. A case of donor-transmitted non-small cell lung cancer after liver transplantation: an unwelcome guest. Oncologist. 2019;24(6):e391–3.
24. Huprikar S, Danziger-Isakov L, Ahn J, et al. Solid organ transplantation from hepatitis B virus-positive donors: consensus guidelines for recipient management. Am J Transplant. 2015;15(5):1162–72.
25. Burton JR Jr, Terrault NA, Goldberg DS, et al. Liver and kidney recipient selection of hepatitis C virus viremic donors: meeting consensus report from the 2019 controversies in transplantation. Transplantation. 2020;104(3):476–81.
26. Crawford DH, Fletcher LM, Hubscher SG, et al. Patient and graft survival after liver transplantation for hereditary hemochromatosis: implications for pathogenesis. Hepatology. 2004;39:1655–62.
27. Adams PC, McAlister V, Chakrabarti S, et al. Is serum hepcidin causative in hemochromatosis? Novel analysis from a liver transplant with hemochromatosis. Can J Gastroenterol. 2008;22(10):851–3.
28. Laurent C, Vallet A, Le Bail B, et al. Extracellular fat globules mimicking dilated sinusoids after grafting steatotic livers. In: Wisse E, Knook DL, de Zanger R, et al., editors. Cells of the hepatic sinusoid. Leiden, The Netherlands: Kupffer Cell Foundation; 2001. p. 26–7.
29. Neil DA, Hubscher SG. Are parenchymal changes in early post-transplant biopsies related to preservation-reperfusion injury or rejection? Transplantation. 2001;71:1566–72.
30. Crowley H, Lewis WD, Gordon F, et al. Steatosis in donor and transplant liver biopsies. Hum Pathol. 2000;31:1209–13.
31. Giorgakis E, Khorsandi SE, Jassem W, et al. DCD consensus and futility in liver transplantation. J Hepatol. 2018;69(1):255–6.
32. Xue W, Tian P, Xiang H, et al. Outcomes for primary kidney transplantation from donation after citizens' death in China: a single center experience of 367 cases. BMC Health Serv Res. 2017;17(1):250.
33. Pan X, Xiang H, LinJuan L, et al. Preliminary results of transplantation with kidneys donated after cardiac death: a path of hope for organ transplantation in China. Nephrol Dial Transplant. 2015;30(9):1590–6.
34. Chen G, Wang C, Zhao Y, et al. Evaluation of quality of kidneys from donation after circulatory death/expanded criteria donors by parameters of machine perfusion. Nephrology (Carlton). 2018;23(2):103–6.
35. Mazzucco G, Magnani C, Fortunato M, et al. The reliability of pre-transplant donor renal biopsies (PTDB) in predicting the kidney state. A comparative single-centre study on 154 untransplanted kidneys. Nephrol Dial Transplant. 2010;25(10):3401–8.
36. Haas M, Segev DL, Racusen LC, et al. Arteriosclerosis in kidneys from healthy live donors: comparison of wedge and needle core perioperative biopsies. Arch Pathol Lab Med. 2008;132(1):37–42.
37. Lu AD, Desai D, Myers BD, et al. Severe glomerular sclerosis is not associated with poor outcome after kidney transplantation. Am J Surg. 2000;180(6):470–4.

38. Sofue T, Inui M, Kiyomoto H, et al. Pre-existing arteriosclerotic intimal thickening in living-donor kidneys reflects allograft function. Am J Nephrol. 2012;36(2):127–35.
39. Woestenburg A, Sennesael J, Bosmans J-L, et al. Vasculopathy in the kidney allograft at time of transplantation: impact on later function of the graft. Transplantation. 2008;85(7 Suppl):S10–8.
40. Woestenburg AT, Verpooten GA, Ysebaert DK, et al. Fibrous intimal thickening at implantation adversely affects long-term kidney allograft function. Transplantation. 2009;87(1):72–8.
41. Liapis H, Gaut JP, Klein C, et al. Banff histopathological consensus criteria for preimplantation kidney biopsies. Am J Transplant. 2017;17(1):140–50.
42. Batra RK, Heilman RL, Smith ML. Rapid resolution of donor-derived glomerular fibrin thrombi after deceased donor kidney transplantation. Am J Transplant. 2016;16(3):1015–20.
43. Gao G, Chen L-X, Brown IE, et al. Donor characteristics, recipient outcomes, and histologic findings of kidney allografts with diffuse donor-derived glomerular fibrin thrombi. Transplantation. 2019;103(9):1921–7.
44. Cima L, Nacchia F, Ghimenton C, et al. Histopathology and long-term outcome of kidneys transplanted from donors with severe acute kidney injury. Prog Transplant. 2019;29(1):36–42.
45. van der Windt DJ, Mehta R, Jorgensen DR, et al. Donor acute kidney injury and its effect on 1-year post-transplant kidney allograft fibrosis .Clin Transplant. 2020;34(2):e13770. https://doi.org/10.1111/ctr.13770. Epub 2020 Feb 11.
46. Pearson R, Asher J, Jackson A, et al. Viability assessment and utilization of declined donor kidneys with rhabdomyolysis using ex vivo normothermic perfusion without preimplantation biopsy. Am J Transplant. 2021;21(3):1317–21.
47. Park KS, Park SJ, Park H, et al. Association of baseline histopathology and kidney donor risk index with graft outcomes in deceased donor kidney transplantation. Clin Nephrol. 2019;91(6):363–9.
48. Frascà GM, D'Errico A, Malvi D, et al. Transplantation of kidneys with tumors. J Nephrol. 2016;29(2):163–8.
49. Lim SY, Kim MG, Park KT, et al. Experiences of renal transplants from donors with renal cell carcinoma after ex vivo partial nephrectomy. Ann Surg Treat Res. 2017;92(5):361–4.
50. Naesens M. Zero-time renal transplant biopsies: a comprehensive review. Transplantation. 2016;100(7):1425–39.
51. Deng R, Dai Y, Zhang H, et al. Higher incidence of renal allograft glomerulonephritis in living-related donor kidney transplantation. Transplant Proc. 2018;50(8):2421–5.
52. Sofue T, Inui M, Hara T, et al. Latent IgA deposition from donor kidneys does not affect transplant prognosis, irrespective of mesangial expansion. Clin Transplant. 2013;27(Suppl 26):14–21.
53. Ji S, Liu M, Chen J, et al. The fate of glomerular mesangial IgA deposition in the donated kidney after allograft transplantation. Clin Transplant. 2004;18(5):536–40.
54. Moriyama T, Nitta K, Suzuki K, et al. Latent IgA deposition from donor kidney is the major risk factor for recurrent IgA nephropathy in renal transplantation. Clin Transplant. 2005;19(Suppl 14):41–8.
55. Mirza MK, Kim L, Kadambi PV, et al. Membranous nephropathy transplanted in the donor kidney: observations of resolving glomerulopathy in serial allograft biopsies. Nephrol Dial Transplant. 2014;29(12):2343–7.
56. Magoon S, Zhou E, Pullman J, et al. Successful transplantation of a donor kidney with diffuse proliferative lupus nephritis and crescents—a case report. Nephrol Dial Transplant. 2010;25(12):4109–13.
57. Truong LD, Suki WN, Gaber LW, et al. Kidney donors with diabetes: renal biopsy findings at time of transplantation and their significance. Transplant Direct. 2019;5(7):e465. https://doi.org/10.1097/TXD.0000000000000903. eCollection 2019 July.
58. Cohen JB, Bloom RD, Reese PP, et al. .National outcomes of kidney transplantation from deceased diabetic donors. Kidney Int. 2015. https://doi.org/10.1038/ki.2015.325. Online ahead of print.
59. Harada S, Ushigome H, Nishimura A, et al. Histological reversibility of diabetic nephropathy after kidney transplantation from diabetic donor to non-diabetic recipient. Nephrology (Carlton). 2015;20(Suppl 2):40–4.
60. Snoeijs MGJ, Buurman WA, Christiaans MHL, et al. Histological assessment of preimplantation biopsies may improve selection of kidneys from old donors after cardiac death. Am J Transplant. 2008;8(9):1844–51.

14 Further Development of Organ Transplantation from Cardiac Death Donors in China

Qiang Zhao and Jinbo Huang

Abstract

Organ transplantation has been a recognized treatment of end-stage organ failure. The development of surgical and anesthesiological techniques as well as progress in immunosuppressive treatment resulted in an increased number of transplantations. Therefore, a significant gap still exists between the number of organ donors and recipients despite efforts to increase the supply pool of suitable organs for transplantation, highlighting the major problem of organ shortage. This was the main reason for a growing interest in donation after circulatory death (DCD). Nearly 136,000 solid organ transplants were performed worldwide in 2017, but WHO estimates that this activity only meets 10% of transplant needs (Manyalich et al. Curr Opin Organ Transplant. 2018;23:136–41). So, over the next few years, there are three main areas of development in DCD that will impact China to improve the number of organs from DCD. These are *technology* which is the most important area, *awareness* and *legislation* with practical guiding significance in the whole process of DCD.

Q. Zhao (✉) · J. Huang
The First Affiliated Hospital of Sun Yat-sen University, Guangzhou, China

14.1 Future Technique Development of DCD

The shortage of organs has resulted in a resurgence of interest in DCD as an effective way to expand the potential donor pool. Nowadays, the World Health Organization (WHO) has encouraged all societies to develop responsible policies concerning DCD and the adoption of DCD worldwide [1]. DCD plays an important role in expanding donor resources and reducing patient mortality. However, upon the utilization of DCD, the organs have to undergo a period of ischemia during the progression to circulatory arrest and after circulatory failure [2]. Such a situation has resulted in that the use of DCD organs is still limited by ischemia-reperfusion syndrome, reduced organ perfusion, hypotension, hypoxia, and so on [3]. In the future, we need to further study how to promote the DCD and overcome the shortcomings like reduced organ perfusion to make full use of the organs from DCD. The following may be the latest achievements or further directions of the DCD.

14.1.1 Further Development of Reducing Organ Injury and Improve Organ Function After DCD

During the process of transplantation, ischemia, which mainly occurs in the organ preservation

X. He (ed.), *Organ Donation and Transplantation after Cardiac Death in China*,
https://doi.org/10.1007/978-981-16-0815-5_14

process, is the main cause of organ damage and organ dysfunction. As a fundamental part of transplantation, the organ preservation process has been a hot area of research for more than half a century. It is broadly defined as "the process by which organs are kept viable outside of the organism from which they were removed" in which the preservation method should ideally mimic the natural state within the organism [4]. In the DCD, the organ will gradually enter a period of ischemia once circulation fails. Therefore, organ preservation in DCD should begin at the moment of circulatory failure. In the clinical practice of DCD, how to limit the adverse influence caused to organs by ischemia is one of the greatest challenges [5]. Any technique that can avoid ischemia and provide postmortem organ reperfusion has the latent capacity to improve transplant outcomes [6]. With the intention of mimicking the physiological environment of the body, normothermic regional perfusion (NRP) in situ (within the donor's body) or ex situ machine perfusion of individual organs (outside the donor's body) can achieve organ reperfusion after death. Both techniques are being increasingly used to improve organ transplant outcomes and have enough potential to get further development.

14.1.1.1 Prior to Organ Recovery: In Situ Normothermic Regional Perfusion

With the aim of improving the outcomes of organs obtained from the DCD, abdominal normothermic regional perfusion was introduced as a method of re-conditioning organs in the donor prior to explantation. It mainly counteracts ischemic damage and improves the recipients' outcome through restoring blood flow (using ECMO-technology) before organ recovery in DCD donors [7–10].

The first step of the NRP is to confirm death. Different countries have different practices regarding the determination of death in DCD. In DCD, as in daily clinical practice, death is generally confirmed according to circulatory criteria at the point of permanent circulation failure. This point means the impossibility of the spontaneous recovery of the circulation, namely the return of the autoresuscitation. After the confirmation of death, organ recovery proceeds with the insertion of an arterial and venous cannula into either the iliac vessels or alternatively the abdominal aorta and inferior vena cava. Above the diaphragm, the descending thoracic aorta is occluded by a vascular clamp or an intraluminal balloon. And then with the help of the ECMO technology, NRP can be established after death to perfuse the abdominal organs with warm, oxygenated, circulating blood. In situ preservation strategies can not only maintain the perfusion of the donor organ but also reserve time for completing consent and authorization requirements, evaluating the individual's suitability for donation. Moreover, NRP can also provide the chance to make an assessment on the organ viability prior to transplantation by parameters that can serve as reflections of the quality of organ preservation, especially in cDCD liver and heart transplantation. The evaluation of organ function prior to transplantation contributes to selecting grafts to minimize the post-transplant outcomes [11–13].

Since first applied in the process of liver transplantation in animal models, NRP has come a long way. Now the NRP has been used in clinical practices like kidney-pancreas, human kidney, and liver DCD organ procurement [14, 15]. In the world, many research teams have published their experience about NRP in the process of DCD, introducing their opinion of the way and outcome of the NRP. Those published series have shown promising results in terms of numbers of organs recovered and transplantation outcomes [16–18]. However, there is still a lack of definitive research outcome that can clearly identify the advantage of NRP. In other words, further development of NRP needs to improve evidence-based medical evidence. Such high quality and abundant evidences are helpful to establish the practice standard of NRP in China and further facilitate the development of DCD.

As an encouraging technique, the use of NRP in DCD is still facing ethical issues. The definition and determination of death in DCD, varying in different countries, is predicated on the cessation of whole-body circulation or circulation to the brain. Therefore, the re-establishment of circulation after the confirmation of death is the most challenging in the process of NRP [19]. Now, some measures like occluding the descending thoracic aorta above the diaphragm with a vascular clamp or an intraluminal balloon have been proposed as ways to respect the dead donor rule. But, with the advent of large-scale controlled, randomized clinical trials and the definitive evidence that NRP greatly contributes to the improvement of transplantation outcomes, such ethical issues are sure to be fully resolved in the near future.

14.1.1.2 After Organ Recovery: Ex-Situ Machine Perfusion

In clinical practice, the common practice of preserving in vitro organs is to save them in a cryogenic container, which is called static cold storage (SCS). SCS has been acceptable and yielded good outcomes for high-quality organs. However, the higher-risk or marginal organs like DCD-derived organs cannot tolerate the SCS. During the process of the SCS, cells are exposed to hypoxia at low temperatures and perform constantly anaerobic metabolism which leading to the accumulation of metabolites. After reperfusion of the organ in the recipient, these metabolites contribute later to the occurrence of ischemia-reperfusion injury (IRI) [20, 21]. This is the key factor limiting the applicability of SCS in DCD-derived organs. But at the same time, it is also the driving force to promote the development of ex-situ machine perfusion (MP).

The biggest difference between MP and SCS is that MP can maintain the cellular metabolism of organs in a dynamic physiological environment. Based on the differences in the single or double portal/arterial perfusion, gravity-fed or pump-driven vessel inflow, pulsatile or continuous perfusion waveform, the temperature of perfusate, substrate additives, and the composition of perfusate, various ex-situ machine perfusion techniques in the liver have been developed [22]. To date, ex situ normothermic perfusion (NMP) (35–38°C) is the only perfusion mode that has shown the potential to considerably extend the preservation period, far exceeding the current possibilities of SCS [23–25].

The greatest advantage of MP is that it provides a dynamic perfusion platform, through which we can improve graft function and assess the viability of DCD grafts. In terms of improving organ function, it tries to create as near a physiologic environment as possible to maintain the complete metabolic state of organs. The preliminary results of the use of NMP in extend criteria liver grafts including DCD are very promising proving that this technique is feasible and well tolerated [26]. In addition, ex situ viability assessment of DCD grafts may be a potential development direction of NMP in the future. This is done by measuring various biomarkers related to the function of the transplanted organs. To be a useful clinical application, those selected predictive markers should be easily accessible, repeatable. Several studies have been conducted to determine combinations of parameters in evaluating graft viability. However, none has been applied in clinical practice, or even clinically validated to date. The establishment of reliable and accurate predictive viability biomarkers which can determine whether a potential graft on ex situ perfusion can actually be transplanted remains an open question.

In addition to the two main aspects above, there are still many potential development points in the process of MP. For example, in the process of NMP, antibody, silencing RNA, or viral manipulative approaches can be used to remove the passenger immunogenic cells of donor origin [27]. On the contrary, it has been reported that immune-regulatory cells such as regulatory T cells, mesenchymal stem cells (MSCs) can regulate immune and inflammatory. Therefore, we can perfuse the grafts with those cells to confer anti-inflammatory or tolerogenic properties to ameliorate graft injury [28].

14.1.2 Further Development of Increasing the Number of Usable DCD Organs

In addition to reducing organ damage and improving organ function, the inclusion criteria of organs from DCD can be relaxed to increase the number of organs from DCD, which is also a further development direction of DCD.

Controlled donation after circulatory death (cDCD) refers to organ donation from patients with a planned withdrawal of life-sustaining treatment (WLST) and subsequent circulatory death [29]. The period from WLST to circulatory arrest highly varies in different areas and may range from a few minutes to many hours, and sometimes even days. As for the observation time of circulatory arrest, most DCD protocols recommend a maximal period of 60–90 min from WLST [30].

This period has a great influence on whether organ donation is likely to occur and on the quality of the organs retrieved for transplantation. If the period is too short, many potential DCD donors will not proceed to organ donation. Inversely, a too-long withdrawal period often means a sustained period of systemic hemodynamic instability and poor oxygenation of organs, leading to a severe ischemic injury to the organs that preclude their use for transplantation. In a word, an appropriate withdrawal period is of great importance. At present, some researches have been carried out to prove that the proper extension of waiting time has a better result than 60–90 min from WLST to circulatory arrest as most DCD protocols recommend. Reid et al. conducted a research on extending the cutoff time for recovery to a minimum of 4 h. Of 173 potential DCD donors, 117 (67.6%) became donors, of which 90 (76.9%) arrested within 1 h and an additional 27 (23.1%) donors arrested after 1 h (8 by 2 h, 11 more between 2 and 4 h, and 8 more after 4 h) [31]. The research proves that longer agonal phases (time from WLST to DOD) could lead to greater donor instability, but increased agonal phase instability or its duration had no affection on transplant outcome.

In the future, an appropriate extension of the waiting combined with the further development of the machine perfusion technology which can reduce graft injury have the potential to enlarge the donor pool. In such a situation, the organ obtained after prolonged waiting time will be repaired by machine perfusion, and then the organ function will be evaluated with the help of machine perfusion technology to determine whether it could be used for further transplantation.

14.2 The Improvement of the Awareness of DCD

With the vigorous development of transplant medicine, the consciousness of organ donation has been significantly improved. According to the Red Cross Society of China (RCSC), China has seen a rise in the number of organ donations since the country began a pilot donation program in 2010. By the end of March 2018, nearly 46,500 organs had been donated in China and nearly 422,000 Chinese had registered for voluntary organ donations, said the RCSC [32]. However, the number of available organs seems to be insufficient to answer the growing demand for organs. Given the large size of China's population, there may be a large space for residents to raise their awareness of organ donation especially in the domain of DCD. Actually, there is a lack of research on DCD cognition in China, so there is still no reliable and objective scientific report showing the awareness of people toward the DCD in China. In India, some cultural similarities are shared with China. Recently, a research conducted in India showed the refusal of family members was the main reason for their poor awareness of organ donation. This warrants that public education plays an important role. An Australian study has illustrated the importance of public education which shows that the altruistic motive of saving lives and improving lives for others highly influences the national's willingness to register as an organ donor. According to the experience of other countries, further education and propaganda in China should better pay close attention to appeal to the altruism of saving others' lives. Such measures can be treated as long-standing and routine campaigns, for the reason that their influence on people attitudes increases over time [33, 34].

14.3 Legislation of Practical Guiding Significance in Whole Process of DCD

For historical reasons, the development of the organ donation system in China has far lagged behind. Nowadays, strict regulations have been developed to ensure transparency, impartiality, fairness, and respect for life during the whole process of organ donation. However, it is undeniable that difficulties still remain in many areas of the current donation practice. For example, some legislation only stays at the theoretical level and lacks the practical guiding significance.

The European experience has revealed that legislative measures are of great value in affecting the donation rate from deceased donors and the success rate of subsequent transplants. Also, the government is developing comprehensive and niche targeting measures to resolve difficulties such as a lack of motivation and significant resistance. In the near future, more attention should be paid to the perfection of legislation and promulgation of legally valid guidelines of donation after circulatory death [35, 36].

References

1. Daemen JW, Kootstra G, Wijnen RM, et al. Nonheart-beating donors: the Maastricht experience. Clin Transp. 1994;7:303.
2. Perera MT. The super-rapid technique in Maastricht category III donors: has it developed enough for marginal liver grafts from donors after cardiac death? Curr Opin Organ Transplant. 2012;17:131.
3. Jadlowiec CC, Taner T. Liver transplantation: current status and challenges. World J Gastroenterol. 2016;22(18):4438–45.
4. Fuller B, Froghi F, Davidson B. Organ preservation solutions: linking pharmacology to survival for the donor organ pathway. Curr Opin Organ Transplant. 2018;23(3):361–8.
5. Manara AR, Murphy PG, Ocallaghan G. Donation after circulatory death. Br J Anaesth. 2012;108(Suppl. 1):i108–21.
6. Watson CJE, Hunt F, Messer S, et al. In situ normothermic perfusion of livers in controlled circulatory death donation may prevent ischemic cholangiopathy and improve graft survival. Am J Transplant. 2019;19(6):1745–58.
7. Minambres E, Suberviola B, Dominguez-Gil B, et al. Improving the outcomes of organs obtained from controlled donation after circulatory death donors using abdominal normothermic regional perfusion. Am J Transplant. 2017;17(8):2165–72.
8. Hessheimer AJ, García-Valdecasas JC, Fondevila C. Abdominal regional in-situ perfusion in donation after circulatory determination of death donors. Curr Opin Organ Transplant. 2016;21(3):322–8.
9. Shapey IM, Muiesan P. Regional perfusion by extracorporeal membrane oxygenation of abdominal organs from donors after circulatory death: a systematic review. Liver Transpl. 2013;19(12):1292–303.
10. Oniscu GC, Randle LV, Muiesan P, et al. In situ normothermic regional perfusion for controlled donation after circulatory death--the United Kingdom experience. Am J Transplant. 2014;14(12):2846–54.
11. Schlegel A, Kalisvaart M, Scalera I, Laing RW, Mergental H, Mirza DF, Perera T, Isaac J, Dutkowski P, Muiesan P. The UK DCD risk score: a new proposal to define futility in donation-after-circulatory-death liver transplantation. J Hepatol. 2018;68:456–64.
12. Dikdan GS, Mora-Esteves C, Koneru B. Review of randomized clinical trials of donor management and organ preservation in deceased donors: opportunities and issues. Transplantation. 2012;94:425–41.
13. Tsui SSL, Oniscu GC. Extending normothermic regional perfusion to the thorax in donors after circulatory death. Curr Opin Organ Transplant. 2017;22:245–50.
14. Farney AC, Singh RP, Hines MH, et al. Experience in renal and extrarenal transplantation with donation after cardiac death donors with selective use of extracorporeal support. J Am Coll Surg. 2008;206:1028.
15. Valero R, Cabrer C, Oppenheimer F, et al. Normothermic recirculation reduces primary graft dysfunction of kidneys obtained from non-heart-beating donors. Transpl Int. 2000;13:303.
16. Oniscu GC, Randle LV, Muiesan P, et al. In situ normothermic regional perfusion for controlled donation after circulatory death–the United Kingdom experience. Am J Transplant. 2014;14:2846.
17. Hessheimer AJ, Coll E, Torres F, et al. Normothermic regional perfusion vs. super-rapid recovery in controlled donation after circulatory death liver transplantation. J Hepatol. 2019;70:658.
18. Valero R, Cabrer C, Oppenheimer F, et al. Normothermic recirculation reduces primary graft dysfunction of kidneys obtained from non-heart-beating donors. Transpl Int. 2000;13:303.
19. Dalle Ave AL, Shaw DM, Bernat JL. Ethical Issues in the use of extracorporeal membrane oxygenation in controlled donation after circulatory determination of death. Am J Transplant. 2016;16:2293–9.
20. Collard CD, Gelman S. Pathophysiology, clinical manifestations, and prevention of ischemia-reperfusion injury. Anesthesiology. 2001;94:1133.
21. Chouchani ET, Pell VR, Gaude E, et al. Ischaemic accumulation of succinate controls reperfusion injury through mitochondrial ROS. Nature. 2014;515:431.

22. Friend PJ, Imber C, Peter SS, Lopez I, Butler AJ, Rees MA. Normothermic perfusion of the isolated liver. Transplant Proc. 2001;33:3436–8.
23. Bral M, Gala-Lopez B, Bigam D, Kneteman N, Malcolm A, Livingstone S, Andres A, Emamaullee J, Russell L, Coussios C, West LJ, Friend PJ, Shapiro AM. Preliminary single-center Canadian experience of human normothermic ex vivo liver perfusion: results of a clinical trial. Am J Transplant. 2017;17(4):1071–80.
24. Vogel T, Brockmann JG, Quaglia A, Morovat A, Jassem W, Heaton ND, Coussios CC, Friend PJ. The 24-hour normothermic machine perfusion of discarded human liver grafts. Liver Transpl. 2017;23:207–20.
25. Butler AJ, Rees MA, Wight DG, Casey ND, Alexander G, White DJ, Friend PJ. Successful extracorporeal porcine liver perfusion for 72 hr. Transplantation. 2002;73:1212–8.
26. van Rijn R, Karimian N, Matton APM, et al. Dual hypothermic oxygenated machine perfusion in liver transplants donated after circulatory death. Br J Surg. 2017;104(7):907–17.
27. Bral M, Gala-Lopez B, Bigam DL, Freed DH, Shapiro AMJ. Ex situ liver perfusion: organ preservation into the future. Transplant Rev (Orlando). 2018;32(3):132–41.
28. Gotts JE, Matthay MA. Mesenchymal stem cells and acute lung injury. Crit Care Clin. 2011;27:719–33.
29. Kotsopoulos AMM, Böing-Messing F, Jansen NE, Vos P, Abdo WF. External validation of prediction models for time to death in potential donors after circulatory death [published correction appears in Am J Transplant]. Am J Transplant. 2018;18(4):890–6.
30. Bernat JL, D'Alessandro AM, Port FK, et al. Report of a national conference on donation after cardiac death. Am J Transplant. 2006;6:281.
31. Reid AW, Harper S, Jackson CH, et al. Expansion of the kidney donor pool by using cardiac death donors with prolonged time to cardio-respiratory arrest. Am J Transplant. 2011;11:995.
32. China sees rise in organ donations [English]. Available at http://english.www.gov.cn/news/top_news/2018/04/01/content_281476098025380.htm. Accessed on April 1, 2018.
33. Kumar V, Ahlawat R, Gupta AK, et al. Potential of organ donation from deceased donors: study from a public sector hospital in India. Transpl Int. 2014;27:1007.
34. Irving MJ, Jan S, Tong A, et al. What factors influence people's decisions to register for organ donation? The results of a nominal group study. Transpl Int. 2014;27:617.
35. Roels L, Rahmel A. The European experience. Transpl Int. 2011;2:350.
36. Huang JF. The key measures promoting the development of organ transplantation projects in China: principal thinking about experimental units for heart death organ donation [Chinese]. Chin J Organ Transplant. 2011;32:1.

GPSR Compliance

The European Union's (EU) General Product Safety Regulation (GPSR) is a set of rules that requires consumer products to be safe and our obligations to ensure this.

If you have any concerns about our products, you can contact us on ProductSafety@springernature.com

In case Publisher is established outside the EU, the EU authorized representative is:

Springer Nature Customer Service Center GmbH
Europaplatz 3
69115 Heidelberg, Germany

Batch number: 09224018

Printed by Printforce, the Netherlands